Medical Terminology
Quick & Concise
A PROGRAMMED LEARNING APPROACH

Medical Terminology
Quick & Concise
A PROGRAMMED LEARNING APPROACH

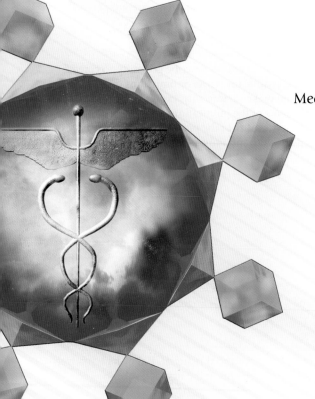

Marjorie Canfield Willis
Program Director
Medical Assisting/Medical Transcription Programs
Orange Coast College
Costa Mesa, California

Wolters Kluwer | Lippincott Williams & Wilkins
Health

Philadelphia · Baltimore · New York · London
Buenos Aires · Hong Kong · Sydney · Tokyo

Senior Publisher: Julie K. Stegman
Senior Managing Editor: Heather A. Rybacki
Developmental Editor: Nancy Peterson
Senior Marketing Manager: Zhan Caplan
Manufacturing Coordinator: Margie Orzech-Zeranko
Cover and Internal Design: Bill Donnelly, WT Design
Compositor: Aptara, Inc.
Printer: RR Donnelley - Shenzhen

Library of Congress Cataloging-in-Publication Data
Willis, Marjorie Canfield.
  Medical terminology quick & concise : a programmed learning approach / Marjorie Canfield Willis.
     p. ; cm.
  Includes flash cards.
  Includes bibliographical references and index.
  ISBN 978-0-7817-6534-3 (alk. paper)
  1. Medicine—Terminology—Programmed instruction. I. Title. II. Title: Medical terminology quick and concise.
  [DNLM: 1. Medicine—Programmed Instruction. 2. Medicine—Terminology—English. W 15 W735mb 2010]
  R123.W477 2010
  610.1′4—dc22

                                                          2008031988

The publishers have made every effort to trace the copyright holders for borrowed material. If they have inadvertently overlooked any, they will be pleased to make the necessary arrangements at the first opportunity.

To purchase additional copies of this book, call our customer service department at **(800) 638-3030** or fax orders to **(301) 223-2400**. International customers should call **(301) 223-2300**.

Visit Lippincott Williams & Wilkins on the Internet: http://www.LWW.com. Lippincott Williams & Wilkins customer service representatives are available from 8:30 am to 5:00 pm, EST.

Dedicated to Gwen Canfield,

my Mom, my best friend

PREFACE

Medical Terminology Quick & Concise: A Programmed Learning Approach provides an introduction to medical terminology. It is designed to give health professions students a basic working knowledge of the language of health care. The focus is on learning the most common medical term components, using these term components to build terms, and analyzing the use of these terms in health records. This text can be used for self-study or classroom instruction with the goal of serving as a basis for individual expansion.

Unique Approach

There are three elements to this original approach: programmed learning, contextual organization, and level of conciseness.

1. **Programmed Learning.** This approach facilitates quick learning and application of information through a self-study system that helps students work easily through the book. It is a self-paced, self-administered form of instruction that is presented in logical sequence with repetition of concepts and positive reinforcement. (Learn more about the programmed approach in Getting Started: A Guide to Student Success, page xxiii.)

2. **Contextual Organization.** The first three chapters explain medical term basics, anatomic structures and terms of reference, and terms and abbreviations used in health records. The following chapters build on this foundational content in a purposeful way, covering symptomatic and diagnostic terms, diagnostic tests and procedures, and operative and therapeutic terms. In all chapters, content is presented *in context*— that is, terms are taught in the context of how they will actually be used in a health care setting. (This is in contrast to many other medical terminology texts, in which terms are taught by body system.) In addition, medical records and related exercises throughout the text help students apply learning to real medical situations.

3. **Concise Level.** *Medical Terminology Quick & Concise* provides the tools needed to successfully develop a working medical vocabulary but without a lot of unessential extras—just the facts. This makes it ideal for busy health professions students and educators.

It's about People

Health care is not just about terms, tests, and procedures. It's about people, and students will eventually use their knowledge of medical terminology to evaluate and assist individuals who may be sick or injured. To help put a face on health care, the following cast of characters is introduced throughout the text:

Dr. SPAULDING

The fictitious Dr. Spaulding is a general practitioner. That is, she sees patients from young to old who have any type of medical complaint. Sometimes, Dr. Spaulding refers her patients to medical specialists for diagnostic tests and treatments that cannot be done in her office. Other times, she admits patients to the hospital for extended care.

PATIENTS

In each chapter, the Meet the Patient vignettes present one or two patients faced with a realistic illness or injury. Often, you will see their course of diagnosis and treatment progress in the form of medical records and Vital Statistics boxes.

⚕ HEALTH CARE PROFESSIONALS

Dr. Spaulding is only one of several types of health care professionals that students learn about in this text. To help students who are choosing their own health care career path, the Health Care Professionals boxes provide brief profiles of many different career choices. Expanded profiles on the 🖸 Student Resource CD-ROM detail educational requirements and explain more fully what each job entails.

Text Features

Unique and engaging features have been designed to assist students' comprehension and retention of information and to spark interest in students and educators alike.

OBJECTIVES

A quick and concise list of key topics is presented first in each chapter.

CHECKLIST

A checklist at the beginning of each chapter serves as the study plan, covering each learning task related to the chapter and its electronic supplements. (Note: Students who are enrolled in the corresponding online course will instead follow the online course Checklist.)

MEET THE PATIENT

This feature introduces patients in realistic situations in the health care setting. Many are linked to Vital Statistics information, medical records, and profiles of health care professionals.

CORE TERM COMPONENTS

This section includes all of the term components featured in the chapter, with their meanings and cross references to corresponding flash card numbers (if applicable). Suffix tables are green, prefix tables are orange, and combining forms tables are purple. (Flash cards are color-coded accordingly.)

SELF-INSTRUCTION AND PROGRAMMED REVIEW SECTIONS

Here, suffixes, prefixes, and combining forms are introduced as term basics in Self-Instruction increments. Next, Programmed Review sections help students quickly take that information and build on it to form new medical terms. Students use the Reveal Card included with the text to hide the answers to the fill-in questions posed in the right column. As part of the programmed approach, students may move at their own pace, given the time allotted.

VITAL STATISTICS

These boxes highlight common diagnostic tests, diseases, or disorders and specific procedures or therapies and are often linked to the patients from the Meet the Patient vignettes and the medical records found in the chapter. This is an opportunity for students to expand on their basic knowledge in a meaningful way.

ON CLOSER INSPECTION

Even in a quick and concise learning environment, some terms or topics require a second look. These boxes give a bit more depth of content to aid in complete understanding.

Rx FOR SUCCESS

Enjoy these snippets that give tips and reminders, as well as specific pitfalls to avoid when analyzing terms.

PRONUNCIATION SUMMARY

Correct and clear pronunciation is critical for success as a health care professional. The key terms introduced in each chapter are listed in this section, each followed by its written pronunciation. Students are directed to listen to the audio pronunciation for each of these terms on the Student Resource CD-ROM and to reinforce each term's meaning by writing out the definition.

EXAMINE YOUR UNDERSTANDING

There's nothing like practice exercises to test comprehension and reinforce newly acquired knowledge. Each chapter ends with a variety of exercises, including word analysis and definitions, matching, multiple choice, fill-in-the blank, word part combinations, and short answer. Answers to Examine Your Understanding questions appear at the end of each chapter.

MEDICAL RECORD EXERCISES

Medical records provide real-world context and a chance to apply knowledge in a practical way. Brief and complete authentic medical records include terms that students have learned. Corresponding questions require students to stretch their thinking and use their new language. Answers to Medical Record Exercises appear at the end of each chapter.

FC FLASH CARDS

A starter set of flash cards covering the core prefixes, suffixes, and combining forms can be found at the back of the text, color coded to match the term components covered in the chapters. A complete set of electronic flash cards are on the Student Resource CD-ROM.

ARTWORK

Full-color medical illustrations and photographs bring the concepts presented in the textbook to life. Students not only learn, for example, what the term "dermatitis" means, but they also see what it looks like.

APPENDICES

Appendix A summarizes medical term components in two easy-to-reference lists: (a) term component to English definition and (b) English definition to term component. Appendix B provides a glossary of abbreviations and symbols. Appendix C is a listing of the 50 most frequently prescribed medications, including their therapeutic uses.

Additional Learning Resources

The interactive learning activities provided on the Student Resource CD-ROM included with this text and online at www.thepoint.lww.com/WillisQC deliver a variety of exercises to reinforce what has been learned in the text, including:

- **Review Exercises** that allow students to choose the types of exercises that best suit their learning style, including *multiple choice, fill-in-the-blank,* and *true/false* questions; *image matching* games; and *figure labeling, spelling bee,* and *medical records* exercises.
- **Scored Chapter Quizzes** and a **Final Assessment** test students' knowledge and prepare them for classroom quizzes and tests.
- **Games** make learning medical terminology fun; try a crossword puzzle or one of the other fast-paced activities.
- The **Audio Pronunciation Glossary** is an electronic glossary of the term components and key terms from the book, organized both from A-to-Z and by chapter. The audio pronunciations may be played individually, or a group of audio pronunciations can be played sequentially as an audio drill. Definitions for the electronic glossary are courtesy of *Stedman's Medical Dictionary, 28th Edition.*

- Interactive **Flash Cards** present all of the term components from the text and can be reviewed electronically by chapter; included is an option to make your own flash cards.

Teaching Resources

Visit thePoint. at **http://thepoint.lww.com/WillisQC** to access resources designed specifically to help instructors teach more effectively and save time. There you will find:

- *Instructor's test generator* with more than 400 questions, encompassing individual chapter tests and a comprehensive exam
- *PowerPoint slides,* with lecture notes, for each chapter
- *Lesson plans* for each chapter
- *Classroom hand-outs*
- *Image bank*
- Customized course content for use with your *learning management system,* such as thePoint CCM (LWW's exclusive learning management system), WebCT, or Blackboard
- And more!

A solid understanding of medical terminology provides an essential foundation for any career in health care. The *Medical Terminology Quick & Concise: A Programmed Learning Approach* product suite makes learning and teaching medical terminology a rewarding and exciting process.

USER'S GUIDE

Medical Terminology Quick & Concise: A Programmed Learning Approach is your creative and interactive introduction to medical terminology. Using a programmed learning approach, contextual organization, and concise level, it will provide you with a basic working knowledge of the language of health care. Along the way, you'll encounter special features and tools that will help you navigate and understand the material presented. This User's Guide explains all of these features. In addition to reading "Getting Started: A Guide to Student Success" on page xxiii, use this guide to get the most out of each chapter, and then take your new language with you into your chosen health care profession!

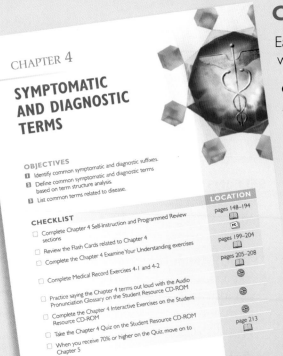

Chapter Opening Elements

Each chapter begins with the following elements, which will help you get off to the right start:

OBJECTIVES
A quick and concise list of need-to-know content.

CHECKLIST
The checklist is your study plan, covering each learning task related to the chapter and its electronic supplements. Use it to set learning goals.

MEET THE PATIENT

Meet patients in realistic situations in the health care setting. Watch for more information on the medical care for each of these patients within the chapter.

CORE TERM COMPONENTS

These tables present the term components featured in the chapter, with their meanings and cross references to flash card numbers (if applicable). Suffix tables are green, prefix tables are orange, and combining forms tables are purple.

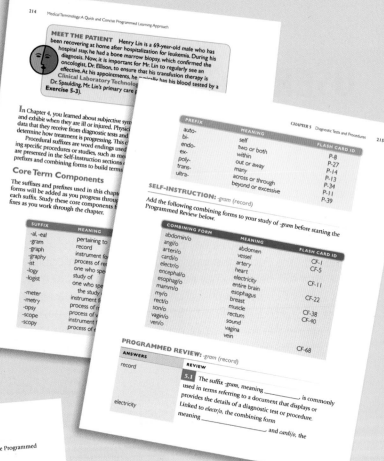

Learning Segments

The programmed learning approach uses two content segments:

SELF-INSTRUCTION FRAMES

Study and memorize the suffixes, prefixes, and combining forms introduced in this section before moving on the next segment.

PROGRAMMED REVIEW FRAMES

Take the information you learned in the Self-Instruction frame and build on it to form new medical terms as the answers to fill-in-the-blank exercises in this section.

REVEAL CARD

Use the Reveal Card to hide the answers in the left column while completing the exercises on the right.

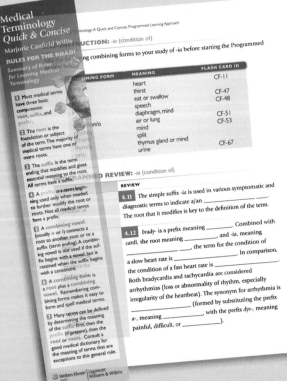

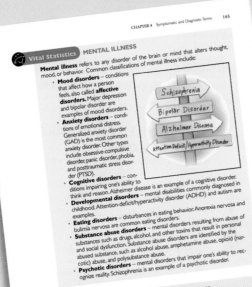

Vital Statistics MENTAL ILLNESS

Mental illness refers to any disorder of the brain or mind that alters thought, mood, or behavior. Common classifications of mental illness include:

- **Mood disorders** – conditions that affect how a person feels, also called **affective disorders.** Major depression and bipolar disorder are examples of mood disorders.
- **Anxiety disorders** – conditions of emotional distress. Generalized anxiety disorder (GAD) is the most common anxiety disorder. Other types include obsessive-compulsive disorder, panic disorder, phobia, and posttraumatic stress disorder (PTSD).
- **Cognitive disorders** – conditions impairing one's ability to think and reason. Alzheimer disease is an example of a cognitive disorder.
- **Developmental disorders** – mental disabilities commonly diagnosed in childhood. Attention-deficit/hyperactivity disorder (ADHD) and autism are examples.
- **Eating disorders** – disturbances in eating behavior. Anorexia nervosa and bulimia nervosa are common eating disorders.
- **Substance abuse disorders** – mental disorders resulting from abuse of substances such as drugs, alcohol, and other toxins that result in personal and social dysfunction. Substance abuse disorders are identified by the abused substance, such as alcohol abuse, amphetamine abuse, opioid (narcotic) abuse, and polysubstance abuse.
- **Psychotic disorders** – mental disorders that impair one's ability to recognize reality. Schizophrenia is an example of a psychotic disorder.

(Schizophrenia / Bipolar Disorder / Alzheimer Disease / Attention-Deficit/Hyperactivity Disorder)

ON CLOSER INSPECTION Anorexia vs. Anorexia Nervosa

Anorexia is a common symptomatic term indicating that one is without an appetite. It is not to be confused with anorexia nervosa, the term for an eating disorder in which the individual has abnormal perceptions about his or her body weight, evidenced by an overwhelming fear of becoming fat that results in a refusal to eat and body weight well below normal.

Special Features

VITAL STATISTICS
These boxes highlight common diagnostic tests, disorders, and specific procedures or therapies. They'll help you expand on your basic knowledge in a meaningful way.

ON CLOSER INSPECTION
Some terms or topics require a second look. These boxes give you a deeper understanding.

ARTWORK
Full-color medical illustrations and photographs bring the concepts to life and appeal to your visual sense.

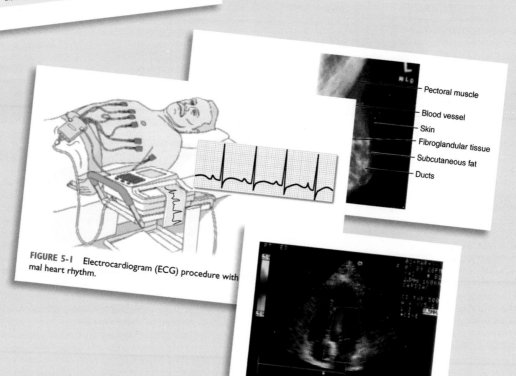

FIGURE 5-1 Electrocardiogram (ECG) procedure with ... mal heart rhythm.

- Pectoral muscle
- Blood vessel
- Skin
- Fibroglandular tissue
- Subcutaneous fat
- Ducts

FIGURE 5-3 Echocardiogram. Normal, two-dimensional, apical four-chamber view of heart.

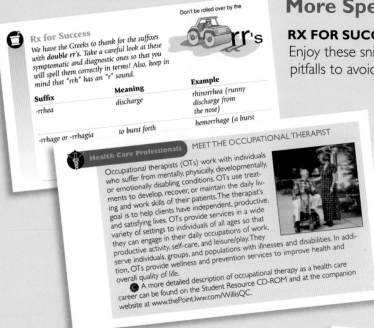

More Special Features

RX FOR SUCCESS

Enjoy these snippets that give tips, reminders, and pitfalls to avoid when analyzing terms.

MEET THE HEALTH CARE PROFESSIONALS

These profiles of different career choices will show you how different health care professionals work together and give you a glimpse of several health care professional opportunities.

Don't miss the expanded profiles on the Student Resource CD-ROM and online at www.thePoint.lww/WillisQC.

PRONUNCIATION SUMMARY

Correct and clear pronunciation is important! The key terms from each chapter are listed in this section with their written pronunciations. Listen to and repeat the audio pronunciation for each of these terms on the Student Resource CD-ROM.

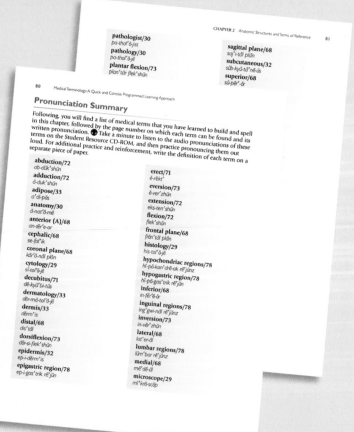

Chapter-Ending Features

EXAMINE YOUR UNDERSTANDING

Put your knowledge to the test with exercises on word analysis and definitions, term building, matching, fill-in-the-blank, multiple choice, short answer, and spelling. Answers appear at the end of the chapter.

MEDICAL RECORD EXERCISES

Medical records provide real-world context and a chance to apply your knowledge in a practical way. Brief and complete actual medical records include terms that you have learned, with corresponding questions that require you to stretch and use your new language. Answers also appear at the end of each chapter.

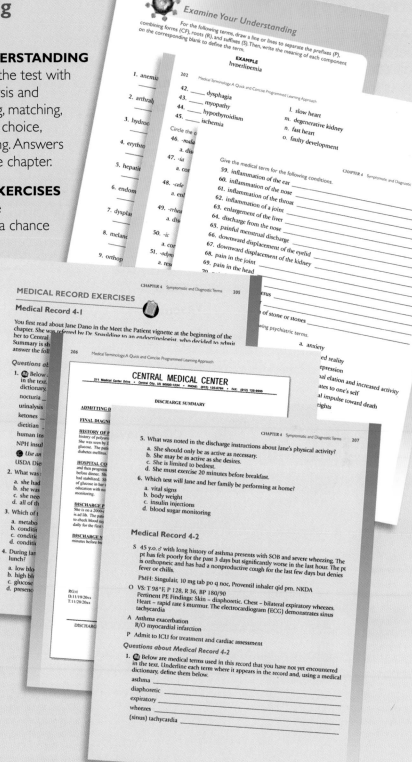

Other Learning Tools

FLASH CARDS

A set of color-coded flash cards can be found at the back of the text to match the prefixes, suffixes, and a select number of combining forms covered in the chapters. Interactive flash cards are included on the Student Resource CD-ROM, along with a Flash Card Generator that allows you to make your own.

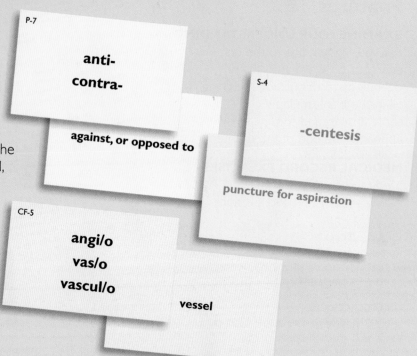

CD-ROM AND WEBSITE

Have fun while you learn with the Student Resource CD-ROM packaged with this text and online at www.thePoint.lww.com/WillisQC! You will find additional exercises for every chapter (including multiple choice questions, figure labeling, fill-in-the-blank questions, spelling bees, case studies, and much more!), an audio pronunciation glossary from Stedman's, and electronic flash cards. Use this interactive learning resource to test your knowledge, assess your progress, and study and review for quizzes and tests.

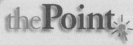

ACKNOWLEDGMENTS

There is only one word that accurately describes my experience writing this text: It was the *best*!

I have been so fortunate to work with the most competent professionals in medical publishing. It started with the opportunity to work with John Goucher, my Acquisitions Editor, and Tom Lochhaas, the Developmental Editor from my first writing experience. They guided me through the early development of this text, and I credit Tom for inspiring its unique approach. They are the best at what they do.

More of the best followed when the project came under the management of Julie Stegman, Senior Publisher, and Heather Rybacki, Senior Managing Editor. It was my second experience working with this "Dynamic Duo," so I already knew I was in good hands, and it was a thrill to work with them again. Added to the mix was the opportunity to work with Nancy Peterson, my Developmental Editor, who has been the best help I could have ever imagined. I credit Julie, Heather, and Nancy for helping me to produce my very best work yet, and we had fun doing it!

Looking back, this project was destined to be the best from the beginning. We had the benefit of the best reviewers, who offered comments and suggestions that were well thought out and helpful. In addition, several contributors wrote and verified the content related to specific health care professions, and several others supplied photos. After editorial development, the designers, artists, copyeditors, and compositors worked tirelessly behind the scenes, and Robin Gardenhire, Loreen MacNichol, Michael Covone, and Patricia O'Brien-Giglia came onboard to assist with development of content for the electronic student and instructor resources.

You are all the best, and I thank you most sincerely!

M.C.W.

REVIEWERS AND CONTRIBUTORS

The author and publisher would like to thank the following reviewers, many of whom provided valuable comments and suggestions throughout development of the manuscript, while others supplied feedback on the design of the book:

Lisa Aberle, BS, RT(R)(CV)
Radiography Program Director
Bloomington-Normal School of
    Radiography
Normal, IL

Huston Brown, BHS, RRT
Assistant Dean
School of Health Sciences
St. Catharine College
St. Catharine, KY

Phyllis A. Clements, MA, OTR
Program Coordinator
Occupational Therapy Assistant Program
Macomb Community College
Clinton Township, MI

Michael P. Covone, EdD (ABD), RT(R), CT
Assistant Professor
School of Health Sciences
Pennsylvania College of Technology
Williamsport, PA

Mary M. Fabick, MSN,
MEd, RN, CEN
Associate Professor
Area of Nursing
Milligan College
Milligan College, TN

Robin Gardenhire, MA, ATC, CSCS
Clinical Instructor
Georgia State University
Atlanta, GA

Nancy Hislop, BSN
Online Instructor
Globe University/Minnesota
    School of Business
Richfield, MN

Cindy Iavagnilio, MSN, CRNA
Assistant Professor
Nursing
Saint Mary's College
Notre Dame, IN

Patti Kalvelage, MS, OTR/L
University Lecturer
Master of Occupational Therapy
   Program
Governors State University
University Park, IL

Diane M. Klieger, RN, MBA, CMA
Program Director/Instructor
Medical Assisting
Pinellas Technical Education Center –
   St Petersburg
St. Petersburg, FL

Robert Kodama
Clinical Ayurvedic Specialist
Jiva Health
San Diego, CA

Tina Lewis, MT(ASCP)(AMT)
Medical Department Co-Director
Spencerian College
Louisville, KY

Judith L. Lichtenberger, CMT, AHDI-F
Adjunct Faculty
Northampton Community College
Bethlehem, PA

Loreen W. MacNichol, CMRS, RMC
Associate Faculty
Allied Health Department
Andover College
South Portland, ME

Peggy Mayo, MEd, MLT (ASCP)
Assistant Professor
Multi-Competency Health Technology
Columbus State Community College
Columbus, OH

Rose Miller, RN, MSN, MPA, LNC, RMA
Nursing and Allied Health
College of Southern Maryland
Leonardtown, MD

Patricia O'Brien-Giglia, CMT

Wanda C. Reygaert, PhD, MS, MT(ASCP)
Assistant Professor
School of Health Sciences
Oakland University
Rochester, MI

Stephanie Roehm, RN, BSN
Instructor
Practical Nursing
MCC-Penn Valley Pioneer
Kansas City, MO

Lorraine E. Schoenbeck, MS, CMA
Associate Professor/Program Director
Medical Assisting Program
Lone Star College – North Harris
Houston, TX

Jackie Lynn Schumacher, RN, BScN, BEd
Instructor
Hospital Unit Clerk/Secretary Program
Red Deer College
Red Deer, Alberta, Canada

Donna Thaler Long, MSM,
RT(R)(M)(QM)
Registered Radiologic Technologist
Radiography Program
Ball State University/Clarian Health-
   Methodist Hospital
Indianapolis, IN

Kathy C. Trawick, EdD, RHIA
Associate Professor and Program Chairman
Department of Health Information
   Management
University of Arkansas for Medical Sciences
Little Rock, AR

Kathy Webb, MS, MEd
Professor
Math, Science, and Technology
Bucks County Community College
Newtown, PA

Dr. Susan Bawell Weber
Psychologist, Music Therapist
Department of Health Professions
Maryville University
St. Louis, MO

We are especially grateful to the contributors who provided the Health Care Professional profiles that appear in the text and on the Student Resource CD-ROM:

Sara D. Brown, MS, ATC
Director, Programs in Athletic Training
Department of Physical Therapy and
    Athletic Training
Boston University
Boston, MA

Mary Ellen Camire, PhD
Professor
Department of Food Science and Human
    Nutrition
University of Maine
Orono, ME

Pamela J. Carter, RN, BSN, MEd, CNOR
Program Coordinator/Instructor
School of Health Professions
Davis Applied Technology College
Kaysville, UT

Diane Gilmore, CMT, FAAMT
Director of Education
Transcription Relief Services
LLC/TRS Institute
Greensboro, NC

Susan J. Jenkins, MS, RDH
Assistant Professor of Dental Hygiene
Forsyth School of Dental Hygiene
Massachusetts College of Pharmacy &
    Health Sciences
Boston, MA

Patti Kalvelage, MS, OTR/L
Professor, Occupational Therapy
Governors State University
University Park, IL

Mary E. Mohr, RPh, MS
Pharmacy Technician Program Director
Health Sciences Education Center
Clarian Health
Indianapolis, IN

Jessica L. Murphy, BS, RRT-NPS,
RDCS, RVT
DCVS Program Director
Alvin Community College
Alvin, TX

S.L. Sherry, CPC
ICBS Program Director
Portland, OR

Ester L. Verhovsek, EdD
Associate Professor (Radiography, Allied
    Health Sciences)
Allied Health Sciences
East Tennessee State University
Johnson City, TN

Ruth Werner, LMP, NCTMB
Massage Therapist, Educator
Layton, UT

TABLE OF CONTENTS

PREFACE, vi

USER'S GUIDE, xi

ACKNOWLEDGMENTS, xvii

REVIEWERS AND CONTRIBUTORS, xviii

GETTING STARTED: A GUIDE TO STUDENT SUCCESS, xxiii

CHAPTER 1   MEDICAL TERMINOLOGY BASICS, I

CHAPTER 2   ANATOMIC STRUCTURES AND TERMS OF REFERENCE, 25

CHAPTER 3   HEALTH CARE RECORDS, 93

CHAPTER 4   SYMPTOMATIC AND DIAGNOSTIC TERMS, 147

CHAPTER 5   DIAGNOSTIC TESTS AND PROCEDURES, 213

CHAPTER 6   OPERATIVE AND THERAPEUTIC TERMS, 269

APPENDIX A   GLOSSARY OF PREFIXES, SUFFIXES, AND COMBINING FORMS, 335

APPENDIX B   ABBREVIATIONS AND SYMBOLS, 347

APPENDIX C   COMMONLY PRESCRIBED DRUGS, 353

FIGURE CREDITS, 357

INDEX, 361

GETTING STARTED: A GUIDE TO STUDENT SUCCESS

To reach the goal of learning the language of health care, you will need a solid plan for completion. Follow the study path that this text and/or your instructor provides, and work the necessary study time into your personal schedule.

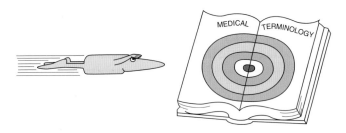

Using Flash Cards

Recognizing their important role in memorization, flash cards for prefixes, suffixes, and a select number of combining forms introduced in this text are provided at the back of the text. Each card is numbered and color coded according to division: prefixes are printed on orange cards, **combining forms** on **purple cards**, and suffixes on green cards. The term component is printed on the front of the card, with its meaning on the back. Remove these cards and stack them according to their type (prefix, suffix, or combining form) and in numbered sequence so that you can access them quickly and easily when studying and completing the programmed review sections within the chapters. Since all the cards are color-coded and in numerical order, it is possible to study the cards for one type of term component and then quickly reorder as needed to retrieve a card for review within a chapter.

ORGANIZING YOUR FLASH CARDS

Choose from the following ideas for organizing your flash cards:

- After separating cards by type and ordering by number, punch a hole in the top of each flash card. Loop the cards through a key chain or ring holder to make a "rotary file." This method keeps groups of cards together and prevents them from becoming lost or scattered.
- Regroup the cards as term components are identified for study in each chapter, and make your own cards for those components for which cards have not been supplied.
- Organize each type of term component into categories. For example, you can organize the prefix cards into components related to position or direction, components related to quantity or measurement, components related to time, and so forth.

MAKING ADDITIONAL FLASH CARDS

Flash cards are provided for most of the key term components in this text. For those components that do not have a preprinted card, you can produce one very simply using 3" × 5" cards. You'll see that the act of creating your cards will give you an added "memory boost." In addition, an electronic flash card generator is offered on the Student Resource CD-ROM as a method of creating new flash cards.

You may also extend the use of flash cards to include abbreviations, symbols, and additional terms and definitions found in the text, such as terms related to medical records, body planes and positions, diseases, diagnostic imaging, lab tests, and drug classifications.

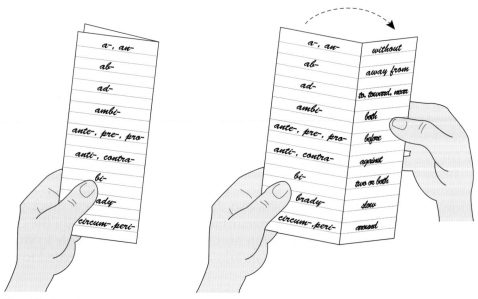

Frugal flash cards.

If you are interested in conserving paper and creating inexpensive flash cards, consider additional reinforcement by making "frugal flash cards":

1. Divide a piece of 8 ½" × 11" lined paper in half lengthwise by folding it down the center, creating two columns.

2. Write the term component, symbol, or medical term on the first line of the first column and its definition on the **same** line in the second column.

3. Skip down a line, and then write the next term component, symbol, or medical term with its definition on the **same** line in the second column. Continue listing any desired series of terms with corresponding definitions on the paper in this fashion until you reach the bottom of the paper.

4. Fold the paper at the lengthwise crease, dividing the columns so that the word component, symbol, or term is listed on one side of the paper, and the definition appears on the same line on the other side of the paper. This allows you to flip from one side to the other, "flashing" and reinforcing the meanings of the terms with the corresponding definitions.

5. Use the other side of the paper in the same way.

Using Programmed Learning Segments

The key to success with programmed learning is taking the time to review the term components listed in the Self-Instruction sections before starting the Programmed Learning segments. Each term component that has a preprinted flash card is identified by type (prefix, suffix, or combining form) and number. Locate and use them for additional reinforcement.

Remove the Reveal Card from the text. Place the card over the left column of the page to hide the correct responses to the questions in the learning material in the right column. Slide the card down the page to reveal the answer only after you've written your response in the fill-in space on the right. Note: Use a pencil so that you can erase any incorrect responses and replace them with the correct ones. Go over all of the correct responses with a highlighter pen for additional reinforcement.

The nice thing about programmed learning is that you can move at your own pace given the time allotted. Between study periods, use the reveal card as a bookmark.

Tips for Learning and Studying

Although you may already have ideas about how you learn and study most effectively, consider the following study tips to enhance your routine.

USING YOUR SENSES

An effective memory depends on intricate processes that recall mental images of sights, sounds, feelings, tastes, and smells. For this reason, try to include as many of your senses as possible in the process of reinforcing learning.

SEE IT	Employ your visual (seeing) sense by making and/or repeatedly reviewing your flash cards.
SAY IT	Pronounce each component out loud three times as you read the text and when using the flash cards to reinforce your auditory (hearing) sense.
WRITE IT	Make use of your kinesthetic (feeling) sense by writing and rewriting responses to programmed review sections and then highlighting the correct answers.
	Add to the preprinted term component flash cards and those that you have created by writing a term example on the back of each, under the definition. Draw lines to separate the components in each term for reinforcement.
	When making your own flash cards, use pleasant-colored paper and ink.

SNATCHING MOMENTS

Like most students, you probably have a busy life! Carry your paper flash cards with you at all times. During most days, there will be times when you can snatch a moment to flash your cards and reinforce what you have learned. You will actually feel less stress when waiting in a line or a waiting room for an appointment when you know that you are making good use of those moments for study time.

MNEMONICS CAN HELP

Named for the goddess of memory in Greek mythology, a mnemonic (pronounced *nē-mon'ik*) is any device for aiding memory. Mnemonic techniques link words and facts with clues for their recall using the stimuli of images, sounds, smell, touch, etc. Consider the following applications:

- Make up rhymes or stories that help to differentiate between meanings. For example: *peri-*, the prefix meaning around, is often confused with *para-*, the prefix meaning along side of. Use the two components in a sentence to compare their meanings, such as: "I sat 'para' (**alongside of**) Sarah on the merry-'peri'-go-**around**." Often the most absurd associations can help you to remember. It doesn't matter if they don't make sense to anyone but you!

- Make up songs and rhythms to help remember facts. Take a song you are familiar with, such as "Row, row, row, your boat..." and insert words with definitions that are in tune with the song.

- Draw pictures depicting term components for reinforcement.

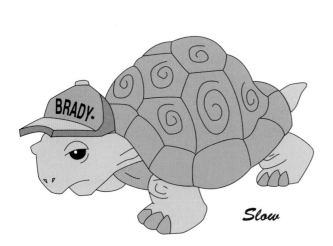

Slow

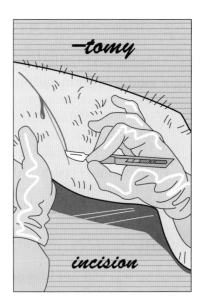

-tomy

incision

MEMORY DRILL

As you work through each chapter, give yourself a memory drill by listing term components, symbols, and medical terms on one side of a piece of paper and then filling in the definitions from memory. Correct your paper by writing out the correct answer over the incorrect one in red ink. Make a list of the incorrectly defined components on a separate piece of paper and repeat the drill. Repeat this process until you have identified a list of the ones most often defined incorrectly, and then spend additional time on those troublesome terms.

Additional Resources

Take advantage of the many fun and interactive learning activities provided on the Student Resource CD-ROM included with this text and online at www.thepoint.lww.com/WillisQC. You'll find a variety of exercises to help you remember medical terminology and to reinforce what you've learned in the text, including:

- **Review exercises and games** – Choose the types of exercises that best suit your learning style:
  - *multiple choice, fill-in-the-blank,* and *true/false* questions support learning
  - *word building* exercises expand your medical vocabulary
  - *figure labeling* exercises and *image matching* games reinforce visual learning
  - *spelling bee* helps you to recognize and correctly spell medical terms
  - *crossword puzzles, timed exercises,* and additional *word building activities* challenge your knowledge
  - *medical records exercises* use actual medical records so you can apply your learning to real-world examples

- **Chapter Quizzes and a Final Assessment** – Prepare for in-class quizzes and exams, or simply check your retention of each chapter's content before moving on to the next section.
- **Audio Pronunciation Glossary** – Listen to the proper audio pronunciation for the term components and key terms in the text. View all of the terms alphabetically, or organize terms by chapter. Use the Pronunciation Drill feature to play a select set of terms sequentially. Definitions are provided by *Stedman's Medical Dictionary, 28th Edition*.
- **Electronic Flash Cards and Flash Card Builder** – Study a complete set of term components from the book, and use the Flash Card Builder to make and print your own flash cards!

Ready, Set, Go!

Everything is laid out for you to proceed with your study, starting with Chapter 1 on the following page. Be creative and enjoy the learning process!

CHAPTER 1

MEDICAL TERMINOLOGY BASICS

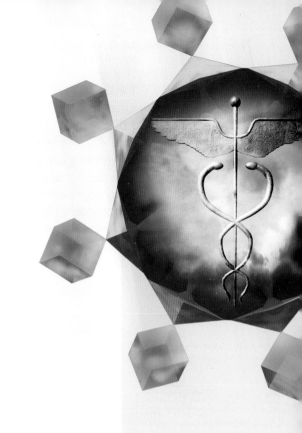

OBJECTIVES

1. Define medical terminology.
2. Describe the origin of medical language.
3. Analyze the component parts of a medical term to determine its meaning.
4. Explain the common rules for proper medical term formation, pronunciation, and spelling.

CHECKLIST | LOCATION

CHECKLIST	LOCATION
☐ Complete Chapter 1 Self-Instruction and Programmed Review sections	pages 2–18 📖
☐ Review the Flash Cards related to Chapter 1	FC
☐ Complete the Chapter 1 Examine Your Understanding exercises	pages 19–21 📖
☐ Practice saying the Chapter 1 terms out loud with the Audio Pronunciation Glossary on the Student Resource CD-ROM	CD-ROM
☐ Complete the Chapter 1 Interactive Exercises on the Student Resource CD-ROM	CD-ROM
☐ Take the Chapter 1 Quiz on the Student Resource CD-ROM	CD-ROM
☐ When you receive 70% or higher on the Quiz, move on to Chapter 2	page 25 📖

MEET THE PATIENT   Anne Stanco has been one of Dr. Spaulding's primary care patients for several years. Although she is diligent about seeing to the needs of her husband and daughter, who are also patients of Dr. Spaulding, Anne needs to take better care of herself. She claims she is "working on it," but still smokes cigarettes and is overweight, despite the history of heart problems in her family. With her 50th birthday approaching, Anne makes an appointment with Dr. Spaulding, who orders blood tests to evaluate her risks for heart disease. Indeed, Anne's lab results show that she has **hyperlipemia**. Information about Anne's condition will be explained in this chapter.

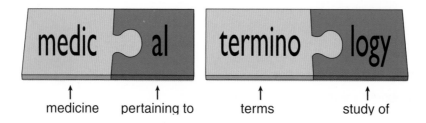

medic | al   termino | logy

↑   ↑   ↑   ↑
medicine   pertaining to   terms   study of

Medical terminology is the study of terms used in medicine and health care. The majority of medical terms have Greek or Latin origins that can be traced back to the founding of modern medicine by the Greeks and the influence of Latin when it was the universal language of the Western world. Other languages, such as German and French, have also influenced medical terms. Today, many new terms are derived from English, which is considered the universal language.

Once you understand the basic structure of medical terms and memorize the key 300 term components covered in this text, you can determine the meaning of most medical terms by simply defining their component parts. Those mysterious words, which are almost frightening at first glance, will soon seem commonplace. With your newfound knowledge and the help of a good medical dictionary, you will be able to analyze and understand each term you encounter.

Start Now

Take time to study the material in each self-instruction frame before starting a review segment. Flash cards for the prefixes, suffixes, and a select number of combining forms presented in this chapter are included at the back of the text and are identified by letter and number. Locate and use them for additional reinforcement. Use the electronic Flash Cards on the Student Resource CD-ROM, or hand write your own cards for those term components for which printed cards are not provided.

Remove the Reveal Card from the text. Place the card over the left column of the Programmed Review sections to hide the answers to the questions posed in the learning material in the right column. Slide the card down the page to reveal the answer only after you have written your response in the fill-in space on the right. Use a pencil so that you can erase any incorrect responses and replace them with the correct answers. You may mark all of the correct responses with a highlighter pen for extra reinforcement.

You can move at your own pace, given the time allotted. Between study periods, use the Reveal Card as a bookmark.

Term Components

Study the following term components to prepare for the Self-Instruction and Programmed Review segments that follow.

TERM COMPONENT	CATEGORY	MEANING	FLASH CARD ID
lip	root	fat	
lip/o	combining form	fat	CF-4
-emia	suffix	blood condition	S-7
hyper-	prefix	excessive	P-21
protein	root	protein	

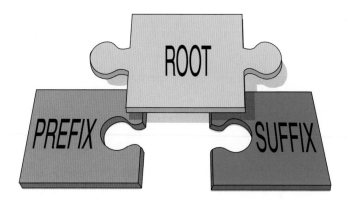

SELF-INSTRUCTION: Basic Term Components

The very first step in the study of medical language is to examine the basic structure of terms. Most medical terms have three **components:** a root, suffix, and prefix.

ROOT AND SUFFIX

The **root** is the foundation or subject of a term. The **suffix** is the word ending that modifies and gives essential meaning to the root. Medical terms are formed by combining one or more roots to a suffix. Consider the term lipemia, for example:

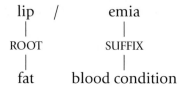

Lip (meaning fat) is the root and the subject of the term. It is modified by the suffix *-emia*, meaning blood condition, to indicate a condition of fat in the blood. Note that each component is dependent on the other to express meaning.

PREFIX

The **prefix** is a term component that is placed at the beginning of a term when needed to further modify the root or roots. Let's look at the term hyperlipemia:

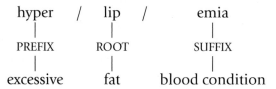

The addition of the prefix *hyper-* (meaning excessive) modifies the root to denote excessive fat in the blood.

ADDITIONAL ROOTS

Often a medical term is formed around two or more roots. For example, in hyperlipoproteinemia:

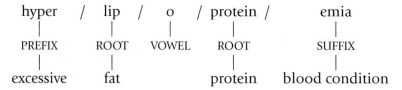

In this term, the second root, *protein* (joined to *lip* by the vowel "o"), further defines the word to indicate an excessive amount of fat and protein in the blood.

COMBINING VOWELS AND COMBINING FORMS

When a medical term contains more than one root, each is joined by a vowel, usually an "o." As shown in the term hyper/lip/o/protein/emia, the "o" links the two roots and fosters easier pronunciation. This vowel is known as a **combining vowel.** Combining vowels are also used to link a root to a suffix. The letter "o" is the most common combining vowel ("i" is the second most common). They are used so frequently that it is common to present them along with the root as a **combining form**:

      lip   root
      lip/o   combining form (root with combining vowel attached)

   This text uses combining forms rather than roots for easier term analysis. Each is presented with a slash between the root and the combining vowel. Hyphens are placed <u>after</u> prefixes to indicate their placement at the beginning of a medical term, and hyphens are placed <u>before</u> suffixes to indicate their placement at the end of a term.

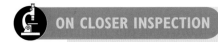
ON CLOSER INSPECTION   *Hem/o, hemat/o,* and *-emia* **Compete for Use in Terms Referring to Blood**

Stemming from the Greek word haima, *hem/o* and *hemat/o* are combining forms that both mean blood.

   The root *hem* was linked to *-ia*, a simple suffix meaning condition of, to form *-emia*, the compound suffix meaning blood condition. The "h" was initially part of the reference but was dropped over time.

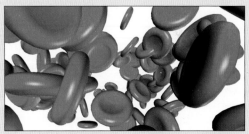
A cluster of erythrocytes (red blood cells).

   hem/o and *hemat/o* are common subjects in medical terms related to blood, and *-emia* is used to modify terms related to blood conditions. For example:

- Hematology is the study of blood.
- Hyperlipemia is a condition of excessive fat in blood.

PROGRAMMED REVIEW: Basic Term Components

ANSWERS	REVIEW
root, suffix, prefix	**1.1** Most medical terms have three basic parts: the _____, _____, and _____.
subject or foundation	**1.2** The root is the _____ of the term.

suffix	**1.3** The _____ is the word ending that modifies and gives essential meaning to the root.
prefix	**1.4** The _____ is a term component at the beginning of a term that further modifies the root.
two	**1.5** Often a medical term is formed from _____ or more roots.
vowel o	**1.6** When a medical term has more than one root, it is joined together by a combining _____ (usually a/an ___).
root vowel	**1.7** A combining form is a/an _____ with a/an _____ attached.
fat subject or foundation blood condition fat, blood	**1.8** In the word lipemia, *lip*, meaning _____, is the root and _____ of the term. It is modified and given essential meaning by the link to the suffix *-emia*, meaning _____ _____. The term refers to a condition of _____ in the _____. Note: Lipemia is synonymous with lipidemia.
prefix beginning modify excessive	**1.9** In the term hyperlipemia, *hyper-* is a/an _____ placed at the _____ of the term to further _____ the meaning of the term to denote above or _____ fat in the blood.
root protein	**1.10** In the term hyperlipoproteinemia, the addition of the _____ protein further defines the word to indicate an excessive amount of fat and _____ in the blood.

root combining form o combining vowel, i	**1.11** In *lip/o*, *lip* is the _____ and *lip/o* is the _____ _____ (root with combining vowel attached). The vowel ___ is the most common _____ _____, and ____ is the second most common combining vowel.

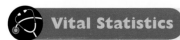

Vital Statistics   HYPERLIPEMIA (hī′per-li-pē′mē-ă)

Origin: *hyper-* (above or excessive) + *lip/o* (fat) + *-emia* (blood condition)

The patient you met at the beginning of this chapter, Anne Stanco, was diagnosed with hyperlipemia. What exactly is that?

Hyperlipemia is an excess of fatty substances called lipids in the blood. It is also called hyperlipoproteinemia because these fatty substances travel in the blood attached to proteins.

Hyperlipemia, along with diabetes, hypertension (high blood pressure), positive family history, and smoking, is a major risk factor for heart disease. It usually has no noticeable symptoms and tends to be discovered during routine examination or evaluation for heart disease. Diagnosis is typically based on medical history, physical examination, and blood tests.

It is necessary to first identify and treat any potential underlying medical problems, such as diabetes or hypothyroidism, that can contribute to hyperlipemia. Treatment of hyperlipemia includes dietary changes, weight reduction, and exercise. If lifestyle modifications cannot bring about optimal lipid levels, then medications may be necessary.

Term Components

The following is a list of term components that are used in this chapter to explain the rules for forming, spelling, and pronouncing medical terms. Study the flash cards for each term component to prepare for the Self-Instruction and Programmed Review segments that follow.

SUFFIX	MEANING	FLASH CARD ID
-al, -ic	pertaining to	S-1
-ectomy	excision or removal	S-6
-emia	blood condition	S-7
-itis	inflammation	S-18
-logy	study of	S-22
-spasm	involuntary contraction	S-45
-stomy	creation of an opening	S-47
-tomy	incision	S-48

PREFIX	MEANING	FLASH CARD ID
hyper-	above or excessive	P-21
hypo-	below or deficient	P-22
para-	alongside of or abnormal	P-31
peri-	around	P-33

COMBINING FORM (ROOT WITH VOWEL)	MEANING	FLASH CARD ID
angi/o, vas/o, vascul/o	vessel	CF-5
cardi/o	heart	CF-11
enter/o	small intestine	CF-23
esophag/o	esophagus	
gastr/o	stomach	CF-26
hem/o, hemat/o	blood	CF-28
lip/o	fat	CF-4
oste/o	bone	
ox/o	oxygen	

SELF-INSTRUCTION: Defining Medical Terms through Word Structure Analysis

You can usually define a term by interpreting the suffix first, then the prefix (if present), and then the succeeding root or roots. Take, for example, the term pericarditis:

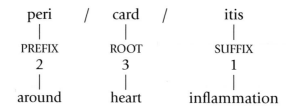

pericarditis = inflammation around the heart

You sense the basic meaning of this term by understanding its components; however, the dictionary further clarifies the fact that pericarditis refers to inflammation of the pericardium, which is the sac that encloses the heart.

Rx for Success

Beginning students often have difficulty differentiating between prefixes and roots (or combining forms) because the root appears first in a medical term when there is no prefix. It is important to memorize the most common prefixes so that you can tell the difference. Also, keep in mind that a prefix is only used as needed to further modify the root or roots, whereas the root is the foundation or subject of the word.

ON CLOSER INSPECTION   **Exceptions to the Rule**

Occasionally, you will come across terms that are formed by a root alone or by a combination of roots. For example:

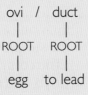

duct
|
ROOT
|
to lead

A duct is a tubular structure that provides for passage.

ovi / duct
| |
ROOT   ROOT
| |
egg   to lead

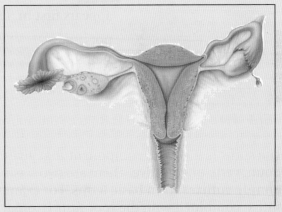

Female reproductive system: ovary, fallopian tube, uterus, and vagina.

An oviduct is the uterine tube that provides for passage of a female egg.

Other times, a term is formed by the combination of a prefix and suffix.

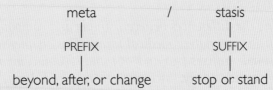

meta   /   stasis
| |
PREFIX   SUFFIX
| |
beyond, after, or change   stop or stand

Metastasis refers to the spread of a disease, such as cancer, from one location to another.

PROGRAMMED REVIEW: Defining Medical Terms through Word Structure Analysis

ANSWERS	REVIEW
suffix, prefix root	**1.12** You can usually define a term by interpreting the _____ first, then the _____ (if present), and then the succeeding _____ or roots.
inflammation around the heart	**1.13** Pericarditis is defined as _____ _____.
combining form prefix	**1.14** Often a root or _____ _____ appears first in a medical term when a/an _____ is not used.

SELF-INSTRUCTION: Role of the Suffix in Defining Medical Terms

The suffix is the word component that gives essential meaning to a term by forming a noun, verb, or adjective. There are two basic types of suffixes: simple and compound. **Simple suffixes** form basic terms. For example, -ic (meaning pertaining to) is a simple suffix; combined with the root *gastr* (stomach), it forms the term gastric (pertaining to the stomach). **Compound suffixes** are formed by a combination of basic term components. For example, the root *tom* (to cut) combined with the simple suffix -y (denoting a process of) forms the compound suffix -tomy (incision). The compound suffix -ectomy (excision or removal) is formed by a combination of the prefix ec- (out) with the root *tom* (to cut) and the simple suffix -y (a process of).

Rx for Success

Noting the differences between simple and compound suffixes will help you analyze medical terms. This chapter introduces two simple suffixes (-al and -ic) and several compound suffixes (-emia, -tomy, -stomy, -ectomy, and -logy). These suffixes, along with others in specific categories, will be highlighted in later chapters to create terms related to anatomy, symptoms, diagnoses, tests, surgeries, and therapies.

Suffixes in this text are divided into four categories, as outlined below:

CATEGORY	FUNCTION	EXAMPLE
Symptomatic suffix	describes the evidence of illness	-spasm
Diagnostic suffix	identifies a medical condition	-emia, -itis
Surgical (or operative) suffix	describes a surgical treatment	-tomy, -stomy, -ectomy
General suffix	has general application, such as to form an adjective or noun	-al, -ic, -logy

PROGRAMMED REVIEW: Role of the Suffix in Defining Medical Terms

ANSWERS	REVIEW
compound, simple	**1.15** There are two basic types of suffixes: simple and _____. -al is an example of a/an _____ suffix.
symptomatic	**1.16** Suffixes that describe the evidence of disease are called _____ suffixes.
diagnostic	**1.17** -emia and -itis are examples of _____ suffixes.
operative

-ectomy | **1.18** Surgical suffixes, also known as _____ suffixes, describe a surgical treatment. -tomy, -stomy, and _____ are examples of surgical suffixes. |
| pertaining to | **1.19** General suffixes, such as -al and -ic, meaning _____ ____, form adjective endings of terms. |

SELF-INSTRUCTION: Rules for Forming and Spelling Medical Terms

Now that you understand the basic term components, the next step is to learn the rules for how to correctly form a medical term. Memorize the following rules and use them to construct terms in the Programmed Review section that follows:

1. A combining vowel (usually an "o" or "i") is used to join a root to another root or to a suffix that begins with a consonant. Example: *gastr/o* + *enter/o* + *-stomy* is spelled gastroenterostomy.

2. A combining vowel is <u>not</u> used before a suffix that begins with a vowel. Example: *vas/o* + *-ectomy* is spelled vasectomy.

3. If the root ends in a vowel and the suffix begins with the same vowel, drop the final vowel from the root and do <u>not</u> use a combining vowel. Example: *cardi/o* + *-itis* is spelled carditis.

4. Occasionally, when a prefix ends in a vowel and the root begins with a vowel, the final vowel is dropped from the prefix. Example: *para-* + *enter/o* + *-al* is spelled parenteral.

 ## Rx for Success

You will encounter exceptions to these rules for forming and spelling medical terms. Follow the basic guidelines set forth in this text, but be prepared to accept exceptions as you encounter them. Rely on your medical dictionary for additional guidance.

PROGRAMMED REVIEW: Rules for Forming and Spelling Medical Terms

ANSWERS	REVIEW
o, i root suffix, consonant	**1.20** A combining vowel (usually a/an ____ or ____) is used to join a root to another _____, or to a/an _____ that begins with a/an _____.
gastroenterostomy creation of an opening (between) the stomach and small intestine	**1.21** *gastr/o* + *enter/o* + *-stomy* is spelled _____ and means _____ _____ _____.

not vowel	**1.22** A combining vowel is _____ used before a suffix that begins with a/an _____.
vasectomy excision or removal of a vessel	**1.23** *vas/o + -ectomy* is spelled _____ and means _____ _____ (the vessel of the vas deferens in the male).
drop do not	**1.24** If the root ends in a vowel and the suffix begins with the same vowel, _____ the final vowel from the root and _____ _____ use a combining vowel.
carditis inflammation of the heart	**1.25** *cardi/o + -itis* is spelled _____ and means _____ _____.
vowel prefix	**1.26** Occasionally, when a prefix ends in a vowel and the root begins with a/an _____, the final vowel is dropped from the _____.
hypoxemia blood condition of below or deficient oxygen	**1.27** *hypo- + ox/o + -emia* is spelled _____ and means _____ _____ _____.
gastrotomy incision in stomach	**1.28** *gastr/o + -tomy* is spelled _____ and means _____.
angitis inflammation of a vessel	**1.29** *angi/o + -itis* is spelled _____ and means _____ _____.

esophagospasm involuntary contraction of the esophagus	**1.30** *esophag/o* + *-spasm* is spelled _____ and means _____ _____.
excision or removal of bone	**1.31** *oste/o* + *-ectomy* is spelled _____ and means _____ _____.
hematology study of blood	**1.32** *hemat/o* + *-logy* is spelled _____ and means _____.
gastric pertaining to the stomach	**1.33** *gastr/o* + *-ic* is spelled _____ and means _____.
parenteral, pertaining to alongside of the small intestine	**1.34** *para-* + *enter/o* + *-al* is spelled _____ and means _____ _____ _____.
pericarditis inflammation around the heart	**1.35** *peri-* + *cardi/o* + *-itis* is spelled _____ and means _____ _____.

SELF-INSTRUCTION: Rules of Pronunciation

When you are learning to pronounce medical terms, the task can seem insurmountable. The first time you open your mouth to say a term is a tense moment for those who want to get it right! The best preparation is to study the basic rules of pronunciation, repeat the words after hearing them pronounced on the CD-ROM that accompanies this text and/or after your instructor has said them, and try to spend time with others who use medical language. There is nothing like the validation you feel when you say something "medical" for the very first time and no one laughs or snarls at you! Your confidence will build with every word you use.

Study the following shortcuts to pronunciation:

Consonant Sounds	Example
c (before a, o, u) = k	cavity, company, cure
c (before e, i) = s	cell, city
ch = k	character
g (before a, o, u) = g	gain, good, guilt
g (before e, i) = j	generic, giant
ph = f	phase
pn = n	pneumonia
ps = s	psychology
pt = t	ptosis
rh, rrh = r	rhythm, diarrhea
x (as first letter) = z	xerosis

The phonetic spelling for the pronunciation of medical terms in this text is provided in summary lists at the end of chapters; these terms are also pronounced on the Student Resource CD-ROM. The phonetic system described here is basic and uses only a few standard rules. The macron and breve are the two diacritical (accent) marks used.

The macron (¯) is placed over vowels that have a long sound:

ā in day
ē in bee
ī in pie
ō in no
ū in unit

The breve (˘) is placed over vowels that have a short sound:

ă in alone
ĕ in system
ĭ in pencil
ŏ in oven
ŭ in sun

The primary accent (′) is placed after the syllable that is stressed when saying the word, for example, x′ray. Monosyllables (words with only one syllable) do not have a stress mark. Other syllables are separated by hyphens.

PROGRAMMED REVIEW: Rules of Pronunciation

ANSWERS	REVIEW
t	**1.36** The "pt" in ptosis has a/an ____ sound.
k	**1.37** The "ch" in the word chronic has a/an ____ sound.
s	**1.38** The "c" in the word citizen has a/an ____ sound.
z	**1.39** The "x" in xiphoid has a/an ___ sound.
j	**1.40** The "g" in genital has a/an ___ sound.
n	**1.41** The "pn" in pneumatic has a/an ___ sound.
r	**1.42** The "rrh" in hemorrhoid has a/an ____ sound.
f	**1.43** The "ph" in pharmacy has a/an ____ sound.
g	**1.44** The "g" in gurney has a/an ____ sound.
s	**1.45** The "ps" in psychic has a/an ____ sound.
k	**1.46** The "c" in cure has a/an ____ sound.

SELF-INSTRUCTION: Singular and Plural Forms

Most often, plurals are formed by adding "s" or "es" to the end of a singular form. The following are common exceptions for forming plurals of terms of Latin and Greek derivation. Study the exceptions in preparation for a review that follows.

Singular Ending	Example	Plural Ending	Example
-a	vertebra *vĕr′ tĕ-bră*	-ae	vertebrae *vĕr′ tĕ-brā*
-is	diagnosis *dī-ag-nō′ sis*	-es	diagnoses *dī-ag-nō′ sēz*

Singular Ending	Example	Plural Ending	Example
-ma	condyloma *kon-di-lō′mă*	-mata	condylomata *kon-di-lō′mah-tă*
-on	phenomenon *fĕ-nom′ĕ-non*	-a	phenomena *fĕ-nom′ĕ-nă*
-um	bacterium *bak-tēr′ē-yŭm*	-a	bacteria *bak-tēr′ē-ă*
-us*	fungus *fŭng′gŭs*	-i	fungi *fŭn′jī*
-ax	thorax *thō′raks*	-aces	thoraces *thō-rā′sēz*
-ex	*apex* *ā′peks*	-ices	apices *ap′i-sēs*
-ix	appendix *ă-pen′diks*	-ices	appendices *ă-pen′di-sēz*
-y	myopathy *mī-op′ă-thē*	-ies	myopathies *mī-op′ă-thēz*

*The terms virus and sinus follow the usual rule of adding "s" or "es" to form the plural (viruses and sinuses) instead of using the Latin ending "i."

PROGRAMMED REVIEW: Singular and Plural Forms

ANSWERS	REVIEW
ovaries ova	**1.47** An ovum is an egg produced by an ovary. There are two _____ in the female that produce eggs, or _____.
metastases	**1.48** The spread of cancer to a distant organ is called metastasis. The spread of cancer to more than one organ is called _____.
verrucae	**1.49** A verruca is a wart. The term for several warts is _____.

condyloma	**1.50** Condylomata are genital warts. One genital wart is a/an _____.
index appendices	**1.51** Indices is a plural form of _____. More than one appendix is termed _____.
thrombi	**1.52** A thrombus is a clot. Several clots are termed _____.
bacteria	**1.53** A bacterium is a single-celled microorganism. The plural form of bacterium is _____.
viruses	**1.54** A virus is an infective agent. The term referring to more than one virus is _____.
thorax	**1.55** Thoraces is a plural form of _____.
a	**1.56** A singular term ending with *-on* is made plural by replacing these letters with a/an ____.

Examine Your Understanding

For the following terms, draw a line or lines to separate the prefixes (P), combining forms (CF), roots (R), and suffixes (S). Then, write the meaning of each component on the corresponding blank to define the term.

EXAMPLE

hyperlipemia

hyper/lip/emia

above or excessive / _fat_ / _blood condition_

P   R   S

1. vasculitis

_____ / _____

R   S

2. osteotomy

_____ / _____

CF   S

3. hematology

_____ / _____

CF   S

4. hypolipoproteinemia

_____ / _____ / _____ / _____

P   CF   R   S

5. hypoxic

_____ / _____ / _____

P   R   S

6. enterostomy

_____ / _____

CF   S

7. periosteal

_____ / _____ / _____

P   R   S

8. gastrectomy

_____ / _____

R   S

9. vasospasm

_____ / _____

CF   S

10. pericarditis

_____ / _____ / _____

P   R   S

Match the following examples of basic term components:

11. _____ -emia   a. root
12. _____ lip/o   b. combining vowel
13. _____ hyper-   c. suffix
14. _____ protein   d. prefix
15. _____ o   e. combining form

Circle the correct meaning for the following term components:

16. *para-*
   a. around   b. deficient   c. alongside of   d. excessive

17. *-al*
   a. condition of   b. study of   c. alongside of   d. pertaining to

18. *angi/o*
   a. heart   b. vessel   c. small intestine   d. blood

19. *hemat/o*
   a. liver   b. blood   c. blood condition   d. enlargement

20. *peri-*
   a. around   b. deficient   c. alongside of   d. excessive

21. *-ic*
   a. pertaining to   b. alongside of   c. around   d. incision

Briefly describe the difference between the following term components:

22. *peri-* vs. *para-* _____

23. *hypo-* vs. *hyper-* _____

24. *hem/o* vs. *-emia* _____

25. *-tomy* vs. *-stomy* vs. *-ectomy* _____

Circle the correct plural form for the following terms:

26. vertebra
   a. vertebray   b. vertebrases   c. vertebrae   d. vertebrus   e. vertebraes

27. speculum
   a. speculata   b. speculumes   c. specula   d. speculae   e. speculuma

28. fungus
   a. fungi   b. fungae   c. funges   d. funguses   e. fungea

29. stoma

    a. stomata   b. stomatae   c. stomes   d. stomatus   e. stomatum

30. diagnosis

    a. diagnosa   b. diagnoses   c. diagnosses   d. diagnosi   e. diagnosae

31. radius

    a. radii   b. radiusos   c. radiuses   d. radia   e. radiis

32. phenomenon

    a. phenomenones b. phenomena c. phenomeni d. phenomenata e. phenomenae

Match the following types of suffixes:

33. _____ symptomatic   a. *-ic*

34. _____ diagnostic   b. *-ectomy*

35. _____ operative   c. *-itis*

36. _____ general   d. *-spasm*

Complete the following statements related to rules of term pronunciation:

37. The "pt" in pterygium has a/an _____ sound.

38. The "c" in the word cell has a/an _____ sound.

39. The "g" in generic has a/an _____ sound.

40. The "pn" in pneumonia has a/an _____ sound.

Combine the following components to correctly form medical terms:

41. *oste/o* + *-tomy* = _____

42. *vascul/o* + *-itis* = _____

43. *gastr/o* + *enter/o* + *-logy* = _____

44. *enter/o* + *-ic* = _____

45. *cardi/o* + *-spasm* = _____

Answers to Examine Your Understanding

1. vascul/itis
   <u>vessel</u> / <u>inflammation</u>
     R   S

2. osteo/tomy
   <u>bone</u> / <u>incision</u>
     CF   S

3. hemato/logy
   <u>blood</u> / <u>study of</u>
     CF   S

4. hypo/lipo/protein/emia
   <u>below or deficient</u> / <u>fat</u> / <u>protein</u> / <u>blood condition</u>
        P   CF   R   S

5. hyp/ox/ic
   <u>below or deficient</u> / <u>oxygen</u> / <u>pertaining to</u>
        P   R   S

6. entero/stomy
   <u>small intestine</u> / <u>creation of an opening</u>
       CF   S

7. peri/oste/al
   <u>around</u> / <u>bone</u> / <u>pertaining to</u>
      P   R   S

8. gastr/ectomy
   <u>stomach</u> / <u>excision or removal</u>
      R   S

9. vaso/spasm
   <u>vessel</u> / <u>involuntary contraction</u>
      CF   S

10. peri/card/itis
    <u>around</u> / <u>heart</u> / <u>inflammation</u>
        P   R   S

11. c	15. b	19. b
12. e	16. c	20. a
13. d	17. d	21. a
14. a	18. b	

22. *peri-* is a prefix meaning around, whereas *para-* is a prefix meaning alongside of or abnormal.

23. *hypo-* is a prefix meaning below or deficient, whereas *hyper-* is a prefix meaning above or excessive.

24. *hem/o* is a combining form meaning blood, whereas *-emia* is a suffix meaning blood condition.

25. *-tomy* is a suffix meaning incision; *-stomy* is a suffix meaning creation of an opening; and *-ectomy* is a suffix meaning excision or removal.

26. c
27. c
28. a
29. a
30. b
31. a
32. b

33. d
34. c
35. b
36. a
37. t
38. s
39. j

40. n
41. osteotomy
42. vasculitis
43. gastroenterology
44. enteric
45. cardiospasm

CHAPTER 2

ANATOMIC STRUCTURES AND TERMS OF REFERENCE

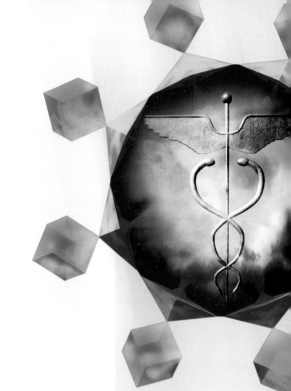

OBJECTIVES

1. Identify anatomic terms common to the following body systems: integumentary, musculoskeletal, cardiovascular, blood and lymph, respiratory, nervous, endocrine, special senses of the eye and ear, gastrointestinal, urinary, and reproductive.

2. Describe the anatomic position.

3. Identify the body planes.

4. Define positional and directional terms, as well as terms related to body movement.

5. List the main body cavities.

6. Name the anatomic and clinical divisions of the abdomen.

CHECKLIST

CHECKLIST	LOCATION
☐ Complete Chapter 2 Self-Instruction and Programmed Review sections	pages 26–79 📖
☐ Review the Flash Cards related to Chapter 2	🃏
☐ Complete the Chapter 2 Examine Your Understanding exercises	pages 82–86 📖
☐ Complete Medical Record Exercise 2-1	pages 87–88 📖

(continued)

☐ Practice saying the Chapter 2 terms out loud with the Audio Pronunciation Glossary on the Student Resource CD-ROM

☐ Complete the Chapter 2 Interactive Exercises on the Student Resource CD-ROM

☐ Take the Chapter 2 Quiz on the Student Resource CD-ROM

☐ When you receive 70% or higher on the Quiz, move on to Chapter 3   page 93

MEET THE PATIENT   Fourteen-year-old Raymond Hauck has been Dr. Spaulding's patient since he was a baby. Last evening, and persisting all night, he had a high fever, headache, and vomiting. In addition, his neck is stiff and painful, and he cannot touch his chin to his chest. Concerned for her son, Mrs. Hauck calls Dr. Spaulding's office the first thing in the morning and explains his symptoms over the telephone. Recognizing that Raymond is experiencing several signs and symptoms of meningitis, Dr. Spaulding makes an immediate referral to Dr. Migeon, a pediatric neurologist. The nature of a pediatric neurology practice requires last-minute adjustments to the schedule for patients who need to be seen immediately, and Jackie Smith, an experienced **Medical Assistant** who has worked for Dr. Migeon for several years, recognizes this urgency when she takes the call from Dr. Spaulding this morning. Jackie arranges for Raymond to be brought to the office immediately so that a lumbar puncture can be performed. Since Jackie performs a variety of administrative and clinical skills in the neurology office, she assists with the procedure by obtaining consent from Raymond's mother, preparing Raymond for the procedure, and assembling the necessary equipment. You will read about the procedure in **Medical Record Exercise 2-1.**

Now that you are familiar with the basic term components and understand the rules for forming and spelling medical terms, the next step in learning the language of health care is to analyze the term components that are used in forming terms related to structures of the body and anatomic reference points.

Term Components

Suffixes and prefixes that are used to form terms related to the anatomic structures of the body and anatomic reference points are listed below. Pertinent combining forms will be added as programmed learning segments are presented. Study the suffixes and prefixes first, and then add the related combining forms as you work through the chapter.

SUFFIX	MEANING	FLASH CARD ID
-al, -ar, -ary, -eal, -ic, -ous	pertaining to	S-1
-e	noun marker	
-genesis	origin or production	S-8
-icle, -ole, -ule	small	S-16
-ist	one who specializes in	S-17
-ium	structure or tissue	S-19
-logist	one who specializes in the study or treatment of	S-21
-logy	study of	S-22
-phil	attraction for	S-33
-poiesis	formation	S-38
-scope	instrument for examination	S-43
-y	condition or process of	S-50

PREFIX	MEANING	FLASH CARD ID
a-, an-	without	P-1
ab-	away from	P-2
ad-	to, toward, or near	P-3
ana-	up, apart	P-5
ante-, pre-, pro-	before	P-6
bi-	two or both	P-27
e-, ex-, exo-	out or away	P-13
endo-	within	P-14
epi-	upon	P-15
hyper-, super-	above or excessive	P-21
hypo-	below or deficient	P-22
inter-	between	P-23
macro-	large	P-24
micro-	small	P-26
mono-, uni-	one	P-27
pan-	all	P-30
para-	alongside of or abnormal	P-31

(continued)

PREFIX	MEANING	FLASH CARD ID
peri-	around	P-33
post-	after	P-35
semi-	half	P-18
sub-	below or under	P-36
trans-	across or through	P-11
tri-	three	P-27

Anatomic Terms Related to Body Structures

Most anatomic terms stem from Latin because it was the language used during the period of the Roman Empire, when early scientific study of the form and structure of the body was conducted. It was common to use everyday terms to describe the structures of the body. For example, the patella (kneecap) was named for its resemblance to a pan, and the tympanic membrane (eardrum) got its name because of its likeness to a tambourine.

Some anatomic terms were named for the person who first discovered or described them. For example, the eustachian tube (also known as the auditory tube), which connects the middle ear to the throat, was named to honor Bartolomeo Eustachio, the anatomist who first discovered the structure. The female uterine tubes are also known as the fallopian tubes, in honor of Gabrielle Fallopius. He compared the ends of each tube to a trumpet (Latin, tuba). The use of proper names (eponyms) is fairly common, but their Latin synonyms were more often used when establishing standard anatomic nomenclature.

SELF-INSTRUCTION: Cells, Tissues, Organs, and Systems

Living things are organized from the simple level to the complex. The **cell** is the simplest living form and the basic unit of life. Cells are specialized and grouped into **tissues**, which are combined to form **organs**. Groups of organs form **body systems**, which work together to perform important functions in the body. The body systems include: integumentary, musculoskeletal, cardiovascular, blood and lymph, respiratory, nervous, endocrine, special senses of the eye and ear, gastrointestinal, urinary, and reproductive.

Study Fig. 2-1 and the following combining forms before starting the Programmed Review section.

COMBINING FORM	MEANING	FLASH CARD ID
cyt/o	cell	CF-19
hist/o	tissue	CF-30
path/o	disease	CF-46
tom/o	to cut	
ur/o, urin/o	urine	CF-67

Levels of organization

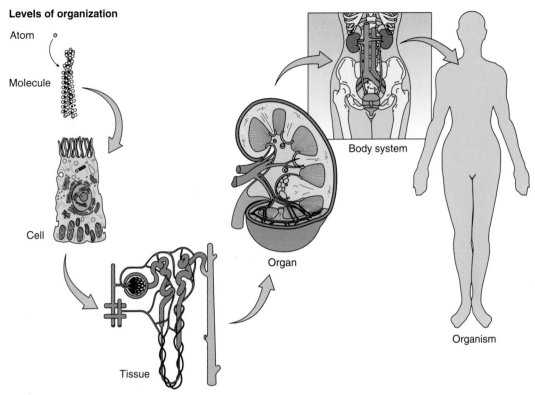

FIGURE 2-1   Levels of organization in the body.

PROGRAMMED REVIEW: Cells, Tissues, Organs, and Systems

ANSWERS	REVIEW
	2.1 The term cell, meaning small room, was used to describe the structures first observed in 1665 by Robert Hooke as he examined cork using a microscope, an
small	instrument to examine something _____. He noted that the small cells were part of a larger web of woven tissue. The study of cells that comprise the human body became
cyto	known as _____logy, and the study of tissue became
histology	known as _____.

	2.2 Body cells combine to form tissues, and combinations of tissues compose the organs necessary for body functions. Organs act together as part of the larger
systems	body _____. For example, the kidneys are
organs	_____ that function to filter blood as part of the
urine	urinary system (*urin/o* means _____, and *-ary*
pertaining to	means _____ ___).

	2.3 Human anatomy is defined as the scientific study of the form and structure of the body. The term was formed
up or apart	by the combination of *ana-*, a prefix meaning _____,
combining form	with *tom/o*, a/an _____ _____ meaning
to cut	___ _____, and *-y*, a simple suffix referring to a
process of	condition or _____ ___. Earliest anatomists performed gross or macroscopic anatomy. Gross refers to something large or visible to the naked eye. *macro-* also
large	refers to something _____. Gross anatomy including dissection is a process of studying the body that has been used since ancient times.

	2.4 Cells and tissues too small to be viewed by the naked eye were analyzed once the microscope was
cytology	invented. This study of cells, or _____,
histology	and study of tissue, or _____, is part of microscopic anatomy. Cytological and histological examinations are part of the medical specialty concerned
pathology	with the study of disease, known as _____. The physician who is a specialist in the study of
pathologist	disease is called a/an _____.

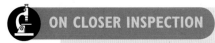

ON CLOSER INSPECTION   **Spelling Medical Terms**

Correct spelling of medical terms is crucial for communication among health care professionals. Careless spelling can cause misunderstandings that have serious consequences. The following are some spelling pitfalls to avoid:

1. Some combining forms have the same meaning but different origins that compete for usage. For example, there are three combining forms that mean uterus:

   hyster/o (Greek)
   metr/o (Greek)
   uter/o (Latin)

2. Other words sound similar but are spelled differently and have different meanings. For example:

   abduction (to draw away from)
   adduction (to draw toward)

3. Some words sound exactly the same but are spelled differently and have different meanings. Context is the clue to spelling. For example:

   cytology (study of cells)   sitology (study of food)
   ileum (part of the intestine)   ilium (part of the hip bone)

SELF-INSTRUCTION: Integumentary System

Study Fig. 2-2 and the following combining forms before starting the Programmed Review section.

COMBINING FORM	MEANING	FLASH CARD ID
adip/o, lip/o	fat	CF-4
derm/o, dermat/o, cutane/o	skin	CF-21
melan/o	black	CF-39
squam/o	scale	

Rx for Success

Take care to note the placement of hyphens when studying the difference between e-, the prefix meaning out or away, and -e, the simple suffix used as a noun marker.

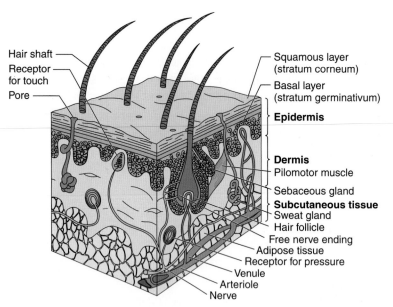

Hair shaft
Receptor for touch
Pore
Squamous layer (stratum corneum)
Basal layer (stratum germinativum)
Epidermis

Dermis
Pilomotor muscle
Sebaceous gland
Subcutaneous tissue
Sweat gland
Hair follicle
Free nerve ending
Adipose tissue
Receptor for pressure
Venule
Arteriole
Nerve

FIGURE 2-2   The skin.

PROGRAMMED REVIEW: Integumentary System

ANSWERS	REVIEW
	2.5 The largest organ of the body, the skin, is part of the integumentary system. Integument is Latin for skin, and
skin	*dermat/o* is Greek, meaning _____. The skin has three layers: the epidermis, dermis, and subcutaneous tissue.
upon	The epidermis is so named because it is _____ the dermis, and the subcutaneous tissue layer is named for
below or under	its location _____ the dermis.
	2.6 The epidermis consists of many layers; the deepest is called the basal layer. Melanocytes are cells in the basal layer responsible for skin color. *melan/o* is a combining form
black, cell	meaning _____, *cyt/o* means _____,
noun marker	and -*e* is a/an _____ _____. The outermost

scale pertaining to	layer of the epidermis is known as the squamous cell layer. *squam/o* means _____, and *-ous* means _____ ____.
      fat	**2.7** The dermis is the connective tissue layer that contains blood vessels, nerves, glands, and hair follicles. The subcutaneous layer contains adipose tissue. *adip/o* and *lip/o* are combining forms meaning _____.
dermatology dermatologist	**2.8** The specialty field involved with the study and treatment of skin diseases is called _____. The specialist in the study and treatment of the skin is called a/an _____.

SELF-INSTRUCTION: Musculoskeletal System

Study Fig. 2-3 and the following combining forms before starting the Programmed Review section.

COMBINING FORM	MEANING	FLASH CARD ID
acr/o	extremity or topmost	CF-2
arthr/o	joint	CF-6
cervic/o	neck	CF-13
chondr/o	cartilage	
cost/o	rib	CF-15
crani/o	skull	CF-16
lumb/o	loin (lower back)	
my/o, muscul/o	muscle	CF-40
myel/o	bone marrow or spinal cord	CF-41
oste/o	bone	
spin/o	thorn	
thorac/o, pector/o	chest	CF-63
vertebr/o, spondyl/o	vertebra	CF-69

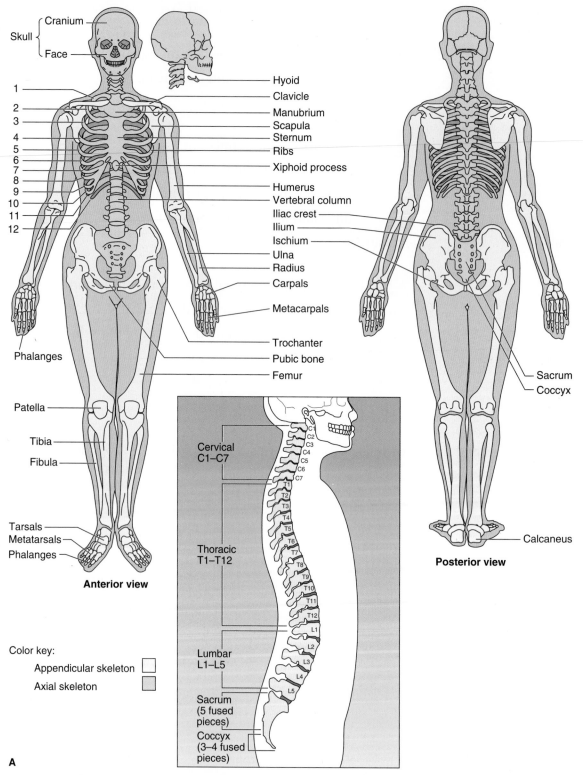

Color key:

Appendicular skeleton ☐

Axial skeleton ☐

FIGURE 2-3 The musculoskeletal system. **A.** The skeleton. Inset shows numbering of the vertebrae. **B.** Skeletal muscles.

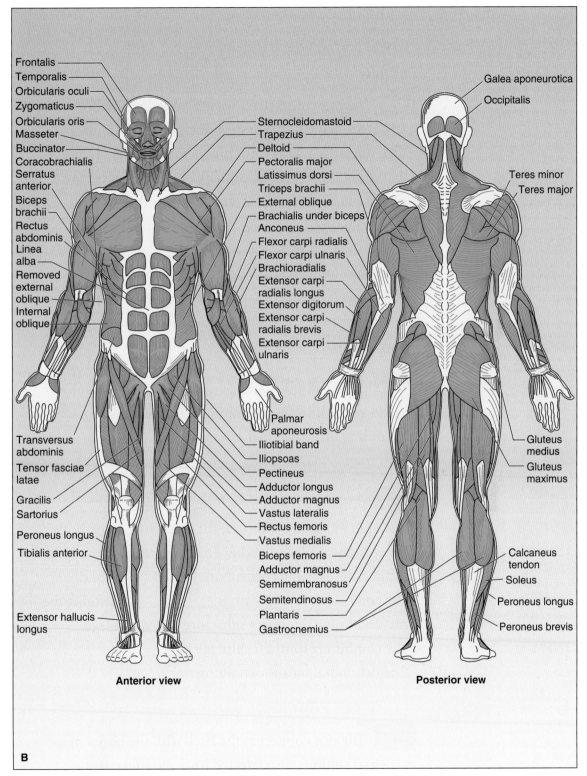

Frontalis
Temporalis
Orbicularis oculi
Zygomaticus
Orbicularis oris
Masseter
Buccinator
Coracobrachialis
Serratus anterior
Biceps brachii
Rectus abdominis
Linea alba
Removed external oblique
Internal oblique

Transversus abdominis
Tensor fasciae latae
Gracilis
Sartorius
Peroneus longus
Tibialis anterior

Extensor hallucis longus

Sternocleidomastoid
Trapezius
Deltoid
Pectoralis major
Latissimus dorsi
Triceps brachii
External oblique
Brachialis under biceps
Anconeus
Flexor carpi radialis
Flexor carpi ulnaris
Brachioradialis
Extensor carpi radialis longus
Extensor digitorum
Extensor carpi radialis brevis
Extensor carpi ulnaris

Palmar aponeurosis
Iliotibial band
Iliopsoas
Pectineus
Adductor longus
Adductor magnus
Vastus lateralis
Rectus femoris
Vastus medialis
Biceps femoris
Adductor magnus
Semimembranosus
Semitendinosus
Plantaris
Gastrocnemius

Galea aponeurotica
Occipitalis

Teres minor
Teres major

Gluteus medius
Gluteus maximus

Calcaneus tendon
Soleus
Peroneus longus
Peroneus brevis

Anterior view

Posterior view

B

FIGURE 2-3 Continued.

PROGRAMMED REVIEW: Musculoskeletal System

ANSWERS	REVIEW
	2.9 The musculoskeletal system provides support and gives shape to the body. Bones, which form the skeleton, are covered with muscle to supply the forces
oste/o	that make movement possible. _____ is the combining form for bone, and *arthr/o* is the combining
joint	form meaning _____ or articulation, the hinge
my/o	between bones. *muscul/o* and _____ are combining forms meaning muscle. There are 206 bones and 600 skeletal muscles in the adult body. The major bones comprise the skull, spine, chest, and upper and lower limbs.
structure or tissue	**2.10** The anatomic term for the skull, the collection of bones of the head, is the cranium. This term is formed by joining the suffix *-ium*, meaning _____,
skull	with *crani/o*, meaning _____.
chest	**2.11** *thorac/o*, a combining form meaning _____, was used to name the thorax, the chest area of the body between the neck and abdomen. The bones of the thorax include the sternum (breastbone) and 12 pairs of ribs.
cost/o	The combining form for rib is _____. Covering the ribs and lining joints is a substance called cartilage.
chondr/o	The combining form for cartilage is _____.
rib	Costochondral means pertaining to _____
cartilage	and _____.
	2.12 The ribs connect at the back with the bones of the vertebral column, also referred to as the spine. *spin/o,*

	which is Latin for thorn, refers to the thorn-like bony processes of the vertebra. There are two combining forms
vertebr/o, spondyl/o	for vertebra: _____ and _____. *vertebr/o*, from Latin, is used in anatomic terms. *spondyl/o*,
vertebra	meaning _____, is Greek in origin and is used in diagnostic and surgical terms that will be covered in upcoming chapters. Note that the plural of vertebra
vertebrae	is _____.

2.13   Each vertebra is named and numbered according to its region and position. The anatomic term for neck is

cervic/o

neck

chest

loin (lower back)

pertaining to

cervix, from the combining form _____. There are 7 cervical vertebrae (C1 to C7), located in the _____. There are 12 thoracic vertebrae (T1 to T12), located in the _____ region. The bones of the spine in the lower back are called lumbar vertebrae (L1 to L5). *lumb/o* means _____, and *-ar* means _____ ____.

2.14   The vertebrae provide protection for the spinal cord and nerves. The combining form for spinal cord (also

myel/o

meaning bone marrow) is _____.

2.15   The bones of the extremities include the arms and legs. *acr/o* is a combining form meaning

extremity

_____. Acral is a term referring to the peripheral parts of the body limbs, such as the fingers. It was formed by the combination of *-al*,

pertaining to, acr/o

meaning _____ ____, and _____, the combining form that means extremity.

Rx for Success

As you learn medical terms, you can have fun experimenting with creating words, such as glyco (sweet) + cardio (heart) = sweetheart! However, in the real medical world, the word must be accepted by the medical community to be considered a legitimate term. Often there seems to be no reason why a particular word form became acceptable. That is why you should check your medical dictionary when in doubt of the spelling, formation, or precise meaning of a term.

SELF-INSTRUCTION: Cardiovascular System

Study Fig. 2-4 and the following combining forms before starting the Programmed Review below.

COMBINING FORM	MEANING	FLASH CARD ID
angi/o, vas/o, vascul/o	vessel	CF-5
aort/o	aorta	
arteri/o	artery	
atri/o	atrium	
cardi/o	heart	CF-11
coron/o	circle or crown	
ven/o, phleb/o	vein	CF-68
ventricul/o	ventricle (belly or pouch)	

PROGRAMMED REVIEW: Cardiovascular System

ANSWERS	REVIEW
angi/o	**2.16** *vas/o, vascul/o,* and _____ are combining forms referring to vessel. The cardiovascular system consists
heart, vessels	of the _____ and _____, which transport blood throughout the body. The heart is a hollow muscular

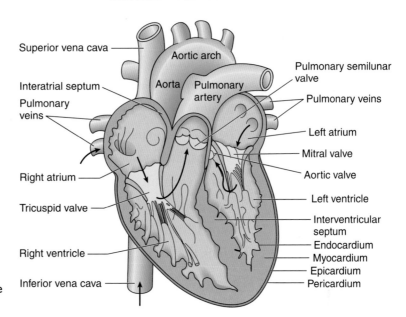

FIGURE 2-4   Structures of the heart.

atrium	organ that has four chambers. *atri/o* is the combing form for _____, stemming from the Latin word for an
atria	entrance hall. The plural form of the word is _____. The right and left atria are the upper chambers of the heart. The ventricles of the heart are the lower chambers, named
ventricul/o	from the combining form _____,
belly, pouch	meaning _____ or _____. The suffix in
small	ventricle refers to something _____.
	2.17 The one-way blood flow from one heart chamber to another, or from a heart chamber to an artery, is regulated by heart valves that open and close as the heart beats. The names of the valves give clues to their structure or function. The valve between the left ventricle and the
aorta	aorta is the aortic valve; *aort/o* means _____
pertaining to	and *-ic* means _____ ____.

three two half	**2.18** Cuspid refers to a tooth-like point. The tricuspid valve, located between the right atrium and right ventricle, was named for its _____ cusps. The bicuspid valve, located between the left atrium and left ventricle, has _____ cusps. It is also known as the mitral valve because its two parallel cusps resemble the shape of a bishop's mitre (headdress of Christian bishops). The pulmonary semilunar valve is between the right ventricle and the pulmonary artery. Semilunar gives clues to its _____-moon shape.
between atria interventricular	**2.19** The term septum refers to an anatomic partition. The interatrial septum is the partition _____ the right and left _____. Between the right and left ventricles is the _____ septum.
within heart tissue -ium	**2.20** You'll recall that the prefix *endo-* means _____. Combined with *cardi/o*, it refers to something within the _____. The endocardium is the structure or _____ lining the cavities of the heart. The suffix denoting structure or tissue is _____.
epi- suffix structure tissue	**2.21** A common prefix that means upon is _____. Combined with *cardi/o* and the _____ -*ium*, it forms the term epicardium, which is the _____ or _____ forming the outer layer of the heart.
muscle myocardium	**2.22** *my/o* is a combining form meaning _____. The term for heart muscle tissue is _____.
around heart	**2.23** *peri-* is a prefix that means _____. The pericardium is a protective sac that encloses the _____.

arteries	**2.24** The names of blood vessels are easy to remember because they are similar to the combining forms. The _____, which carry blood from the heart, are named from *arteri/o*. The veins, which carry blood to the heart, are named from _____. *phleb/o*, the second combining form meaning _____, is Greek in origin. The arterioles, also from *arteri/o*, are the small vessels that receive blood from the arteries. The blood then flows to the capillaries, the tiniest vessels. The blood is then gathered from the capillaries into the venules, which are small vessels that connect to the veins. The suffixes -*ole* and -*ule* are used to indicate something _____.
ven/o	
vein	
small	
	2.25 Circulation refers to the flow of the blood through the vessels. The blood flow through the body (except the lungs) is called the systemic circulation. The pulmonary circulation is the blood flow through the _____. The blood flow to the heart muscle, based on the combining form *coron/o*, meaning _____, is the _____ circulation.
lungs	
circle or crown, coronary	

SELF-INSTRUCTION: Blood and Lymph Systems

Study Figs. 2-5 and 2-6 and the following combining forms before starting the Programmed Review below.

COMBINING FORM	MEANING	FLASH CARD ID
cyt/o	cell	CF-19
erythr/o	red	CF-24
hem/o, hemat/o	blood	CF-28
immun/o	safe	
leuk/o	white	CF-35
lymph/o	clear fluid	
splen/o	spleen	
thromb/o	clot	CF-64
thym/o	thymus gland or mind	

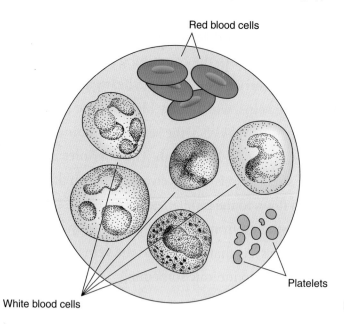

Red blood cells

White blood cells

Platelets

FIGURE 2-5   Components of the blood.

PROGRAMMED REVIEW: Blood and Lymph Systems

ANSWERS	REVIEW
hemat/o blood, hematology formation, blood	**2.26** Blood provides transport for oxygen, nutrients, and waste. *hem/o* and _____ are combining forms meaning _____. The study of blood is _____. Hemopoiesis refers to the _____ of _____. Plasma, the liquid part of the blood, has three cellular components: red cells, white cells, and platelets.
cell red suffix noun, erythrocyte	**2.27** *cyt/o* is the combining form meaning _____, and *erythr/o* is the combining form meaning _____. When combined and modified by -*e*, the _____ used as a/an _____ marker, the term _____ is formed. Erythrocytes, also known as red blood cells (RBC), are responsible for the transport of oxygen and carbon dioxide in the blood.

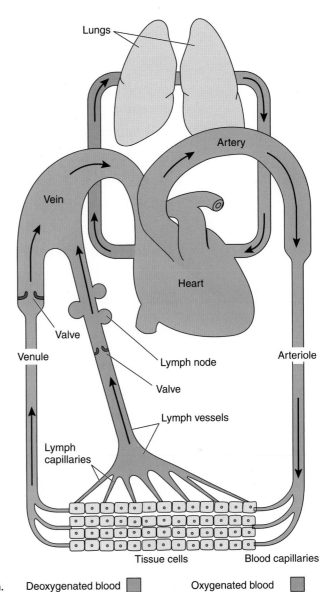

FIGURE 2-6 Blood and lymph circulation. Deoxygenated blood ▉ Oxygenated blood ▉

white	**2.28** The combining form *leuk/o* means _____;
leukocyte	thus a white blood cell (WBC) is a/an _____.
	Leukocytes are the cells that fight infection and protect the
	body from invasion of harmful substances. There are five
white blood	types of leukocytes or _____ _____
cells	_____. Three types, classified as granulocytes because

suffix attraction for	they contain granules in their cytoplasm, were named for the distinct attraction each had for the dye used to stain them for microscopic examination. Using the _____ -phil, meaning _____ _____, the basophil was named for its granules' attraction for the dark base color in the stain. The leukocyte with granules that took
combining form	to a neutral stain uses the _____ _____ neutr/o, meaning neither, modified by -phil to make the term
phil	neutro_____. Similarly, eosin/o, a combining form meaning rose-colored, was used to name the
phil	eosino_____, due to the attraction of its granules to the rose color in the dye.
without leukocytes without one cell noun marker clear fluid	**2.29** Using the prefix a-, meaning _____, the other two types of white blood cells, or _____, are known as agranulocytes because they are _____ granules: monocytes and lymphocytes. The name monocyte was formed by linking mono-, a prefix meaning _____, with cyt/o, a combining form meaning _____, and -e, a suffix referring to a/an _____ _____. lymph/o is a combining form meaning _____ _____.
clot, cell	**2.30** Platelets were named for their plate-like, fragmented structure. They are also known as thrombocytes because of their function in the clotting process; thromb/o means _____, and cyte refers to a/an _____.
	2.31 The lymph system protects the body by filtering microorganisms and foreign particles from the lymph and supporting the activities of the lymphocytes in the immune response. Immune is a term formed from immun/o, a

safe noun	combining form meaning _____, and -*e*, a suffix used as a/an _____ marker.
thym/o, splen/o lymph/o	**2.32** The two organs of the lymph system are the thymus and the spleen. The combining form for thymus is _____; _____ is the combining form for spleen. Lymph, the fluid that is circulated by lymph vessels, is filtered by lymph nodes. The combining form for lymph is _____, meaning clear fluid.

SELF-INSTRUCTION: Respiratory System

Study Fig. 2-7 and the following combining forms before starting the Programmed Review below.

COMBINING FORM	MEANING	FLASH CARD ID
alveol/o	alveolus (air sac)	
bronch/o	bronchus (airway)	
laryng/o	larynx (voice box)	
nas/o, rhin/o	nose	CF-43
pharyng/o	pharynx or throat	
pneum/o, pneumon/o	air or lung	CF-51
pulmon/o	lung	CF-54
trache/o	trachea (windpipe)	

PROGRAMMED REVIEW: Respiratory System

ANSWERS	REVIEW
air lung	**2.33** *pneum/o* and *pneumon/o*, meaning _____ or _____, are the key combining forms of the respiratory system, which is responsible for the exchange of gases (oxygen and carbon dioxide) within the body.

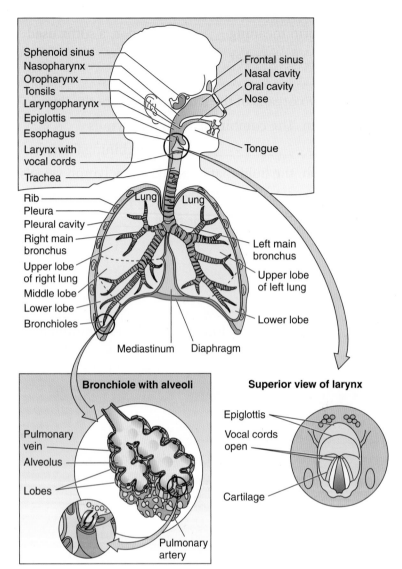

FIGURE 2-7   The respiratory system.

	2.34 The nose is the first structure to receive oxygen.
nose	*nas/o* is the Latin combining form meaning _____. The other combining form that means nose is Greek in
rhin/o	origin: _____. *pharyng/o* is the combining form for
pharynx, throat	_____ or _____, the next structure to receive air. Beneath the pharynx is the larynx (voice box),
laryng/o	from the combining form _____. The windpipe,

trachea, trache/o	or _____, from the combining form _____, is the structure that connects with two main airways into the lungs: the right bronchus and the left bronchus.
bronch/o, bronchi small singular alveol/o	**2.35** The combining form for bronchus (airway) is _____. The plural of bronchus is _____. These airways split into smaller branches, the smallest of which are the bronchioles. The suffix *-ole* means _____. At the ends of the bronchioles are thin-walled microscopic sacs known as alveoli. Alveolus is the _____ term, the combining form for which is _____.
lung, study of	**2.36** Pulmonology, the medical specialty concerned with the study and treatment of the lungs, is formed by *pulmon/o*, meaning _____, and *-logy*, meaning _____ _____.

SELF-INSTRUCTION: Nervous System

Study Fig. 2-8 and the following combining forms before starting the Programmed Review below.

COMBINING FORM	MEANING	FLASH CARD ID
cerebr/o	largest part of the brain	
encephal/o	entire brain	CF-22
mening/o	membrane (meninges)	
myel/o	bone marrow or spinal cord	CF-41
neur/o	nerve	

PROGRAMMED REVIEW: Nervous System

ANSWERS	REVIEW
nerve	**2.37** The nervous system is a complicated network of nerves and fibers that control all functions of the body. *neur/o* is the combining form for _____.

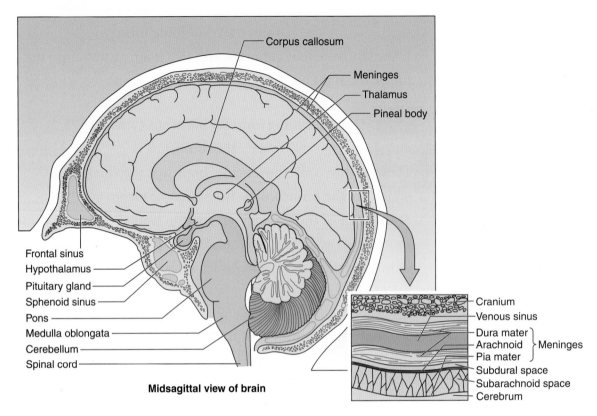

Midsagittal view of brain

FIGURE 2-8   Midsagittal view of the brain.

	2.38 The central nervous system (CNS) is composed of the brain and spinal cord. *cerebr/o* is the Greek combining
cerebrum	form for _____, the largest part of the brain.
combining form	*encephal/o* is another Greek _____ _____
brain	referring to the entire _____. The vertebrae house the spinal cord, a bundle of nerves coming from the brain and ultimately connecting to all areas of the body. *mening/o,*
membrane	a combining form meaning _____, is used to name the protective coverings around the brain and spinal
meninges	cord known as the _____. *myel/o* is the combining form referring to either bone marrow
spinal cord	or _____ _____.

neurology neur/o suffix, study of	**2.39** The study of the nervous system is _____, from _____, the combining form for nerve, and *-logy*, the _____ meaning _____ ____.

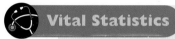 **Vital Statistics**   **MENINGITIS** (*men-in-jī′tis*)

Origin: *mening/o* (membrane) + G. *-itis* (inflammation)

Our patient at the beginning of this chapter had classic symptoms of meningitis. Meningitis is an infection of the meninges, which are the coverings around the brain and spinal cord (see Fig. 2-8). The infection occurs most often in children, teens, and young adults. Also at risk are older adults and people who have long-term health problems, such as a weakened immune system.

There are two main kinds of meningitis, both of which share the same symptoms:

- Viral meningitis is fairly common. It usually does not cause serious illness.
- Bacterial meningitis is not as common but is very serious. It needs to be treated right away to prevent brain damage and death.

Viral meningitis is caused by viruses, and bacterial meningitis is caused by bacteria. Meningitis can also be caused by other organisms and some medicines, but this is rare.

Meningitis is contagious. The germs that cause it can be passed from one person to another through coughing and sneezing and through close contact.

The most common symptoms are:

- A stiff and painful neck
- Fever
- Headache
- Vomiting
- Trouble staying awake
- Seizures

Lumbar puncture, or spinal tap, is the most important lab test for meningitis (see **Vital Statistics: Lumbar Puncture** and **Medical Record Exercise 2-1**).

Treatment depends on the cause. Bacterial meningitis is treated in a hospital with antibiotics and close observation to prevent serious problems such as hearing loss, seizures, or brain damage. Individuals with viral meningitis most commonly receive home treatment and typically get better within a few weeks.

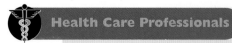
Health Care Professionals   MEET THE MEDICAL ASSISTANT

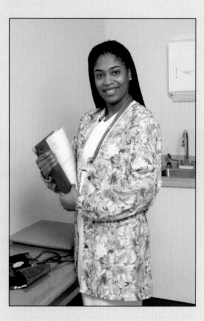

The medical assistant who assisted with Raymond Hauck's lumbar puncture worked for a neurologist, but medical assistants can work in a variety of settings. Following is a brief description of this health care profession.

Medical assistants are multiskilled health professionals who perform administrative and clinical procedures in medical offices, clinics, and outpatient care facilities. Examples of administrative duties include scheduling appointments and filing insurance forms. Clinical duties typically involve direct patient care, such as obtaining vital signs and assisting physicians and other health care providers with examinations and treatments. Some medical assistants are trained on the job, but many complete one-year or two-year education programs.

(CD-ROM) A more detailed description of medical assisting as a health care career can be found on the Student Resource CD-ROM and at www.thePoint.lww.com/WillisQC.

SELF-INSTRUCTION: Endocrine System

Study Fig. 2-9 and the following combining forms before starting the Programmed Review section.

COMBINING FORM	MEANING	FLASH CARD ID
aden/o	gland	CF-3
adren/o, adrenal/o	adrenal gland	
crin/o	to secrete	CF-17
hormon/o	hormone	
ovari/o	ovary	
pancreat/o	pancreas	
test/o, orchi/o, orchid/o	testis or testicle	CF-61
thym/o	thymus gland or mind	
thyr/o, thyroid/o	thyroid gland (shield)	

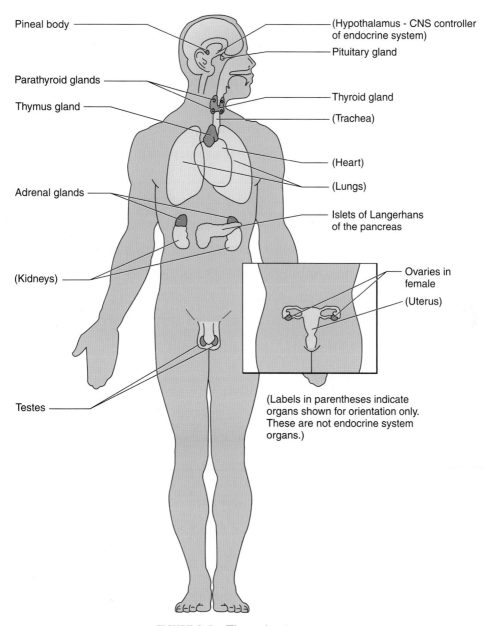

FIGURE 2-9   The endocrine system.

PROGRAMMED REVIEW: Endocrine System

ANSWERS	REVIEW
secrete within endocrine gland hormon/o adjective	**2.40** The combining form *crin/o*, meaning to _____, plus the prefix *endo-*, meaning _____, and *-e* (the suffix used as a noun marker) form the term for the system of glands that secretes hormones within the body known as the _____ system. The endocrine system helps regulate and maintain various body functions by secreting hormones and other substances from ductless glands. *aden/o* is a combining form meaning _____. The combining form for hormone is _____, from a Greek word meaning "an urging on" (a hormone is a substance that urges an action to occur). Hormonal is the _____ form.
adrenal near	**2.41** The combining forms *adren/o* and *adrenal/o* mean _____ gland. The prefix *ad-* used in these combining forms gives a clue that the gland is to, toward, or _____ the kidney.
thymus	**2.42** The combining form *thym/o* means _____ gland. It was named for its resemblance to a bunch of the herb thyme.
thyr/o, thyroid/o shield	**2.43** The two combining forms meaning thyroid gland are _____ and _____. The Greek term at the origin of these combining forms means shield, and the thyroid gland is so named because it resembles a/an _____.
all	**2.44** The prefix *pan-*, meaning _____, and *creas*, a root meaning flesh, were combined to name the pancreas

because of its "all flesh" appearance when first examined. The pancreas performs an endocrine function by secreting insulin.

alongside of parathyroid	**2.45** Recall that the prefix *para-* means _____ ____ or abnormal. Located alongside of the thyroid glands in the neck are the _____ glands.
below	**2.46** The pituitary gland, located at the base of the brain, secretes a long list of hormones. It is also called the hypophysis, a term using the prefix *hypo-*, meaning _____ (or deficient), because it hangs below the hypothalamus part of the brain.
testis testicle testes, testicles testis testicle	**2.47** *test/o*, a Latin combining form meaning _____ or _____, is used to name the glands in males that are located on both sides within the scrotum and secrete testosterone, a hormone that affects masculinization and reproduction. These glands are called the _____ or _____. *orchi/o* and *orchid/o* are Greek combining forms meaning _____ or _____.
ovary ovaries	**2.48** *ovari/o*, a combining form meaning _____, was used to name the female glands responsible for regulation of reproduction by secretion of estrogen and progesterone. These glands are called the _____.

SELF-INSTRUCTION: The Special Senses: Eye and Ear

Study Fig. 2-10 and the following combining forms before starting the Programmed Review section.

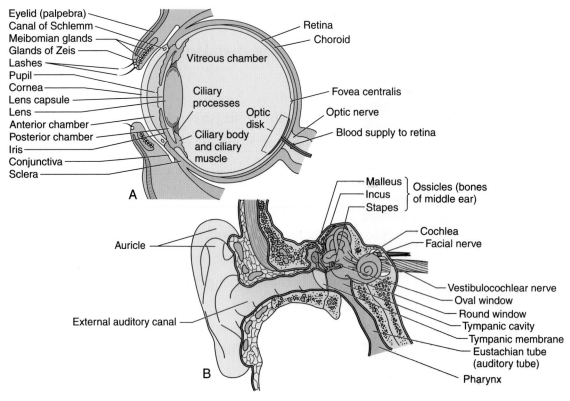

FIGURE 2-10   The special senses. **A.** The eye. **B.** The ear.

COMBINING FORM	MEANING	FLASH CARD ID
ocul/o, opt/o, ophthalm/o	eye	
aur/i, ot/o	ear	CF-8
conjunctiv/o	conjunctiva	
corne/o, kerat/o	cornea	
ir/o, irid/o	iris (colored circle)	
lacrim/o, dacry/o	tear	CF-34
retin/o	retina	
scler/o	hard or sclera	CF-58
tympan/o, myring/o	eardrum or tympanic membrane	CF-66

PROGRAMMED REVIEW: The Special Senses: Eye and Ear

ANSWERS	REVIEW
ocul/o, opt/o, ophthalm/o eye pertaining to	**2.49** There are three combining forms meaning eye: _____, _____, and _____. Ophthalmic, optic, and ocular are examples of adjectives referring to the _____. They are modified by suffixes meaning _____ ____.
cornea kerat/o	**2.50** *corne/o* is the Latin combining form used to name the transparent outer covering of the eye called the _____. The second combining form meaning cornea, from the Greek word kera meaning horn or hard tissue, is _____.
lacrim/o dacry/o	**2.51** There are two combining forms for tears, one based on a Latin word and one from Greek. The lacrimal gland (tear gland) comes from the combining form _____. The term dacryocyst means the lacrimal sac (cyst = sac), where tears are collected before they flow to the nose. The second combining form for tears is _____.
conjunctiv/o scler/o retin/o ir/o	**2.52** Many combining forms are very similar to the terms that express their meaning. For example, the combining form meaning the conjunctiva, the mucous membrane that lines the eyelids and outer surface of the eyeball, is _____. The combining form for the sclera, the tough, white outer layer of the eye, is _____. The combining form for retina, the innermost, light-sensitive layer at the back of the eye, is _____. Similarly, the two combining forms for the iris, the colored circle of the eye that surrounds the pupil, are *irid/o* and _____.

ot/o	**2.53** The two combining forms for ear are *aur/i* and _____. Medical study of the ear is called otology.
otologist	The physician who specializes in the study and treatment of the ear is a/an _____. Otology is a subspecialty of otorhinolaryngology (otolaryngology), involving study
ear	and treatment of the _____, nose, and throat, more commonly known as ENT.
aur/i	**2.54** The other combining form meaning ear is _____. The auricle, for example, is the outer, visible part of the ear.
tympan/o	**2.55** A kind of drum used in symphony orchestras is called a tympany, from the Greek word for drum. The combining form for the eardrum is _____. A second combining form for eardrum comes from the Latin word for drum membrane, myringa. That combining
myring/o	form is _____.

MEET THE PATIENT   Tenille Jovian has been a candy lover for as long as she can remember. She blames this affinity, along with the fact that she grew up in an area where fluoride was not added to drinking water, for the multiple dental cavities she had as a child and young adult. Over the years, she has learned a great deal about dental health and the importance of seeing the dentist every six months for a check up and teeth cleaning. Her **Dental Hygienist,** Jacob Kaplan, spends time during each of her visits educating her about healthy dental practices and disease prevention. Tenille has called the office for an earlier appointment because she is experiencing some tooth sensitivity.

SELF-INSTRUCTION: Gastrointestinal System

Study Fig. 2-11 and the following combining forms before starting the Programmed Review section.

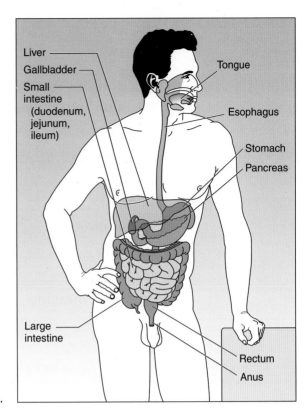

FIGURE 2-11   The gastrointestinal system.

COMBINING FORM	MEANING	FLASH CARD ID
an/o	anus	
chol/e, bil/i	bile	CF-14
col/o, colon/o	colon (large intestine)	
dent/i, odont/o	teeth	CF-20
enter/o	small intestine	CF-23
esophag/o	esophagus	
gastr/o	stomach	CF-26
hepat/o	liver	CF-29
lingu/o, gloss/o	tongue	CF-36
or/o, stomat/o	mouth	
pancreat/o	pancreas	
rect/o	rectum	

PROGRAMMED REVIEW: Gastrointestinal System

ANSWERS	REVIEW
	2.56 The gastrointestinal (GI) system provides for digestion and elimination. Combining forms related to key structures of the digestive tract are: *or/o* and *stomat/o*,
mouth	meaning _____; *dent/i* and *odont/o*,
teeth	meaning _____, *gloss/o* and *ling/o*,
tongue, esophagus	meaning _____; *esophag/o*, meaning _____;
stomach	*gastr/o*, meaning _____; *enter/o*,
small	meaning _____ intestine; *col/o* and *colon/o*,
large, anus	meaning _____ intestine; *an/o*, meaning _____;
rectum	and *rect/o*, meaning _____.
liver	**2.57** *hepat/o* is the combining form for _____, the organ that produces bile necessary for digestion. *chol/e*
bil/i, bile	and _____ are combining forms meaning _____. Cholecyst is a term used to refer to the gallbladder, the
bile	sac-like structure that stores _____.
	2.58 *pancreat/o* is the combining form meaning
pancreas, within	_____. *endo-*, the prefix meaning _____,
out, away	and *exo-*, the prefix meaning _____ or _____, are used to explain the complex functions of the pancreas. As noted earlier in this chapter, the endocrine function of the pancreas is to secret insulin. Its exocrine function is to secrete pancreatic enzymes delivered out through ducts into the small intestine during digestion.

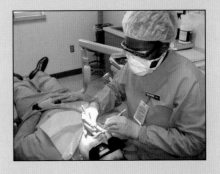

Dental hygienists are licensed dental professionals who perform routine teeth cleaning, which is referred to as "oral prophylaxis." Dental hygienists are also trained to take dental x-rays, place dental sealants, take alginate impressions, administer local anesthesia, and, in some states, place and carve dental amalgam (fillings). As you learned in Tenille Jovian's story earlier, dental hygienists also play an important role in providing patient education about dental health and preventing oral disease.

📀 A more detailed description of dental hygiene as a health care career can be found on the Student Resource CD-ROM and at www.thePoint.lww.com/WillisQC.

SELF-INSTRUCTION: Urinary System

Study Fig. 2-12 and the following combining forms before starting the Programmed Review section.

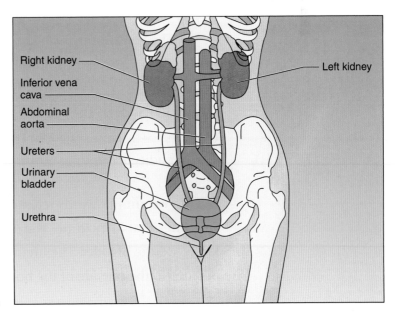

FIGURE 2-12   The urinary system.

COMBINING FORM	MEANING	FLASH CARD ID
abdomin/o	abdomen	CF-1
cyst/o, vesic/o	bladder or sac	CF-18
ren/o, nephr/o	kidney	CF-45
ur/o, urin/o	urine	CF-67
ureter/o	ureter	
urethr/o	urethra	

PROGRAMMED REVIEW: Urinary System

ANSWERS	REVIEW
abdomen	**2.59** *abdomin/o* is a combining form meaning _____. The abdominal cavity houses several organs in the body. Among the most vital are the kidneys, the two structures on each side of the lumbar (lower back) region of the abdomen that filter blood and secrete impurities, forming
urine, noun	urine (*urin/o* means _____ and *-e* is a/an _____
kidney	marker). *ren/o* is the Latin combining form for _____,
nephr/o	and _____ is the Greek combining form. Renal is
pertaining to	a common adjective, meaning _____ _____
kidney	the _____.
bladder	**2.60** The combining form *cyst/o* means sac or _____. Another combining form meaning bladder
vesic/o	or sac is _____ (from the Latin word vesica, meaning bladder). The sac that holds urine is called
urinary	the _____ bladder (combining *urin/o* with *-ary*,
pertaining to	another adjective ending meaning _____ ___).
	2.61 Two similar words refer to different urinary system structures that carry urine. The ureters carry urine from the kidney to the bladder. The urethra carries urine from the bladder to the outside of the body. The combining form for

ureter/o urethr/o	ureter is _____. The combining form for urethra is _____.
urine urology urologist nephro	**2.62** *ur/o* is another combining form meaning _____. The medical specialty concerned with study of the urinary tract is _____. The physician who specializes in the study and treatment of the urinary system is called a/an _____. The physician who particularly specializes in the study and treatment of the kidneys is known as a/an _____logist.

SELF-INSTRUCTION: Male Reproductive System

Study Fig. 2-13 and the following combining forms before starting the Programmed Review section.

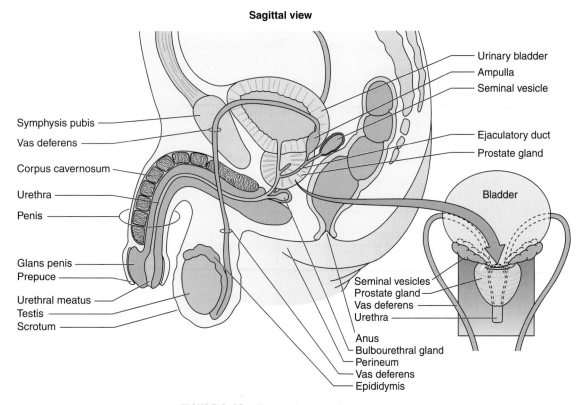

FIGURE 2-13 The male reproductive system.

COMBINING FORM	MEANING	FLASH CARD ID
prostat/o	prostate gland	
sperm/o, spermat/o	sperm	
test/o, orch/o, orchi/o, orchid/o	testis or testicle	CF-61
vas/o	vessel	CF-5

PROGRAMMED REVIEW: Male Reproductive System

ANSWERS	REVIEW
testicles orch/o orchi/o, orchid/o	**2.63** Stemming from *test/o*, a Latin combining form, the testis, or testicle, is one of the two glands that produce sperm and the male hormone testosterone. The plural forms are testes and _____. There are three different Greek combining forms meaning testis (the names are due to the resemblance of the gland to an orchid bulb): _____, _____, and _____.
sperm/o, spermat/o sperm pertaining to	**2.64** The Greek word sperma means seed, and thus, sperm is the male's reproductive "seed." The two combining forms for sperm are _____ and _____. Spermatic is an adjective formed by combining *spermat/o*, meaning _____, and *-ic*, meaning _____ ____.
vas/o	**2.65** The Latin word vas refers to vessel, which includes ducts and blood vessels. The combining form for vessel is _____. The vas deferens is the vessel (duct) that carries sperm from the testicle.
	2.66 The Latin term prostata has its origins in a Greek word meaning one who stands before. Perhaps the prostate gland

prostat/o	was so named because it stands before the opening for sperm leaving the body to exit through the penis. The combining form for prostate gland is _____.

SELF-INSTRUCTION: Female Reproductive System

Study Fig. 2-14 and the following combining forms before starting the Programmed Review section.

COMBINING FORM	MEANING	FLASH CARD ID
gynec/o	female	CF-27
mast/o, mamm/o	breast	CF-38
ovari/o, oophor/o	ovary	
ov/i, ov/o	egg	
salping/o	uterine or fallopian tube	CF-56
uter/o, hyster/o, metr/o	uterus	
vagin/o, colp/o	vagina	
vulv/o, episi/o	vulva	CF-70

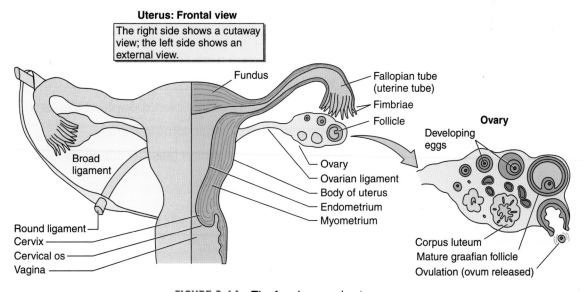

FIGURE 2-14   The female reproductive system.

PROGRAMMED REVIEW: Female Reproductive System

ANSWERS	REVIEW
	2.67 The uterus is the hollow organ (the womb) where females carry a fetus before childbirth. The Latin combining
uter/o	form used to name the uterus is _____. There are two
hyster/o	other Greek combining forms that mean uterus: _____
metr/o	and _____. *metr/o* is one of the Greek combining
uterus	forms meaning _____. When combined with the
structure or tissue	suffix -*ium*, meaning _____, and *my/o*, the
muscle	combining form meaning _____, it forms the term
myometrium	for the muscular wall of the uterus: _____.
within	Recall that the prefix *endo-* means _____. Within
	the uterus is a tissue that forms its lining, which is shed
endometrium	during menstruation, called the _____.
	2.68 An ovum is the female's egg produced in the ovary.
ov/i	The two combining forms for egg are very similar: _____
ov/o, origin	and _____. Ovigenesis refers to the _____
production, ovum (egg)	or _____ of the _____.
	2.69 Once again, the two combining forms for the ovary come from Latin and Greek roots. The adjective ovarian is
ovari/o	built from the combining form _____, from the Latin word for the ovary. The Greek word oophoros means
oophor/o	egg-bearing, giving rise to the combining form _____. You'll find *oophor/o* used in terms related to diagnosis and treatment in later chapters.
	2.70 The Greek word salpinx means trumpet or tube. It
salping/o	gives rise to the combining form _____, which refers to the uterine or fallopian tube (which carries the

	ovum from the ovary to the uterus). The uterine tubes, which resemble a trumpet or tube, were first described by the anatomist Gabrielle Fallopius, thus the reference to
fallopian	_____ tube. The Latin word for trumpet or tube is tuba.

2.71 The Latin word cervix means neck; the cervix in the female is like a neck between the vagina and the uterus.

cervic/o   The combining term for cervix is _____.
The common adjective form, using the suffix -*al*

pertaining to, cervical   (meaning _____ ____), is _____.

2.72 There are two combining forms for vagina, as often happens: one from a Latin word and one from a Greek word. The Latin word vagina means sheath (as the vagina sheaths the penis during intercourse); this combining form

vagin/o   is _____. The Greek word kolpos means a hollow;

colp/o   this combining form is _____.

2.73 The Greek term episeion, meaning pubic region, is the origin for this combining form for the vulva

episi/o   (the external female genitalia): _____. The Latin combining form for which the vulva was named

vulv/o   is _____.

2.74 Recall that the two combining forms for breast

mast/o, mamm/o   are _____ and _____. The combination of

breast   *mamm/o*, meaning _____, with -*ary*, an adjective

pertaining to   ending meaning _____ ____, forms the
term for the glands in the female breast that make

mammary   milk: _____ glands.

gynecology	**2.75** Treatment of the female reproductive system involves two medical specialties: obstetrics (OB) and _____ (GYN) (study of female).

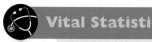 **Vital Statistics   LUMBAR PUNCTURE**

Origin: *lumb/o* (loin or lower back) + -*ar* (pertaining to) + puncture (to prick)

Returning to our patient Raymond Hauck, who was introduced at the beginning of the chapter, the procedure performed by Dr. Migeon to definitively diagnose his condition was a **lumbar puncture.** Also called a spinal tap, this is a procedure that is used to collect and look at the fluid (cerebrospinal fluid) surrounding the brain and spinal cord.

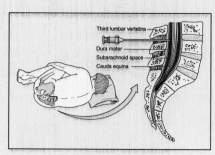

Be sure to note the patient's position and placement of the needle in the figure above; we'll be learning more about body planes, positions, and anatomic reference points next.

During a lumbar puncture, a needle is carefully inserted into the spinal canal low in the back (lumbar area). Samples of cerebrospinal fluid are collected. The samples are studied for color, blood cell counts, protein, glucose, and other substances. Some of the sample may be put into a special culture cup to see if any infection, such as bacteria or fungi, grows. The pressure of the cerebrospinal fluid also is measured during the procedure.

A lumbar puncture is done to:

- Find a cause for symptoms possibly caused by an infection (such as meningitis), inflammation, cancer, or bleeding in the area around the brain or spinal cord.
- Diagnose certain diseases of the brain and spinal cord, such as multiple sclerosis or Guillain-Barré syndrome.
- Measure the pressure of cerebrospinal fluid (CSF) in the space surrounding the spinal cord. If the pressure is high, it may be causing certain symptoms.

SELF-INSTRUCTION: Anatomic Position, Body Planes, and Directional Terms

To communicate effectively about the body, health care professionals use terms with specific meanings to refer to body parts and locations. These terms of reference are based on the body being in **anatomic position**, in which the person is visualized

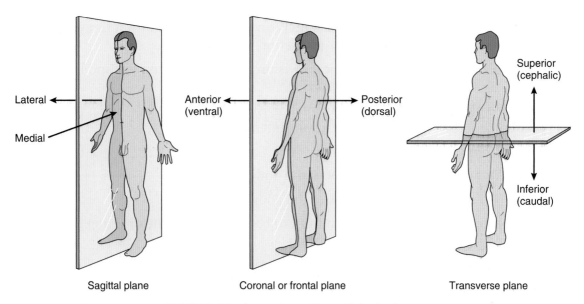

Lateral

Medial

Anterior
(ventral)

Posterior
(dorsal)

Superior
(cephalic)

Inferior
(caudal)

Sagittal plane   Coronal or frontal plane   Transverse plane

FIGURE 2-15   Anatomic position with body planes.

standing upright (erect), facing forward, with feet pointed forward and slightly apart, and arms at the sides with palms facing forward. No matter how the patient presents for care, he or she is pictured in this pose before applying any other term of reference. With the body in an anatomic position, three different imaginary lines divide the body in half, forming **body planes** (Fig. 2-15). In addition to the three body planes, **positional** and **directional** terms are used to indicate the location or direction of body parts with respect to each other.

Memorize the meanings of the terms related to the anatomic position, body planes, and directional terms defined below in preparation for a Programmed Review that follows.

TERM	MEANING
anatomic position	the position of the body to which health care professionals refer when noting body planes, positions, and directions: the person is assumed to be standing upright (erect), facing forward, feet pointed forward and slightly apart, with arms at the sides with palms facing forward; the patient is visualized in this pose before applying any other term of reference
body planes	three different imaginary lines dividing the body in half; used as a reference for indicating the location or direction of body parts

coronal or frontal plane	vertical division of the body into front (anterior) and back (posterior) portions
sagittal plane	vertical division of the body into right and left portions
transverse plane	horizontal division of the body into upper (superior) and lower (inferior) portions
Directional Terms	
anterior (A), *syn.* ventral	front of the body
posterior (P), *syn.* dorsal	back of the body
anterior-posterior (AP)	from front to back; such as in the direction of an x-ray beam
posterior-anterior (PA)	from back to front; such as in the direction of an x-ray beam
superior, *syn.* cephalic	situated above another structure, toward the head
inferior, *syn.* caudal	situated below another structure, toward the feet (toward the tail in veterinary medicine)
proximal	toward the beginning or origin of a structure, i.e., the proximal aspect of the femur (thigh bone) is the area closest to where it attaches to the hip
distal	away from the beginning or origin of a structure, i.e., the distal aspect of the femur (thigh bone) is the area at the end of the bone near the knee (*dist/o* = far)
medial	toward the middle (midline) (*medi/o* = middle)
lateral	toward the side

PROGRAMMED REVIEW: Anatomic Position, Body Planes, and Directional Terms

ANSWERS	REVIEW
	2.76 Health care professionals describe body part
anatomic	locations relative to the _____ position, in which
erect, forward	one is standing upright or _____, facing _____,

sides, forward	feet pointed forward and slightly apart, with the arms at the _____ and palms facing _____.

2.77   Body planes are imaginary lines that divide the body into portions. The body is vertically divided into front (anterior) and back (posterior) portions by the _____,

coronal

or frontal, plane. The _____ plane divides the

sagittal

body vertically into right and left portions. *trans-* is a prefix

across, through

meaning _____ or _____. The transverse

horizontally

plane divides the body _____ into upper and lower portions.

2.78   Recall that the prefix *ante-* means _____,

before

and the prefix *post-* means _____. Using these word

after

parts, the front of the body is _____, and the

anterior

back of the body is _____. The synonym for

posterior

anterior is _____ (from ventralis, a Latin word for

ventral

belly). The synonym for posterior is _____

dorsal

(from dorsalis, a Latin word meaning back).

2.79   The direction of an x-ray beam from front to back is

anterior-posterior

designated _____-_____,
whereas the direction from back to front

posterior-anterior

is _____-_____.

above or excessive

2.80   *super-*, a prefix meaning _____, is used in
the term referring to that which is situated above another

superior

structure, toward the head: _____. *cephal/o,*

head

a combining form meaning _____, linked to *-ic*, a/an

suffix, pertaining to

_____ meaning _____ ____, forms

cephalic

the synonym for superior: _____. That which is

below superior inferior caudal	inferior is situated _____ another structure, toward the feet. Therefore, the head is _____ to (above) the shoulders, whereas the feet are _____ to (below) the knees. The synonym for inferior is _____ (a term used more often in veterinary medicine pertaining to toward the cauda or tail).
before proximal distal proximal end	**2.81** *pro-*, the prefix meaning _____, gives a clue to the meaning of the term that describes the area of a structure that is closest to its beginning or origin: _____. In contrast, the area of a structure that is away from its origin or attachment is _____. The _____ aspect of the femur (thigh bone) is the area closest to where it attaches to the hip. The distal aspect of the femur (thigh bone) is the area at the _____ of the bone near the knee (*dist/o* = far).
pertaining to medial side one side two or both	**2.82** *medi/o* is a combining form meaning middle. Combined with *-al*, the suffix meaning _____ ____, the term pertaining to the middle or midline is _____. Lateral pertains to that which is toward the _____. Unilateral refers to _____ _____, whereas bilateral refers to _____ sides.

SELF-INSTRUCTION: Body Positions

The anatomic position is the reference point that is visualized when referring to specific body parts and locations, but there are also terms that describe the actual position that the patient is in or how the patient is placed when receiving care. Memorize the meanings of the basic body positions in preparation for a Programmed Review that follows.

TERM	MEANING
erect	normal standing position
decubitus	lying down, especially in a bed, i.e., lateral decubitus is lying on the side (*decumbo* = to lie down)
prone	lying face down and flat
recumbent	lying down
supine	horizontal recumbent; lying flat on the back ("on the spine")

 ### Rx for Success

Use these tricks to help you remember the difference between supine and prone:
Supine *is on your* **spine**; *therefore,* **prone's** *the "other" one.*
Also, **prone** *to suffocate in the* **prone** *position.*

PROGRAMMED REVIEW: Body Positions

ANSWERS	REVIEW
erect	**2.83** The normal standing position is _____ (as in the anatomic position). Several terms describe different ways the body lies down. The general term for lying down is
recumbent	_____. Lying down, especially in bed,
decubitus	is called _____. A patient lying on one side
lateral	in bed is in a/an _____ decubitus position.
face, supine	Prone means lying _____ down flat, whereas _____ means lying face up, flat on the back.

SELF-INSTRUCTION: Body Movements

Many different terms are used to describe body movements at joints, as shown in Fig. 2-16. Study Fig. 2-16 and memorize the meanings of the body movements in preparation for a Programmed Review that follows.

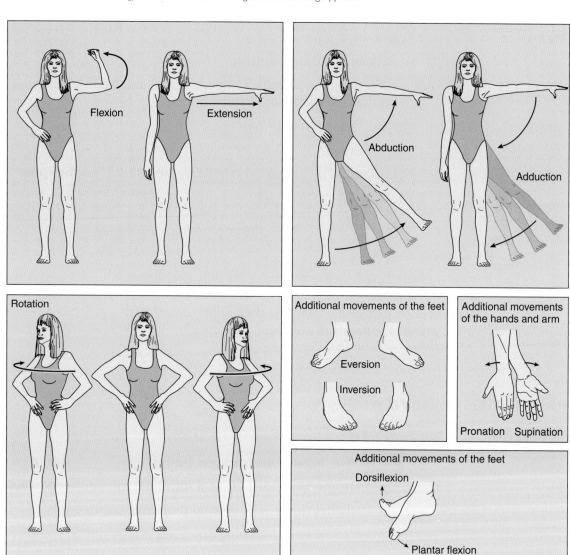

FIGURE 2-16   Body movements.

TERM	MEANING
flexion	bending at the joint so that the angle between the bones is decreased
extension	straightening at the joint so that the angle between the bones is increased
abduction	movement away from the body
adduction	movement toward the body

rotation	circular movement around an axis
eversion	turning outward, e.g., a foot
inversion	turning inward, e.g., a foot
supination	turning upward or forward of the palmar surface (palm of the hand) or plantar surface (sole of the foot)
pronation	turning downward or backward of the palmar surface (palm of the hand) or plantar surface (sole of the foot)
dorsiflexion	bending of the foot or the toes upward
plantar flexion	bending of the sole of the foot by curling the toes toward the ground

Rx for Success

Use these tricks to help you remember the difference between supination and pronation:

*"**SOUP**ination": Supination is to turn your with the arm palm up, as if you are holding a bowl of soup.*

*"**POUR**-nation": Pronation is to turn your arm with the palm down, as if you are **pour**ing out whatever is in your bowl.*

*Alternatively, **pronation donation**: **Pronation** is palm facing downward, as if making a donation.*

PROGRAMMED REVIEW: Body Movements

ANSWERS	REVIEW
	2.84 To flex is to bend. Flexing a joint (flexion)
decreases	_____ the angle between the bones; the opposite
extension	movement (increasing the angle) is _____.
away	Movement _____ from the body is called abduction
away from	(the prefix *ab-* means _____ _____); the opposite
adduction	movement is _____ (the prefix *ad-*
toward	means _____).

out, away eversion	**2.85** A circular movement turning around an axis is called rotation. For example, you can rotate your feet inward and outward. The term for inward rotation is inversion. The prefix *e-*, meaning _____ or _____, is used in the term for outward rotation: _____.
supination pronation	**2.86** Turning the palm of the hand upward or forward is called _____; the opposite movement is _____. Note the relationship of these terms to the terms for the body lying supine or prone.
dorsiflexion plantar flexion	**2.87** The foot and toes bend upward in _____ and downward in _____ _____.

SELF-INSTRUCTION: Body Cavities

Five body cavities house the organs and other vital structures of the body (Fig. 2-17). Memorize the meanings of the each of them in the table below in preparation for the Programmed Review that follows.

TERM	MEANING
cranial cavity	space within the skull that houses the brain
vertebral (spinal) cavity	contains the spinal cord
thoracic cavity	contains the heart and lungs
abdominal cavity	contains the stomach, small and large intestines, liver, gallbladder, spleen, and kidneys
pelvic cavity	contains the urinary tract and male and female reproductive organs

PROGRAMMED REVIEW: Body Cavities

ANSWERS	REVIEW
skull	**2.88** The nervous system is comprised of the brain and spinal cord. *crani/o*, a combining form meaning _____, is used to name the bones of the head that house the brain.

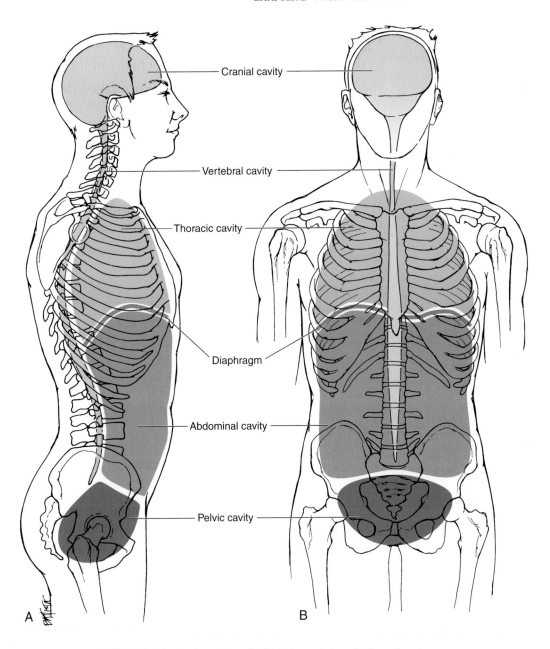

FIGURE 2-17   Body cavities. **A.** Right lateral view. **B.** Anterior view.

pertaining to cranial	Formed by linking -*al*, a suffix meaning _____ _____, to the combining form for skull, the name of the hollow space that encloses the brain is therefore called the _____ cavity.
vertebral	**2.89** Continuous with the cranial cavity, the thorn-like bones of the back provide a canal for the spinal cord. This space is called the spinal cavity, or _____ cavity (using the combining form meaning vertebra).
chest pertaining to thoracic cavity	**2.90** *thorac/o*, a combining form meaning _____, linked to -*ic*, a suffix meaning _____ _____, is used to name the space that houses the vital organs of the heart and lungs called the _____ _____.
abdomen pertaining to abdominal cavity	**2.91** *abdomin/o*, a combining form meaning _____, is linked with -*al*, a suffix meaning _____ _____, to name the cavity that contains the stomach, small and large intestines, liver, gallbladder, spleen, and kidneys: _____ _____.
pertaining to pelvic cavity	**2.92** *pelv/i*, a combining form meaning basin, is linked to -*ic*, the suffix meaning _____ _____, in the term describing the space formed by the bones of the pelvis that contains the urinary tract, male and female reproductive organs, and lower portions of the intestine: _____ _____.

SELF-INSTRUCTION: Anatomic and Clinical Divisions of the Abdomen

The abdomen is divided into several regions for reference purposes. There are nine specific anatomic divisions (Fig. 2-18) and four general clinical divisions (Fig. 2-19). All references are based on the <u>patient's</u> right or left. Study the illustrations and

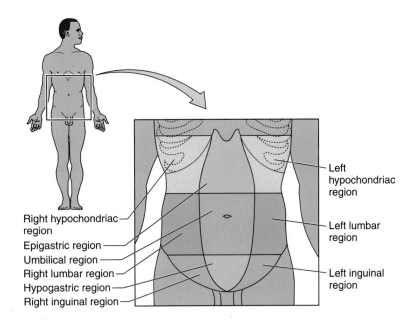

Right hypochondriac region
Epigastric region
Umbilical region
Right lumbar region
Hypogastric region
Right inguinal region

Left hypochondriac region
Left lumbar region
Left inguinal region

FIGURE 2-18   Anatomic divisions of the abdomen.

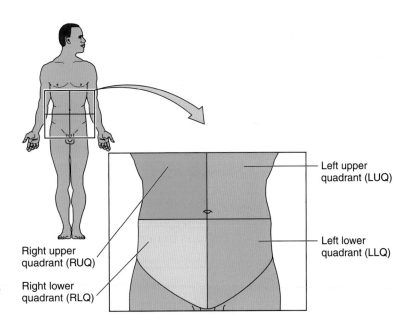

Right upper quadrant (RUQ)
Right lower quadrant (RLQ)

Left upper quadrant (LUQ)
Left lower quadrant (LLQ)

FIGURE 2-19   Clinical divisions of the abdomen.

memorize the meanings of the terms describing the anatomic and clinical divisions of the abdomen in preparation for the Programmed Review that follows.

REGION	LOCATION
Anatomic Divisions of Abdomen	
hypochondriac regions	upper lateral regions beneath the ribs
epigastric region	upper middle region below the sternum
lumbar regions	middle lateral regions
umbilical region	region of the navel
inguinal regions	lower lateral groin regions
hypogastric region	region below the navel
Clinical Divisions of Abdomen	
right upper quadrant (RUQ)	upper right one-fourth of abdomen
left upper quadrant (LUQ)	upper left one-fourth of abdomen
right lower quadrant (RLQ)	lower right one-fourth of abdomen
left lower quadrant (LLQ)	lower left one-fourth of abdomen

PROGRAMMED REVIEW: Anatomic and Clinical Divisions of the Abdomen

ANSWERS	REVIEW
below hypochondriac	**2.93** The abdomen is divided into a number of anatomic regions for reference purposes. Recall that the prefix *hypo-* means _____ or deficient. The upper lateral regions beneath the ribs (*chondr/o* = cartilage) are the _____ regions.
upon gastr/o epigastric	**2.94** The prefix *epi-* means _____. You'll recall that the combining form meaning stomach is _____. Thus, the name for the upper middle region below the sternum and lying approximately upon the stomach is the _____ region.

lumbar	**2.95** The middle lateral areas of the abdomen, to each side of the lumbar spine, are the _____ regions.
pertaining to umbilical	**2.96** *umbilic/o* is the combining form for umbilicus, the navel. When linked to *-ic*, the suffix meaning _____ ____, it forms the terms for the anatomic area in the region of the navel called the _____ region.
suffix pertaining to inguinal	**2.97** The combining form for groin is *inguin/o*. When linked to *-al*, the _____ meaning _____ ____, it forms the term describing the lower lateral groin areas of the abdomen known as the _____ regions.
below suffix, pertaining to hypogastric	**2.98** *hypo-* is the prefix meaning _____ or deficient. Linked to the combining form for stomach and *-ic*, the _____ meaning _____ ____, it forms the term naming the area of the abdomen below the navel, approximately below the stomach, known as the _____ region.
left upper quadrant LLQ right lower quadrant right upper quadrant patient's	**2.99** The clinical divisions of the abdomen consist of four sections called quadrants. LUQ refers to the patient's _____ _____ _____, whereas the left lower quadrant is abbreviated _____. The appendix is located in the RLQ or _____ _____ _____, and the liver is located in the RUQ or _____ _____ _____. All references are based on the _____ right or left.

Pronunciation Summary

Following, you will find a list of medical terms that you have learned to build and spell in this chapter, followed by the page number on which each term can be found and its written pronunciation. 🎧 Take a minute to listen to the audio pronunciations of these terms on the Student Resource CD-ROM, and then practice pronouncing them out loud. For additional practice and reinforcement, write the definition of each term on a separate piece of paper.

abduction/72
ab-dŭk'shŭn

adduction/72
ă-duk'shŭn

adipose/33
a'di-pōs

anatomy/30
ă-nat'ō-mē

anterior (A)/68
an-tēr'e-or

cephalic/68
se-fal'ik

coronal plane/68
kōr'ŏ-năl plān

cytology/29
sī-tol'ŏ-jē

decubitus/71
dē-kyū'bi-tūs

dermatology/33
dĕr-mă-tol'ŏ-jē

dermis/33
dĕrm'is

distal/68
dis'tăl

dorsiflexion/73
dōr-si-flek'shūn

epidermis/32
ep-i-dĕrm'is

epigastric region/78
ep-i-gas'trik rē'jŭn

erect/71
ĕ-rĕkt'

eversion/73
ē-ver'zhŭn

extension/72
eks-ten'shŭn

flexion/72
flek'shŭn

frontal plane/68
frŏn'tăl plān

histology/29
his-tol'ŏ-jē

hypochondriac regions/78
hī-pō-kon'drē-ak rē'jŭnz

hypogastric region/78
hī-pō-gas'trik rē'jŭn

inferior/68
in-fēr'ē-ŏr

inguinal regions/78
ing'gwi-năl rē'jŭnz

inversion/73
in-vĕr'zhŭn

lateral/68
lat'er-ăl

lumbar regions/78
lŭm'bar rē'jŭnz

medial/68
mē'dē-ăl

microscope/29
mī'krō-scōp

pathologist/30
pa-thol'ŏ-jist

pathology/30
pa-thol'ŏ-jē

plantar flexion/73
plan'tăr flek'shŭn

posterior (P)/68
pos-tēr'ē-ŏr

pronation/73
prō-nā'shŭn

prone/71
prōn

proximal/68
prok'si-măl

recumbent/71
rē-kŭm'bĕnt

rotation/73
rō-tā'shŭn

sagittal plane/68
saj'i-tāl plān

subcutaneous/32
sŭb-kyū-tā'nē-ŭs

superior/68
sŭ-pēr'-ŏr

supination/73
sū'pi-nā'shŭn

supine/71
sū-pīn'

transverse plane/68
trans-vĕrs'plān

umbilical region/78
ŭm-bil'i-kăl rē'jŭn

urinary/60
yūr'i-nār-ē

ventral/68
ven'trăl

Examine Your Understanding

For the following terms, draw a line or lines to separate the prefixes (P), combining forms (CF), roots (R), and suffixes (S). Then, write the meaning of each component on the corresponding blank to define the term.

EXAMPLE

hyper/lip/emia

above or excessive / *fat* / *blood condition*

      P   R   S

1. anatomy

   _____ / _____ / _____

       P   R   S

2. mammary

   _____ / _____

       R   S

3. histology

   _____ / _____

       CF   S

4. subcutaneous

   _____ / _____ / _____

       P   R   S

5. ovigenesis

   _____ / _____

       CF   S

6. cranium

   _____ / _____

       R   S

7. pathologist

   _____ / _____

       CF   S

8. costochondral

   _____ / _____ / _____

       CF   R   S

9. colonic

   _____ / _____

       R   S

10. cardiovascular

   _____ / _____ / _____

       CF   R   S

11. myocardium

_____ / _____ / _____
          CF   R   S

12. epigastric

_____ / _____ / _____
          P   R   S

13. coronary

_____ / _____
          R   S

14. venous

_____ / _____
          R   S

15. arterial

_____ / _____
          R   S

16. hematology

_____ / _____
          CF   S

17. splenic

_____ / _____
          R   S

18. endocrine

_____ / _____ / _____
          P   R   S

19. parathyroidal

_____ / _____ / _____
          P   R   S

20. esophageal

_____ / _____
          R   S

21. tympanic

_____ / _____
          R   S

22. hepatobiliary

_____ / _____ / _____
          CF   CF   S

23. rectovaginal

_____ / _____ / _____
          CF   R   S

24. myometrium

_____ / _____ / _____
 CF   R   S

25. lacrimal

_____ / _____
 R   S

Match the combining form in the first column with its synonym in the second column.

26. _____ vertebr/o   a. vesic/o

27. _____ dacry/o   b. oophor/o

28. _____ mamm/o   c. episi/o

29. _____ nas/o   d. myring/o

30. _____ vulv/o   e. lingu/o

31. _____ ovari/o   f. colp/o

32. _____ ven/o   g. rhin/o

33. _____ gloss/o   h. lacrim/o

34. _____ or/o   i. phleb/o

35. _____ vagin/o   j. mast/o

36. _____ tympan/o   k. spondyl/o

37. _____ adip/o   l. metr/o

38. _____ dermat/o   m. bil/i

39. _____ uter/o   n. pector/o

40. _____ dent/i   o. kerat/o

41. _____ angi/o   p. orchid/o

42. _____ thorac/o   q. stomat/o

43. _____ test/o   r. nephr/o

44. _____ corne/o   s. odont/o

45. _____ chol/e   t. cutane/o

46. _____ cyst/o   u. lip/o

47. _____ ren/o   v. vas/o

Circle the prefix that corresponds to the meaning given.

48. to, toward or near   _bi-_   _ad-_   _para-_

49. half   _pan-_   _semi-_   _bi-_

50. small	*macro-*	*sub-*	*micro-*
51. before	*pro-*	*post-*	*epi-*
52. up, apart	*semi-*	*ana-*	*trans-*
53. around	*peri-*	*para-*	*epi-*
54. above or excessive	*hypo-*	*macro-*	*super-*
55. across or through	*trans-*	*peri-*	*ad-*
56. two	*tri-*	*mono-*	*bi-*
57. below or deficient	*hyper-*	*endo-*	*hypo-*
58. out or away	*ex-*	*a-*	*ad-*
59. between	*para-*	*inter-*	*semi-*

Give the plural for the following terms.

60. testis _____

61. vertebra _____

62. atrium _____

63. bronchus _____

Identify the color associated with the following cells.

64. melanocyte _____

65. leukocyte _____

66. erythrocyte _____

Write the correct medical term for each definition.

67. plane that divides the body into right and left portions_____

    _____

68. plane that divides the body into front and back portions _____

    _____

69. lying flat on the back _____

    _____

70. horizontal plane that divides the body into superior and inferior portion

    _____

71. turning the palm of the hand or sole of the foot downward or backward

    _____

72. toward the beginning of a structure_____

73. above another structure or toward the head_____

74. bending of the foot or the toes upward _____

75. lying face down and flat _____

Match the following terms with the appropriate body movements.

76. _____ flexion   a. movement toward the body
77. _____ inversion   b. straightening
78. _____ adduction   c. bending
79. _____ extension   d. to turn inward
80. _____ abduction   e. to turn outward
81. _____ eversion   f. movement away from the body

Match the following body cavities with the structures they contain.

82. _____ cranial   a. stomach, intestines, and liver
83. _____ vertebral   b. urinary tract and reproductive organs
84. _____ thoracic   c. spinal cord
85. _____ abdominal   d. brain
86. _____ pelvic   e. heart and lungs

Name the anatomic divisions of the abdomen.

87. lower lateral groin regions _____

88. upper lateral regions beneath the ribs _____

89. upper middle region below the sternum _____

90. region below the navel _____

91. middle lateral regions _____

92. region of the navel _____

Identify the combining form(s) for the following body parts.

93. head _____

94. eye(s) _____

95. ear(s) _____

96. nose _____

97. throat _____

98. neck _____

99. chest _____

100. abdomen _____

MEDICAL RECORD EXERCISES

Medical Record 2-1

The following is an example of a medical record, which you will learn much more about in the next chapter. Read it and then answer the following questions—you will be surprised by how much you can already discern because of your growing knowledge of medical terminology.

Questions about Medical Record 2-1

1. The indication, or reason, for the lumbar puncture is to determine if Raymond has (a) _____. The link of -*itis*, a (b) _____ meaning (c) _____, with *mening*, the root meaning (d) _____, provides the basic meaning of this term. The meninges are the coverings of the (e) _____ and (f) _____. This test will show whether these coverings are (g)_____.

2. Look back in Chapter 1 and give the rule used to form the term meningitis. _____

    _____

3. In your own words, not using medical terminology, describe the position in which the patient was placed for this procedure. _____

4. Identify the places along the vertebrae where the needles were inserted. _____

    _____

5. The abbreviation CSF is used several times in this record. Look up this abbreviation in your dictionary, and write the sentence that is used to define it. _____

    _____

    _____

CENTRAL MEDICAL CENTER

211 Medical Center Drive • Central City, US 90000-1234 • PHONE: (012) 125-6784 • FAX: (012) 125-9999

Department of Pediatric Neurology

REPORT OF PROCEDURE

PATIENT: HAUCK, RAYMOND

DATE OF BIRTH: 11/25/20xx

DATE OF PROCEDURE: 02/03/20xx

PROCEDURE PERFORMED: LUMBAR PUNCTURE

INDICATIONS: Rule out meningitis.

PROCEDURE IN DETAIL:

The patient was placed on a warmer and was held in a right lateral decubitus position. The spine was bent and after preparing the area with Betadine and draping in a sterile fashion, a $1^1/_2$-inch long 22-gauge spinal needle with a stylet was introduced at the level of L4-L5. There was a small amount of clear CSF, which was collected in one tube. There was no further dripping of CSF, so another spinal needle was introduced at the level of L3-L4 with good CSF dripping back, which was collected in the first tube plus into other tubes. Total amount of CSF was about 3 mL, which was clear with some red blood cells noted in it. After collection of the tubes, the spinal needle was removed.

After cleaning with alcohol, the puncture wound was covered with a Band-Aid. The patient tolerated the procedure well with no complications. There was a drop of blood at the puncture wounds.

CSF will be sent in three separate tubes. Tube 1 will be for Gram stain, culture, and Bactigen panel. Tube 2 will be for chemistries, glucose, and protein. Tube 3 will be for cell count with differential.

E. Migeon MD
_____
Edward Migeon, M.D.

EM:bst
D: 02/03/20xx
T: 02/03/20xx

REPORT OF PROCEDURE

PT. NAME:	HAUCK, RAYMOND
ID NO:	OPS-167480621
SURGEON:	E. MIGEON, M.D.

Answers to Examine Your Understanding

1. ana/tom/y
   <u>up, apart</u> / <u>to cut</u> / <u>condition or process of</u>
      P   R   S

2. mamm/ary
   <u>breast</u> / <u>pertaining to</u>
      R   S

3. histo/logy
   <u>tissue</u> / <u>study of</u>
      CF   S

4. sub/cutane/ous
   <u>below or under</u> / <u>skin</u> / <u>pertaining to</u>
         P   R   S

5. ovi/genesis
   <u>egg</u> / <u>origin or production</u>
      CF   S

6. cran/ium
   <u>skull</u> / <u>structure or tissue</u>
      R   S

7. patho/logist
   <u>disease</u> / <u>one who specializes in the study or treatment of</u>
      CF   S

8. costo/chondr/al
   <u>rib</u> / <u>cartilage</u> / <u>pertaining to</u>
      CF   R   S

9. colon/ic
   <u>colon (large intestine)</u> / <u>pertaining to</u>
            R   S

10. cardio/vascul/ar
    <u>heart</u> / <u>vessel</u> / <u>pertaining to</u>
       CF   R   S

11. myo/card/ium
    <u>muscle</u> / <u>heart</u> / <u>structure or tissue</u>
       CF   R   S

12. epi/gastr/ic
    <u>upon</u> / <u>stomach</u> / <u>pertaining to</u>
       P   R   S

13. coron/ary
    <u>circle or crown</u> / <u>pertaining to</u>
          R   S

14. ven/ous
    <u>vein</u> / <u>pertaining to</u>
       R   S

15. arteri/al
    <u>artery</u> / <u>pertaining to</u>
       R   S

16. hemato/logy
   <u>blood</u> / <u>study of</u>
    CF   S

17. splen/ic
   <u>spleen</u> / <u>pertaining to</u>
    R   S

18. endo/crin/e
   <u>within</u> / <u>to secrete</u> / <u>noun marker</u>
    P   R   S

19. para/thyroid/al
   <u>alongside of or abnormal</u> / <u>thyroid gland (shield)</u> / <u>pertaining to</u>
    P   R   S

20. esophag/eal
   <u>esophagus</u> / <u>pertaining to</u>
    R   S

21. tympan/ic
   <u>eardrum</u> / <u>pertaining to</u>
    R   S

22. hepato/bili/ary
   <u>liver</u> / <u>bile</u> / <u>pertaining to</u>
    CF   CF   S

23. recto/vagin/al
   <u>rectum</u> / <u>vagina</u> / <u>pertaining to</u>
    CF   R   S

24. myo/metr/ium
   <u>muscle</u> / <u>uterus</u> / <u>structure or tissue</u>
    CF   R   S

25. lacrim/al
   <u>tear</u> / <u>pertaining to</u>
    R   S

26. k	42. n	58. ex-
27. h	43. p	59. inter-
28. j	44. o	60. testes
29. g	45. m	61. vertebrae
30. c	46. a	62. atria
31. b	47. r	63. bronchi
32. i	48. ad-	64. black
33. e	49. semi-	65. white
34. q	50. micro-	66. red
35. f	51. pro-	67. sagittal plane
36. d	52. ana-	68. coronal or frontal plane
37. u	53. peri-	69. supine or horizontal recumbent
38. t	54. super-	
39. l	55. trans-	70. transverse plane
40. s	56. bi-	71. pronation
41. v	57. hypo-	

72. proximal
73. superior or cephalic
74. dorsiflexion
75. prone
76. c
77. d
78. a
79. b
80. f
81. e
82. d
83. c
84. e
85. a
86. b
87. inguinal regions
88. hypochondriac regions
89. epigastric region
90. hypogastric region
91. lumbar regions
92. umbilical region
93. cephal/o
94. opt/o, ophthalm/o, or ocul/o
95. aur/i or ot/o
96. nas/o or rhin/o
97. pharyng/o
98. cervic/o
99. thorac/o or pector/o
100. abdomin/o

ANSWERS TO MEDICAL RECORD EXERCISE 2-1

1. (a) meningitis; (b) suffix; (c) inflammation; (d) membrane (meninges); (e) brain; (f) spinal cord; (g) inflamed
2. A combining vowel is *not* used before a suffix that begins with a vowel.
3. The patient was lying down on the right side (right lateral decubitus position).
4. The first needle was inserted between the 4th and 5th lumbar vertebrae. The second needle was inserted between the 3rd and 4th lumbar vertebrae.
5. CSF = cerebrospinal fluid—See medical dictionary for definition.

CHAPTER 3

HEALTH CARE RECORDS

OBJECTIVES

1 Define the basic terms and abbreviations used in documenting a history and physical and a progress note.

2 Recognize common hospital records.

3 Identify common abbreviations and symbols related to medical facilities and patient care.

4 List common units of measure and their related abbreviations.

5 Identify drug forms, routes of medication administration, and their related abbreviations and symbols.

6 Identify a drug prescription, and explain the differences between chemical, generic, and trade (brand) names of drugs.

7 Define common prescription abbreviations and symbols.

8 Recognize medical abbreviations and symbols that are deemed to be error prone.

9 Record military dates and times.

CHECKLIST

CHECKLIST	LOCATION
☐ Complete Chapter 3 Self-Instruction and Programmed Review sections	pages 94–131 📖
☐ Complete the Chapter 3 Examine Your Understanding exercises	pages 132–136 📖

(continued)

☐ Complete Medical Record Exercises 3-1, 3-2, and 3-3	pages 137–142 📖
☐ Complete the Chapter 3 Interactive Exercises on the Student Resource CD-ROM	(CD-ROM)
☐ Take the Chapter 3 Quiz on the Student Resource CD-ROM	(CD-ROM)
☐ When you receive 70% or higher on the Quiz, move on to Chapter 4	page 147 📖

MEET THE PATIENT   Mr. Michael Marsi called Dr. Spaulding's office first thing in the morning with new symptoms. He has had chronic health problems for the past two years, including **hypertension,** for which Dr. Spaulding treats him with medication. This morning, he woke up with numbness in his left leg and hand, and he is extremely worried. Fortunately, Dr. Spaulding was able to see him right away. She uses problem-orientated medical records and writes a new SOAP progress note at each patient visit. One step Dr. Spaulding takes toward diagnosing Mr. Marsi's problem is to order a chest x-ray, which is performed by a **Radiologic Technologist**. Read ahead to learn more about Mr. Marsi's condition and the documents used by medical professionals to evaluate and treat patients. Dr. Spaulding's notes regarding Mr. Marsi's visit are included in **Medical Record 3-1.**

To put your knowledge of medical terminology into use, you need to see how this language is used in everyday communication about patients. In this chapter, you will learn the common abbreviations, symbols, forms, and formats used to record all aspects of patient care. This knowledge will help you to comprehend medical record documentation within the health care industry.

Common Patient Care Records

Patient care records vary somewhat from setting to setting. For example, the medical records used in a physician's office are different from those used in a hospital. Some common records that you will encounter regardless of the setting are the history and physical report and progress notes. Common hospital records are introduced later in the chapter.

THE HISTORY AND PHYSICAL

The record that serves as a cornerstone of patient care is the **history and physical (H&P)** (Fig. 3-1). The H&P documents the patient's medical history and the findings from the

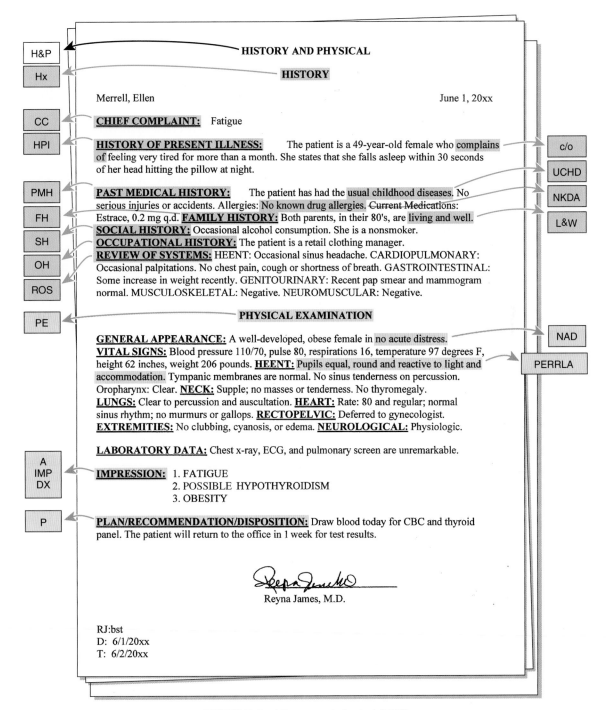

HISTORY AND PHYSICAL

H&P

Hx

HISTORY

Merrell, Ellen   June 1, 20xx

CC   **CHIEF COMPLAINT:**   Fatigue

HPI   **HISTORY OF PRESENT ILLNESS:**   The patient is a 49-year-old female who complains   c/o
of feeling very tired for more than a month. She states that she falls asleep within 30 seconds
of her head hitting the pillow at night.   UCHD

PMH   **PAST MEDICAL HISTORY:**   The patient has had the usual childhood diseases. No   NKDA
serious injuries or accidents. Allergies: No known drug allergies. Current Medications:
FH   Estrace, 0.2 mg q.d. **FAMILY HISTORY:** Both parents, in their 80's, are living and well.   L&W
SOCIAL HISTORY: Occasional alcohol consumption. She is a nonsmoker.
SH   **OCCUPATIONAL HISTORY:** The patient is a retail clothing manager.
REVIEW OF SYSTEMS: HEENT: Occasional sinus headache. CARDIOPULMONARY:
OH   Occasional palpitations. No chest pain, cough or shortness of breath. GASTROINTESTINAL:
Some increase in weight recently. GENITOURINARY: Recent pap smear and mammogram
ROS   normal. MUSCULOSKELETAL: Negative. NEUROMUSCULAR: Negative.

PE   **PHYSICAL EXAMINATION**

GENERAL APPEARANCE: A well-developed, obese female in no acute distress.   NAD
VITAL SIGNS: Blood pressure 110/70, pulse 80, respirations 16, temperature 97 degrees F,
height 62 inches, weight 206 pounds. **HEENT:** Pupils equal, round and reactive to light and   PERRLA
accommodation. Tympanic membranes are normal. No sinus tenderness on percussion.
Oropharynx: Clear. **NECK:** Supple; no masses or tenderness. No thyromegaly.
LUNGS: Clear to percussion and auscultation. **HEART:** Rate: 80 and regular; normal
sinus rhythm; no murmurs or gallops. **RECTOPELVIC:** Deferred to gynecologist.
EXTREMITIES: No clubbing, cyanosis, or edema. **NEUROLOGICAL:** Physiologic.

LABORATORY DATA: Chest x-ray, ECG, and pulmonary screen are unremarkable.

A
IMP   **IMPRESSION:**   1. FATIGUE
DX   2. POSSIBLE HYPOTHYROIDISM
                               3. OBESITY

P   **PLAN/RECOMMENDATION/DISPOSITION:** Draw blood today for CBC and thyroid
panel. The patient will return to the office in 1 week for test results.

Reyna James, M.D.

RJ:bst
D: 6/1/20xx
T: 6/2/20xx

FIGURE 3-1   History and physical (H&P).

physical examination. It is usually the first document generated when a patient presents for care and is most often recorded at a new patient visit or as part of a consultation.

The first portion of the H&P, the **history (Hx)**, documents **subjective information** from the patient's personal statements about his or her medical history, including information regarding past injuries, illnesses, operations, defects, and habits. It begins with the **chief complaint (CC)**, which is the patient's reason for seeking medical care. The chief complaint is usually brief and is often recorded in the patient's own words, which are indicated by quotation marks (e.g., CC: "feeling sick and tired, like the flu"). Often, especially in handwritten notes, the abbreviation **c/o (complains of)** is used. Details of the complaint are amplified in the **present illness (PI)** or **history of present illness (HPI)** section of the H&P report, noting the duration and severity of the complaint (e.g., how long the patient has had the complaint, and how bad it is).

Notations about the patient's **symptoms (Sx)**, which describe subjective evidence of illness, indicate what the patient is experiencing. For example, the patient may feel overly tired, congested, achy, and nauseated—these are feelings that the patient can describe, but they cannot necessarily be seen or examined by a physician.

Information about the patient's **past history (PH)** or **past medical history (PMH)** is recorded next. This includes information about the patient's past illnesses, starting with childhood, as well as surgical operations, injuries, physical defects, medications, and allergies. The abbreviation **UCHD (usual childhood diseases)** is used here to record that the patient had the "usual" or commonly contracted illnesses during childhood. The abbreviation **NKDA (no known drug allergies)** indicates that the patient has had no known allergic reaction to a previously administered drug. The **family history (FH)** includes the state of health of the immediate family members (mother, father, and siblings). A&W and L&W are abbreviations used interchangeably to note that the relative is alive (living) and well. The **social history (SH)** notes the patient's recreational interests, hobbies, and use of tobacco and drugs, including alcohol. A record of work habits that may involve health risks is included in the **occupational history (OH)**.

The history is complete after documenting the patient's answers to questions related to the **review of systems (ROS)** or **systems review (SR)**, which is a head-to-toe review of the functions of all body systems. This review makes it possible to evaluate other symptoms that may not have been previously mentioned.

After the subjective data are recorded, the provider begins a **physical examination (PE)** or a **physical (Px)** to obtain **objective information**. Different from symptoms, this refers to facts that can be seen or detected by testing. Examples of **signs**, or objective evidence of disease, include swelling, skin color changes, visible response to pain, deformation, and abnormal vital signs, among others. After signs are documented, selected diagnostic tests are performed or ordered when further evaluation is necessary. Several abbreviations are used to document the findings of physical examination, such as **HEENT (head, eyes, ears, nose, and throat)**, **PERRLA (pupils equal, round, and reactive to light and accommodation)**, **NAD (no acute distress)**, and **WNL (within normal limits)**.

The identification of a disease or condition is recorded in the **Impression (IMP)**, **Diagnosis (Dx)**, or **Assessment (A)** section of the H&P. This determination is made after the physician evaluates all subjective and objective data. Often, when the diagnosis is uncertain, a **differential diagnosis** is made, using the abbreviation **R/O (rule out)**. Differential diagnoses are the possible conditions that require further investigation, often through diagnostic tests and procedures, in order to **rule out** or eliminate each suspected diagnosis and to verify the final diagnosis.

Final notations include the health care provider's **plan (P)** for treating the patient, which is also called the **recommendation** or **disposition**. Here, the provider outlines strategies designed to remedy the patient's condition, including instructions to the patient and orders for medications, diagnostic tests, or therapies.

Often, physicians are required to submit a current H&P report before admitting a patient to the hospital (e.g., for elective surgery). When the patient is to have surgery, this report is called a **preoperative H&P**.

 Health Care Professionals   MEET THE RADIOLOGIC TECHNOLOGIST

Radiologic technologists, also referred to as radiographers, use radiographic and fluoroscopic equipment to produce images of the tissues, organs, bones, and vessels of the human body with ionizing radiation. These x-ray images are usually ordered by physicians to assist in the diagnosis of disease or injury. Some therapeutic procedures also require the application of x-rays and other ionizing radiations.

A more detailed description of the radiographic technologist health care career can be found on the Student Resource CD-ROM and at the companion website at www.thePoint.lww.com/WillisQC.

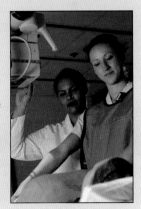

PROGRESS NOTES

After the initial H&P is recorded, progress notes are used to document the patient's continued care. The SOAP method of documenting a patient's progress is most common. The letters represent the order in which progress is noted as each complaint or problem is addressed (Fig. 3-2):

S:	Subjective	that which the patient describes
O:	Objective	observable information (e.g., test results, blood pressure readings)
A:	Assessment	patient's progress and evaluation of the plan's effectiveness; any newfound problem or diagnosis is also noted here
P:	Plan	decision to proceed or to alter the plan strategy

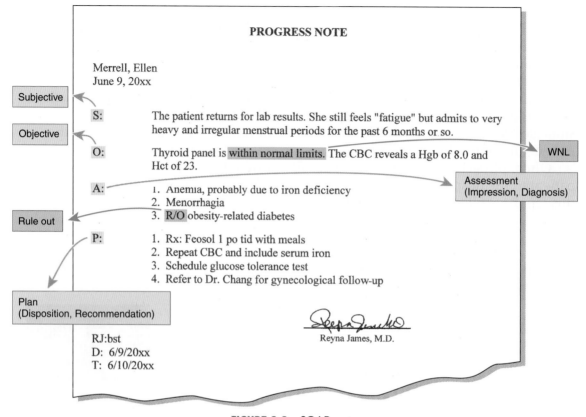

FIGURE 3-2   SOAP note.

Rx for Success

Make flash cards for and memorize the following abbreviations used in documenting a history and physical examination and progress notes so that you will recognize them in the health records found throughout this text.

SELF-INSTRUCTION: Common Abbreviations Used in the History and Physical and Progress Notes

ABBREVIATION	EXPANSION
A	assessment
A&W; L&W	alive and well; living and well
CC	chief complaint
c/o	complains of

Dx	diagnosis
FH	family history
HEENT	head, eyes, ears, nose, and throat
H&P	history and physical
HPI; PI	history of present illness; present illness
Hx	history
IMP	impression
NAD	no acute distress
NKDA	no known drug allergies
O	objective information
OH	occupational history
P	plan (*also* recommendation, disposition)
PE; Px	physical examination
PERRLA	pupils equal, round, and reactive to light and accommodation
PH; PMH	past history; past medical history
R/O	rule out
ROS; SR	review of systems; systems review
S	subjective information
SH	social history
Sx	symptom
UCHD	usual childhood diseases
WNL	within normal limits

PROGRAMMED REVIEW: Common Abbreviations Used in the History and Physical and Progress Notes

ANSWERS	REVIEW
history and physical	**3.1** The H&P, or _____ _____ _____, is the first document generated in the care of a patient. It is divided into two categories: the Hx,
history, subjective	or _____, which provides all _____

physical

physical examination

objective

information obtained from the patient, including his or her own perceptions; and the Px, or _____,
or PE, or _____ _____,
which records all _____ information that can be seen or verified by the examiner.

chief complaint

complains of

3.2 The first thing that is noted in the history is the CC, or _____ _____, or what the patient c/o, or _____ _____. It is a brief explanation of why the patient is seeking medical care. Further details about the complaint are noted in

present illness

history, present

illness

the PI, or _____ _____,
or HPI, or _____ of _____
_____, to report how long the patient has had the complaint and how bad it is. All subjective evidence of disease that the patient reports is noted as Sx,

symptoms

or _____.

past history, past

medical history

usual childhood

diseases

no known drug

allergies

3.3 The history continues by gathering information regarding past injuries, illnesses, operations, physical defects, medications, and allergies in the PH, or _____ _____, or PMH, or _____ _____ _____. UCHD notes that the patient had the _____ _____ _____, or commonly contracted illnesses during childhood. NKDA, or ____ _____ _____ _____, indicates that the patient has had no known allergic reactions to a previously administered drug.

family

history

3.4 "Father, age 58, mother, age 54, brother, age 32, all L&W" is an example of an FH, or _____ _____. Notes about recreational interests, hobbies,

social history	and use of tobacco and drugs, such as alcohol, are noted in the SH, or _____ _____. Work habits that may involve health risks are included in the OH,
occupational history	or _____ _____. The history is complete after the patient answers questions related to a review of the functions of the body systems in
review of systems	the ROS, or _____ ____ _____,
systems review	or SR, or _____ _____.

3.5 The second portion of the H&P is the Px,

physical, physical examination	or _____, or PE, or _____ _____. Objective evidence of disease,
signs	called _____, are documented; then, selected tests are ordered and the findings recorded. Common
head	abbreviations include HEENT, which means _____,
eyes, ears, nose, throat	_____, _____, _____, and _____;
pupils equal	PERRLA, which means _____ _____,
round, reactive, light	_____, and _____ to _____
accommodation	and _____; WNL, which
within normal limits	means _____ _____ _____; and
no acute distress	NAD, which indicates ____ _____ _____.

3.6 The identification of a disease or condition is recorded

impression	in the IMP, or _____; the Dx,
diagnosis, assessment	or _____; or the A, or _____. This is made after all subjective and objective data are evaluated. When the diagnosis is uncertain, a differential diagnosis is made using the abbreviation R/O,
rule out	or _____ _____.

3.7 An outline of strategies designed to remedy the

plan	patient's condition is noted in the provider's P, or _____,

recommendation	which is also called a/an _____
disposition	or _____. This section includes the provider's instructions to the patient and orders for medications, diagnostic tests, and therapies.
progress	**3.8** After the initial history and physical is recorded, _____ notes are used for further documentation of the patient's care. The letters "SOAP" represent the order in which progress is noted:
subjective	S: _____; that which the patient describes
objective	O: _____; observable information (e.g., test results or blood pressure readings)
assessment	A: _____; patient's progress and an evaluation of the effectiveness of the plan
plan	P: _____; decision to proceed or to alter the plan strategy

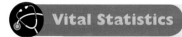 **Vital Statistics**   **HYPERTENSION (HTN)** (hī′pĕr-ten′shŭn)

Origin: *hyper-* (above or excessive) + L. *tensio* (tension)

Hypertension is commonly referred to as high blood pressure, a medical condition in which the blood pressure is persistently elevated. Hypertension can be classified as either essential (primary) or secondary. Essential hypertension indicates that no specific medical cause can be found to explain a patient's condition. Secondary hypertension indicates that the high blood pressure is a result of (i.e., secondary to) another condition, such as kidney disease. Persistent hypertension is one of the risk factors for strokes, heart attacks, heart failure, and arterial aneurysm and is a leading cause of chronic renal failure. Because of its wide prevalence and its impact on cardiovascular health, hypertension is recognized as a major cause of disease and death in industrialized societies.

SELF-INSTRUCTION: Hospital Records

The **history and physical** (Fig. 3-3) is often the first document entered into the patient's hospital record on admission, and it is commonly required before elective admission for surgery. **Physician's orders** (Fig. 3-4) list the directives for care prescribed by the doctor attending to the patient (the doctor who admits the patient to the hospital is the "attending physician"). The **nurse's notes** (Fig. 3-5) and **physician's progress notes** chronicle the care throughout the patient's stay.

In many cases, a specialist is called in by the attending physician; after he or she examines the patient, a **consultation report** is filed. If surgery is necessary, a narrative **operative report** (Fig. 3-6) is required of the primary surgeon. In this report, a detailed description of the operation is given, including the method of incision, technique, instruments used, types of suture, method of closure, and the patient's responses during the procedure and at the time of transfer to recovery. The anesthesiologist, who is in charge of life support during surgery, must file an **anesthesiologist's report**, which covers the anesthesia details, including the drugs used, the dose and time given, and monitoring of the patient's vital signs throughout the procedure. When a surgery or procedure involves a reasonable risk to the patient, an **informed consent** form must be signed by the patient to show that he or she has been advised of the risks and benefits of the proposed treatment as well as any alternatives. **Ancillary reports** note any additional procedures and therapies, including **diagnostic tests** and **pathology reports.**

The final hospital document, which is recorded at the time of discharge, is the **discharge summary** (also termed **clinical resume**, **clinical summary**, or **discharge abstract**) (Fig. 3-7). It is a summary of the patient's hospital care, including the date of admission, preliminary diagnoses, diagnostic tests, course of treatment, final diagnoses, and date of discharge.

MEET THE PATIENT   Carleen Perron, a 28-year-old female, normally sees Dr. Spaulding for check-ups on a yearly basis, but she has been treated for a sore throat and cold-like symptoms every month now for at least six months. On her last visit, Dr. Spaulding noted that her condition had become chronic and recommended that Carleen be seen in consultation by Dr. Patrick Rodden, an ear, nose, and throat (ENT) specialist. The referral was made, and Dr. Rodden's recommendation was that Carleen undergo surgery.

The medical records in Figures 3-3 through 3-7 chronicle Carleen's hospital care. Later, you'll refer to some of these documents again when completing interactive exercises that are provided for Chapter 3 on the Student Resource CD-ROM. Medical records like Carleen's are also used by **Medical Billers/Coders,** who assign diagnostic and procedural codes to the patient's health insurance claim form and then process the claim so the hospital and health care professionals can be reimbursed.

CENTRAL MEDICAL CENTER

211 Medical Center Drive • Central City, US 90000-1234 • PHONE: (012) 125-6784 • FAX: (012) 125-9999

PREOPERATIVE HISTORY AND PHYSICAL

HISTORY

DATE OF ADMISSION: June 3, 20xx

HISTORY OF PRESENT ILLNESS:
The patient is a 28-year-old white female with a chief complaint of frequent, recurrent, suppurative tonsillitis. She has had some eight infections over the last 6 months and is admitted at this time for elective tonsillectomy. The surgery has been discussed with the patient and family, including risks and complications. The patient's internist is C. Camarillo, M.D.

MEDICATIONS: None.

ALLERGIES: None known.

PAST SURGICAL HISTORY: None.

PAST MEDICAL HISTORY: UCHD (usual childhood diseases).

REVIEW OF SYSTEMS: CARDIOVASCULAR: No high blood pressure, heart murmurs, or shortness of breath. PULMONARY: No chronic lung disease; no asthma. GASTRO-INTESTINAL: No hepatitis. RENAL HISTORY: Negative for infections. ENDOCRINE: No diabetes or thyroid disease. MUSCULOSKELETAL: Negative for arthritis. HEMATOLOGIC: No history of anemia or bleeding tendencies.

FAMILY HISTORY: Grandmother has history of diabetes.

GYNECOLOGICAL HISTORY: Regular menses.

SOCIAL HISTORY: The patient is a nonsmoker. Alcohol use was denied, and drug use was denied.

(continued)

P. Rodden MD
PATRICK RODDEN, M.D.

JR:bst

D: 6/1/20xx
T: 6/2/20xx

HISTORY AND PHYSICAL Page 1	PT. NAME: PERRON, CARLEEN ID NO: 672894017 ROOM NO: ATT. PHYS: PATRICK RODDEN, M.D.

FIGURE 3-3 Preoperative history and physical (H&P) submitted to the hospital before surgical admission.

CENTRAL MEDICAL CENTER

211 Medical Center Drive • Central City, US 90000-1234 • PHONE: (012) 125-6784 • FAX: (012) 125-9999

PREOPERATIVE HISTORY AND PHYSICAL

PHYSICAL EXAMINATION

VITAL SIGNS: Afebrile, alert, oriented, normotensive. Blood Pressure: 124/80. Pulse: 84. Respirations: 18.

HEENT: PERRLA (pupils equal, round, and reactive to light and accommodation). Tympanic membranes are clear. Light reflex is present. No sinus tenderness on percussion. Oropharynx: Clear. Hypertrophic tonsils. No exudates. Nasopharynx: No masses. Larynx: Clear.

NECK: Supple; no masses or tenderness. No cervical adenopathy.

LUNGS: Clear to percussion and auscultation.

HEART: Rate: 84 and regular; normal sinus rhythm; no murmurs or gallops.

RECTOPELVIC: Deferred.

EXTREMITIES: No peripheral edema. No ecchymoses.

NEUROLOGICAL: Physiologically intact.

IMPRESSION: Chronic, recurrent tonsillitis. The patient is admitted for an elective tonsillectomy.

P. Rodden MD
PATRICK RODDEN, M.D.

JR:bst
D: 6/1/20xx
T: 6/2/20xx

HISTORY AND PHYSICAL PAGE 2	PT. NAME:	PERRON, CARLEEN
	ID NO:	672894017
	ROOM NO:	
	ATT. PHYS:	PATRICK RODDEN, M.D.

FIGURE 3-3   Continued.

CENTRAL MEDICAL CENTER

211 Medical Center Drive • Central City, US 90000-1234 • PHONE: (012) 125-6784 • FAX: (012) 125-9999

DOCTOR: PLEASE STATE PERTINENT CLINICAL INFORMATION WHEN ORDERING RADIOLOGY PROCEDURES

WRITE WITH BALLPOINT INK PEN; PRESS HARD

DATE	TIME	
6-3-xx	10⁰⁰	Post-op
		1) VS q⅟₄ h x 4 then q 2h x 4,
		then q 4h
		2) bed rest c̄ BRP when alert
		3) continue IV's 80 mL/hr
		until taking fluids well
		4) Vicodin (7.5 mg/500 mg) elixir
		15 mL p.o. q 4h p.r.n. mild to mod pain
		5) hydromorphone 4 mg IM
		q 4h p.r.n. severe pain
		6) ice & liquids at bedside
		& encourage P Rodden MD
		noted W. Cliff RN. 6-3-xx 1130
		M 6/3/xx 1145

PERRON, CARLEEN
DOB 07/20/xx
67289417
Rodden, Patrick MD

6/3/20xx
F 284
SURG 312

WRITE WITH BALLPOINT INK PEN; PRESS HARD

DATE	TIME	
6-3-XX	12³⁰	1) full liquids requiring
		soft diet
		2) admit
		3) ambien 5 mg p.o. q hs
		p.r.n. sleep mRx10p.r.n.
		P Rodden MD
		noted W. Cliff RN 12:38
		M 6/3/xx 123

PERRON, CARLEEN
DOB 07/20/xx
67289417
Rodden, Patrick MD

6/3/20xx
F 284
SURG 312

PHYSICIAN'S ORDERS

FIGURE 3-4 Physician's orders: orders written by the surgeon and noted by the nursing staff during the patient's surgical care.

DATE	TIME	REMARKS
6/3/xx	0615	admitted & oriented to room 312. In no acute distress. VS stable. Afebrile NPO maintained. Condition stable K. Brown RN
6/3/xx	0800	To OR via gurney - awake & oriented accompanied by her mother - condition stable K. Brown RN
6/3/xx	1110	Returned from PACU drowsy but arouses easily Skin warm & dry. Color pink - VS stable - Throat dry unable to take sips of water very well - no nausea - c/o severe sore throat medicated $\bar{x}$ with IM pain medication with desired effect - mother very supportive & remains @ bedside - Using a bedpan but unable to urinate - IV infusing well K. Brown RN

CENTRAL MEDICAL CENTER **PATIENT'S PROGRESS NOTES** **GENERAL CARE & TREATMENT**	**PT. NAME:** PERRON, CARLEEN **ID NO:** 672894017 **ROOM NO:** 312 **ATT. PHYS:** PATRICK RODDEN, M.D.

FIGURE 3-5 Nurse's notes: a recording by the nursing staff of the patient's progress made during general care and treatment.

CENTRAL MEDICAL CENTER

211 Medical Center Drive • Central City, US 90000-1234 • PHONE: (012) 125-6784 • FAX: (012) 125-9999

OPERATIVE REPORT

DATE OF OPERATION: June 3, 20xx.

PREOPERATIVE DIAGNOSIS: Chronic tonsillitis.

POSTOPERATIVE DIAGNOSIS: Frequent, recurrent tonsillitis.

SURGEON: Patrick Rodden, M.D.

ASSISTANT SURGEON: None

ANESTHESIOLOGIST: Robert Jung, M.D.

ANESTHESIA: General.

SURGERY PERFORMED: Tonsillectomy.

DESCRIPTION OF OPERATION: After general anesthesia induction, with intubation, the McGivor mouth gag and tongue retractor were utilized for exposure of the oropharynx. Local anesthetic consisting of 6 mL of 0.5% Xylocaine with 1:100,000 epinephrine was utilized. Tonsillectomy was carried out using dissection and air technique. The right tonsillectomy electrocoagulation Bovie suction was utilized for hemostasis. Examination of the nasopharynx was normal.

The patient tolerated the procedure well and went to the recovery room in good condition.

P. Rodden MD
_____
PATRICK RODDEN, M.D.

JR:as
D: 6/3/20xx
T: 6/4/20xx

OPERATIVE REPORT	PT. NAME:	PERRON, CARLEEN
	ID NO:	672894017
	ROOM NO:	312
	ATT. PHYS:	PATRICK RODDEN, M.D.

FIGURE 3-6 Operative report: surgeon's account of surgical procedure.

THAT CONDITION WHICH AFTER STUDY IS DETERMINED TO BE THE REASON FOR ADMISSION TO THE HOSPITAL

	MEDICAL RECORDS USE
PRINCIPAL DIAGNOSIS - *Chronic tonsillitis*	474.00
FINAL DIAGNOSIS - NO ABBREVIATIONS	474.00
Same	

SECONDARY DIAGNOSIS:

—

COMPLICATIONS AND/OR COMORBIDITY:

—

PRINCIPAL OPERATION/PROCEDURES(S)/TREATMENT RENDERED:

Tonsillectomy

SECONDARY OPERATIONS/PROCEDURES:

CONDITION ON DISCHARGE   *Stable*

☐ DISCHARGE INSTRUCTIONS   ☐ PRE-PRINTED INSTRUCTIONS GIVEN

MEDICATIONS   *Tylenol*

PHYSICAL ACTIVITY   *Bed rest*

DIET   *full liquid*

FOLLOW-UP   *office in 48 h*

DATE OF SUMMARY IF DICTATED:

DATE ADMITTED: 6/3/XX	DATE DISCHARGED: 6/4/XX	ATTENDING PHYSICIAN *P. Rodden* M.D.
		06/03/20XX

FOR MED. RECORDS USE ONLY	ASSEMBLY	ANALYSIS	CODED	KEYED	FINAL CHECK
	SL	*ML/39*	*NX*	*L*	

CONSULTANTS:			
		AA	1
		DP	R48
		SC	1212

CENTRAL MEDICAL CENTER

DIAGNOSIS RECORD/
DISCHARGE SUMMARY

FIGURE 3-7   Discharge summary (abstract): final report documented at the time of discharge.

Health Care Professionals   MEET THE MEDICAL BILLER/CODER

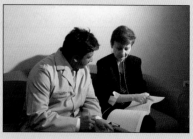

Medical billers and medical coders (medical billers/coders) evaluate medical records and documentation concerning patient diagnoses and services rendered in order to accurately and completely bill for those services. Medical billers/coders must comply with legal standards and guidelines as they interpret medical information and assign and sequence the correct diagnostic (ICD-9-CM) and procedural (CPT) codes. They also review insurance claims before submission for completeness and accuracy in order to minimize claim denial by the insurance carriers.

Medical billers/coders work in a variety of health care settings with multiple health professionals.

A more detailed description of the medical biller/coder health care career can be found on the Student Resource CD-ROM and at the companion website at www.thePoint.lww.com/WillisQC.

PROGRAMMED REVIEW: Hospital Records

ANSWERS	REVIEW
history physical	**3.9** A recent H&P, or _____ and _____, is usually the first document entered into the patient's hospital record on admission. The attending physician, the doctor who makes arrangements for the patient to be hospitalized, makes a list of the directives for care. These orders are
physician's orders	called _____ _____. The notes that chronicle the care throughout the patient's stay
nurse's	are made by the nursing staff in _____
notes, physician's	_____ and by the physician in the _____ progress notes.

3.10   If the attending physician calls in a specialist to evaluate the patient's condition, the record that is documented after such an evaluation is called a/an

consultation
_____ report.

3.11   If surgery is necessary, a narrative report is required of the primary surgeon, giving a detailed account of the operation. This document is known as the

operative report
_____ _____.

3.12   The anesthesiologist, who is in charge of life support during surgery, must file the _____

anesthesiologist's
_____, which includes details of anesthesia during

report
surgery.

3.13   When a surgery or procedure involves a reasonable

informed
risk, the patient must sign a/an _____

consent
_____ form, advising him or her of the risks and benefits of the proposed treatment, as well as alternatives.

3.14   Diagnostic tests and pathology reports are examples

ancillary reports
of _____ _____ that document various procedures and therapies.

3.15   The final hospital document recorded at the time of discharge, which summarizes the patient's hospital care,

discharge summary
is called the _____ _____

clinical
(also termed the _____ resume,

summary, discharge
clinical _____, or _____ abstract).

Medical Facilities and Patient Care Abbreviations and Symbols

The following table introduces additional medical abbreviations that are commonly used in patient care documentation. They represent the "acceptable" abbreviations that are used in medical records found in this text. Individual medical facilities provide their own list of acceptable terms and abbreviations that may not be used elsewhere. Memorize the terms and abbreviations in this list, and plan on adapting them to the various settings you encounter in the health care field.

Rx for Success

Medical errors caused by illegible writing and misinterpretations of medical abbreviations and symbols have led health care agencies, such as the Joint Commission on Accreditation of Healthcare Organizations (JCAHO), to require that medical facilities publish lists of authorized abbreviations and symbols for use by all personnel, including a list of those abbreviations and symbols that are unacceptable.

In this text, the abbreviations and symbols that have been identified as error prone are in red, with the preferred use noted in brackets ([ ]). Depending on the medical facility, use of these abbreviations and symbols may or may not be deemed to be acceptable; therefore, it is very important to study them so that you can properly interpret their meaning if they are used in a medical record. Those included on the official JCAHO "Do Not Use" list are marked by an asterisk (*).

A sampling of these error-prone abbreviations and symbols, including the risk for misinterpretation and the preferred use, is provided in the following list. A comprehensive list of error-prone abbreviations, symbols, and dose designations is available through the Institute for Safe Medication Practices (www.ismp.org). JCAHO provides the official "Do Not Use" list on their website (www.jointcommission.org).

Error Prone Abbreviation	Meaning	Risk	Preferred Use
AD, AS, AU	right ear, left ear, both ears	mistaken as OD, OS, OU (right eye, left eye, both eyes)	spell out *right ear, left ear,* or *both ears*
OD, OS, OU	right eye, left eye, both eyes	mistaken as AD, AS, AU (right ear, left ear, both ears)	spell out *right eye, left eye,* or *both eyes*

cc	cubic centimeter	mistaken as units	use the metric equivalent *mL*
DC, D/C	discharge, discontinue	mistaken for "discontinue" when followed by medications prescribed at the time of discharge	spell out *discontinue* or *discharge*
h.s.	bedtime	mistaken as "half-strength"	spell out bedtime
q.d. (*)	every day	mistaken for q.i.d. when the period after the "q" is sloppily written to look like an "i"	NEVER USE – spell out *every day* or *daily*
q.o.d. (*)	every other day	mistaken for q.d. when the "o" is mistaken for a period	NEVER USE – spell out *every other day*
SC, SQ, sub-Q	subcutaneous	mistaken for SL (sublingual) or 5Q ("5 every")	spell out *subcut* or *subcutaneously*
s̄s̄	one-half	mistaken as "55"	use *one-half* or ½
>, <	greater than, less than	mistaken for each other	spell out *greater than* or *less than*

SELF-INSTRUCTION: Medical Facilities and Patient Care Abbreviations and Symbols

ABBREVIATION	EXPANSION
Medical Care Facilities	
CCU	coronary (cardiac) care unit
ECU	emergency care unit
ER	emergency room
ICU	intensive care unit

IP	inpatient (a patient who is admitted to the hospital for care and assigned a bed)
OP	outpatient (a patient who is treated in an ambulatory [walk-in] facility in an office, clinic, or hospital who goes home after treatment and is not admitted to the hospital for an overnight stay)
OR	operating room
PACU	postanesthesia care unit
PAR	postanesthesia recovery
post-op or postop	postoperative (after surgery)
pre-op or preop	preoperative (before surgery)
RTC	return to clinic
RTO	return to office
Patient Care	
BRP	bathroom privileges
CP	chest pain
DC or D/C	discharge; discontinue [spell out "discharge" or "discontinue"]
ETOH	ethyl alcohol
Ⓛ	left
Ⓡ	right
ⓜ	murmur
Pt	patient
RRR	regular rate and rhythm
SOB	shortness of breath
Tr	treatment
Tx	treatment; traction
VS	vital signs (temperature, pulse, respiration, and blood pressure)
T	temperature
P	pulse
R	respiration
BP	blood pressure

Ht	height
Wt	weight
WDWN	well-developed and well-nourished
y/o or y.o.	year old
#	number or pound; if before a numeral, it means number (e.g., #2 = number 2); if after the numeral, it means pound (e.g., 150# = 150 pounds)
C	Celsius, centigrade
F	Fahrenheit
♀	female
♂	male
°	degree; hour
↑	increased
↓	decreased
∅	none; negative

PROGRAMMED REVIEW: Medical Facilities and Patient Care Abbreviations and Symbols

ANSWERS	REVIEW
	3.16 The patient seeking emergency care is often seen in
emergency care unit	the ECU, or _____ _____ _____,
ER	most commonly known as the hospital _____.
	Depending on the circumstances of the accident or illness,
outpatient	the patient is treated as an OP, or _____,
inpatient	or admitted as an IP, or _____. Sometimes,
	in a critical case, the patient is transferred directly to the
intensive care unit	ICU, or _____ _____ _____.
	Some hospitals have a special unit to care for critically ill
coronary (cardiac) care	coronary patients: _____ _____
unit	_____ (CCU). If surgery is necessary, it is performed
operating room	in the OR, or _____ _____, after which

postanesthetic care unit	a period of recovery is made in the PACU, or _____ _____ _____.
patient	**3.17** While hospitalized, the pt, or _____, is seen by the attending physician and is cared for by the nursing staff. The doctor writes orders for all Tx,
treatment	or _____, including how often the VS,
vital signs	or _____ _____, are to be taken. Vital signs
temperature, pulse	include: T, or _____; P, or _____;
respiration, blood	R, or _____; and BP, or _____
pressure	_____. A notation as to whether the patient
bathroom privileges	is to have BRP, or _____ _____, should also be made. The nurses must document the care and report any abnormal findings, such as CP,
chest pain, shortness	or _____ _____, and SOB, or _____
of breath	____ _____. The doctor usually asks the patient
return to office	to RTO, or _____ ____ _____, within a
discharge	few days of DC, or _____, from the hospital.

Pharmaceutical Abbreviations and Symbols

Pharmaceutical abbreviations and symbols are frequently used in documenting patient care. They are found throughout the medical record. Efficient medical record keeping and effective communication among health care workers depends on knowledge of commonly used pharmaceutical abbreviations and symbols.

UNITS OF MEASURE

Both metric and apothecary systems are used to express pharmaceutical units of measure. Consult your medical dictionary for a complete listing of units of measurement and conversion formulas.

Metric System

Metric is the most commonly used system of measurement in health care. It is a decimal system based on the following units:

Unit	Measure	Equivalent
meter (m)	length	39.37 inches
liter (L)	volume	1.0567 U.S. quarts
gram (g or gm)	weight	15.432 grains

The Apothecary System

The apothecary system is a method of liquid and weight measures that was used by the earliest chemists and pharmacists. The liquid measure was based on one drop, and the weight measure was based on one grain of wheat. Although the small apothecary measures are rarely used, the larger ones (e.g., fluid ounces) are still common.

SELF-INSTRUCTION: Abbreviations and Symbols related to Units of Measure

ABBREVIATION	EXPANSION
Metric	
cc	cubic centimeter; 1 cc = 1 mL [use the metric equivalent mL]
cm	centimeter; 2.5 cm = 1 inch
g or gm	gram
kg	kilogram; equal to 1,000 grams or 2.2 pounds
L	liter
mg	milligram; equal to one-thousandth (0.001) of a gram
mL or ml	milliliter; equal to one-thousandth (0.001) of a liter
mm	millimeter; equal to one-thousandth (0.001) of a meter
cu mm or mm^3	cubic millimeter
Apothecary	
fl oz	fluid ounce
gr	grain
gt	drop (L. *gutta* = drop)
gtt	drops

oz	ounce
lb or #	pound; equal to 16 ounces
qt	quart; equal to 32 ounces

PROGRAMMED REVIEW: Units of Measure

ANSWERS	REVIEW
Metric	**3.18** _____ is the most commonly used system of measurement in health care.
gm kg, one mg gram	**3.19** Gram, abbreviated g or _____, is a weight measure. *kilo-* is a prefix meaning one thousand. Therefore, a kilogram, or _____, contains _____ thousand grams (2.2 pounds). Body weight is often measured in kilograms instead of pounds. *milli-* is a prefix signifying one-thousandth. Therefore, a milligram, or _____, is one-thousandth of a/an _____.
L quart mL liter	**3.20** Liter, abbreviated _____, is a volume measure. One liter is equal to 1.0567 U.S. qt, or _____. A milliliter, which is abbreviated as ml or _____, is one-thousandth of a/an _____.
length mm, meter cm centimeters	**3.21** Meter is a measure of _____. There are 39.37 inches in a meter. A millimeter, which is abbreviated as _____, is one-thousandth of a/an _____. *centi-* is a prefix meaning one hundred. A centimeter, which is abbreviated as _____, is one-hundredth of a meter. There are 2.5 cm or _____ in an inch. The diameter of a lesion is commonly measured in centimeters.

cubic centimeter, 1 milliliter, 3 cu mm	**3.22** The measure 1 cc, or __________ ____________________, is equal to ____ mL, or ____________________. A 3-cc syringe holds ____ mL. Cubic millimeter is abbreviated _____ _____ or mm^3.
drop drops, fluid ounce quart, grain pound	**3.23** Measures of the apothecary system that are still commonly used include gt, or ________; gtt, or __________; fl oz, or ___________ ___________; qt, or __________; gr, or __________; and # (also lb), or __________.

DRUG FORMS AND ROUTES OF MEDICATION ADMINISTRATION

Prescribed medications can be administered to a patient in various ways, depending on the indication for the drug and the patient's status. The following table gives an overview of drug forms and routes of administration, including abbreviations and symbols.

SELF-INSTRUCTION: Drug Forms and Routes of Medication Administration

DRUG FORM	ROUTE OF ADMINISTRATION	MEANING
Solid and Semisolid Forms		
tablet (tab) capsule (cap)	oral (per os [p.o.]) sublingual (SL) buccal	by mouth under the tongue in the cheek
suppository (suppos)	vaginal (per vagina [PV]) rectal (per rectum [PR])	inserted in the vagina inserted in the rectum
Liquid Forms		
fluid	inhalation	inhaled through the nose or mouth
	aerosol	spray
	nebulizer	device used to produce a fine spray or mist, often in a metered dose

parenteral (Fig. 3-8)	by injection	
	intradermal (ID)	within the skin
	intramuscular (IM)	within the muscle
	intravenous (IV)	within the vein
	subcutaneous (SC, SQ, or sub-q)	under the skin [write out "subcut" or "subcutaneous"]
cream, lotion, ointment	topical	applied to the surface of the skin
other delivery systems	transdermal	absorption of drug through unbroken skin
	implant	a drug reservoir imbedded in the body to provide continual infusion of a medication (e.g., insulin pump)

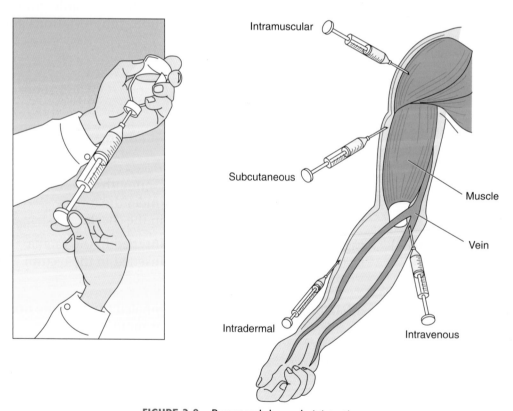

FIGURE 3-8   Parenteral drug administration.

PROGRAMMED REVIEW: Drug Forms and Routes of Medication Administration

ANSWERS	REVIEW
tablet by mouth sublingual buccal through rectum, through vagina	**3.24** Drugs are administered in many ways. The most common form is the tab, or _____, which is usually taken p.o., or _____ _____, under the tongue, or _____ (SL), and sometimes in the cheek, or _____. The word *per* means by or through. Suppositories are inserted PR, or _____ _____, or PV, or _____ _____.
injection, intradermal intramuscular intravenous subcutaneous subcut	**3.25** The parenteral route of administration is by _____: ID, or _____; IM, or _____; IV, or _____. Since the abbreviations SC, SQ, and sub-q, meaning _____, have been identified as error-prone, it is recommended that the words subcutaneous or _____ be spelled out.
surface through, implant	**3.26** Topical administration of a drug is applied to the _____ of the skin. Transdermal pertains to penetration _____ the skin. A/an _____ refers to a drug reservoir imbedded in the body to provide continual infusion of a medication.

THE PRESCRIPTION (Rx) AND DRUG NAMES

The Rx symbol, meaning recipe, is commonly used to identify a **prescription**, which is a written direction by a physician to dispense or administer a medication to a patient. It is an order to supply a named patient with a particular drug of a specific strength and quantity along with the **Sig:** (specific instructions for administration) (Fig. 3-9).

```
CENTRAL MEDICAL GROUP, INC.
Patrick Rodden, M.D.
DEA #:  AR 0000000
201 Medical Center Drive
Central City, US  90000-1234


Name of Patient  Carleen Perron        Date  6/4/xx

Address _____


Rx    Tylenol c codeine No. 3      #24
       Sig: tab i q 4 h  p r n pain




_____  M.D.      Patrick Rodden  M.D.
    SUBSTITUTION PERMITTED                 DISPENSE AS WRITTEN


May refill  3  times
```

FIGURE 3-9   Sample prescription.

DRUG NAMES

Medications have several names. The **chemical name** is assigned to a drug in the laboratory at the time it is invented. It is the formula for the drug, which is written exactly according to its chemical structure. The **generic name** is the official, nonproprietary name given a drug. The **trade** or **brand name** is the manufacturer's name for a drug. Health care providers tend to use the names interchangeably, but the distinction between generic and trade name is critical for pharmacists and Pharmacy Technicians to ensure that patients get exactly what their physician prescribes. For example:

chemical name	1-[[3-(6,7-dihydro-1-methyl-7-oxo-3-propyl-1H-pyrazolo[4,3-d]pyrimidin-5-yl)-4-ethoxyphenyl]sulfonyl]-4-methylpiperazine citrate
generic name	sildenafil
trade or brand name	Viagra

Over-the-counter (OTC) drugs do not require a prescription for individuals to purchase. For example:

Generic Name	Trade or Brand Name
acetylsalicylic acid (ASA) or aspirin	Bufferin, Ascriptin
ibuprofen	Advil, Motrin

See Chapter 6 for coverage of classifications of drugs and Appendix C for a list of commonly prescribed drugs, including their classification and common therapeutic uses.

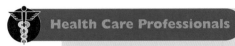

Health Care Professionals   MEET THE PHARMACY TECHNICIAN

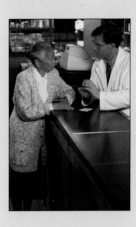

The prescription that Dr. Rodden gave Carleen as she left the hospital (see Fig. 3-9) was received at her local pharmacy by a pharmacy technician. Pharmacy technicians are health care professionals who assist pharmacists in providing medications and services to meet the needs of patients. Pharmacy technicians can work in outpatient and inpatient pharmacies in a variety of capacities, such as:

- Accepting and evaluating prescriptions
- Entering information into the computerized patient profile
- Retrieving the correct medication and placing it in an appropriately labeled container
- Filling unit dose medication carts and delivering them to patient floors
- Stocking and maintaining automated medication dispensing machines located on patient floors
- Using aseptic technique to mix intravenous medications

Since the technician is the first person to greet the patient in a pharmacy, excellent communication skills are vital, as is the ability to differentiate between the types of questions that can be answered by a technician and those that must be referred to the pharmacist.

A more detailed description of the pharmacy technician health care career can be found on the Student Resource CD-ROM and at the companion website at www.thePoint.lww.com/WillisQC.

PROGRAMMED REVIEW: The Prescription (Rx) and Drug Names

ANSWERS	REVIEW
	3.27 Rx is a symbol meaning recipe or
prescription	_____. A prescription is a direction
drug or medication	by a physician for dispensing a/an _____.
	It includes the name, strength, and quantity of a drug, along
	with the indication for its use (e.g., as needed for pain),
	and the Sig:, or the label that provides
instruction	specific _____ for administration.
	Brand and generic names must be provided on all

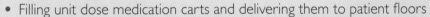

generic	medication orders. The _____ name is the official, nonproprietary name for a drug, and the trade
brand	or _____ name is given to a drug by the manufacturer. Related to drug formulation, 8-chloro-1-methyl-6-phenyl-4H-s-triazolo[4,3-a] [1,4]
chemical	benzodiazepine is a/an _____ name. Ibuprofen
generic	is a/an _____ name. Bufferin is an example of
brand or trade	a/an _____ name. The generic name for Motrin
ibuprofen	is _____.

PRESCRIPTION ABBREVIATIONS

Historically, prescriptions were written in Latin, and the words were abbreviated for convenience. For example, "quarter in die," which is Latin for four times a day, is abbreviated as q.i.d. The periods indicated the abbreviation of three words. In health care practice today, you will find variations that include or exclude the periods and that use uppercase instead of lowercase letters (e.g., QID vs. qid). To assist with readability and recognition, the periods are included in the Latin prescription abbreviations in this text. The trend, however, is to discourage their use, especially in handwritten documentation, because they can be misinterpreted. Roman numerals were used exclusively in the early days and are still being used today, but most pharmacy organizations now promote the use of Arabic numerals only.

SELF-INSTRUCTION: Common Prescription Abbreviations and Symbols

ABBREVIATION	EXPANSION	LATIN†
Time and Frequency		
$\bar{a}$	before	ante
a.c.	before meals	ante cibum
a.m.	before noon	ante meridiem
b.i.d.	twice a day	bis in die
d	day	
h	hour	hora

h.s.	at the hour of sleep (bedtime) [spell out *bedtime*]	hora somni
noc	night	noctis
p̄	after	post
p.c.	after meals	post cibum
p.m.	after noon	post meridiem
p.r.n.	as needed	pro re nata
q	every	quaque
q.d. (*)	every day [NEVER USE; spell out "every day" or "daily"]	quaque die
qh	every hour	quaque hora
q2h	every two hours	
q.i.d.	four times a day	quarter in die
q.o.d. (*)	every other day [NEVER USE; spell out "every other day"]	quaque altera die
STAT	immediately	statium
t.i.d.	three times a day	ter in die
wk	week	
yr	year	

Other Prescription Abbreviations and Symbols

AD	right ear [spell out "right ear"]	auris dextra
ad lib.	as desired	ad libitum
AS	left ear [spell out "left ear"]	auris sinistra
AU	both ears [spell out "both ears"]	auris unitas
c̄	with	cum
NPO	nothing by mouth	non per os
OD	right eye [spell out "right eye"]	oculus dexter
OS	left eye [spell out "left eye"]	oculus sinister
OU	both eyes [spell out "both eyes"]	oculi unitas
per	by or through	
p.o.	by mouth	per os
PR	through rectum	per rectum

PV	through vagina	per vagina
Rx	recipe; prescription	
$\overline{s}$	without	sine
Sig	label; instruction to the patient	signa
$\overline{ss}$	one-half [spell out "one-half" or use "1/2"]	semis
×	times or for; ×6 means "six times," and ×2d means "for two days"	
>	greater than [spell out "greater than"]	
<	less than [spell out "less than"]	
ī	one (modified lowercase Roman numeral i)	
īī	two (modified lowercase Roman numeral ii)	
īīī	three (modified lowercase Roman numeral iii)	
īv	four (modified lowercase Roman numeral iv)	
I, II, III, IV, V, VI, VII, VIII, IX, X	uppercase Roman numerals from 1 to 10	

†The original Latin is supplied when deemed helpful.

PROGRAMMED REVIEW: Common Prescription Abbreviations and Symbols

ANSWERS	REVIEW
	3.28 The most common abbreviations used in
Latin	prescription writing stem from _____ words. Ante,
before, $\overline{a}$	meaning _____, is abbreviated as ____.
a.m.	Before noon is abbreviated _____, and a.c. stands
before meals	for _____ _____. Post,
after, $\overline{p}$	meaning _____, is abbreviated ____. After noon is
p.m., after	abbreviated _____, and p.c. stands for _____

meals, d, noc	_____. Day is abbreviated ____, night as _____,
h.s.	and bedtime as _____. Some medications must be taken
STAT	immediately or _____. If a medication is taken p.r.n.,
as needed	it is taken _____ _____. If the patient can have as
lib	much as desired, the abbreviation is ad _____. Sometimes,
	such as before surgery, the doctor wants the patient to take
NPO	nothing by mouth, or _____. Some drugs are taken twice
b.i.d., t.i.d.	a day, or _____; three times a day, or _____; or
four, wk	q.i.d., or _____ times a day. Week is abbreviated _____,
yr	and year is abbreviated _____. The abbreviation for
q, qh	every is ____. Every hour is abbreviated _____. Every 2 hours
q2h	is abbreviated _____. The symbol ×, meaning times
for	or _____, is used to abbreviate the words "for seven days"
×7d, ×10	as _____, and "ten times" as _____. q.d.,
every day	meaning _____ _____, and q.o.d.,
every other day	meaning _____ _____ _____, are error-prone
Do Not Use	abbreviations on the official "_____ _____ _____" list
NEVER	provided by JCAHO and should _____ be used.
spelled	They should be _____ out instead.

I	**3.29** Roman numerals 1 through 10 are written as ____,
II, III, IV, V, VI, VII, VIII, IX	____, ____, ____, ____, ____, ____, ____, ____,
X	and ____, respectively. The modified lowercase Roman
i, ii	numeral that means one is ____. Two is _____,
iii, iv	three is _____, and four is _____. The symbol for one-half
s̄s̄, c̄, s̄	is _____, for with is ____, and for without is ____.

	3.30 Sinister, meaning left, and dexter, meaning right,
	are referenced in abbreviations for the eyes and ears.
OD	The right eye, or oculus dexter, is abbreviated _____.
OS	The left eye, or oculus sinister, is abbreviated _____.

OU	Oculi unitas, referring to both eyes, is abbreviated _____.
AD	Auris refers to ear. The right ear is abbreviated as _____,
AS, AU	the left ear as _____, and both ears as _____. Because
	abbreviations related to the eyes and ears have been
	misinterpreted, it is recommended that they
spelled	be _____ out instead. The symbols for
>, <	greater than (____) and less than (____) have also
	been confused with each other, and it is recommended
spelled	that they also be _____ out instead.

Regulations and Legal Considerations

Medical record documentation is created by physicians who treat patients and by other authorized health care professionals who are involved with patient care. State, federal, and private accrediting agencies (e.g., JCAHO) provide specific guidelines that regulate how medical records are stored and maintained, including proper format for all forms, use of appropriate terminology and accepted abbreviations, protocol for personnel having access to records, and responsibilities for documentation.

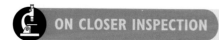 **ON CLOSER INSPECTION**   **Electronic Health Records**

Health records have been recorded on paper for decades, but the advancement of computers and information technology, and the ability to produce and share documents in digital format, have led to the emergence of electronic health records (EHR) and systems that manage and exchange medical information.
     Key features of electronic health records include:
- Improved documentation – Problems with illegibility are eliminated, decreasing errors. Touch screens make input easy, and drop-down menus take less time than handwriting notes; this improves quality and productivity in charting.
- Medication management – Computerized prescription order entry helps prevent medication errors by providing warnings about patient allergies, contraindications, and possible interactions. It also avoids problems at the pharmacy due to poor handwriting by the prescriber.
- Assistance with clinical decision making – Alerts, reminders, and patient care recommendations give providers valuable information at their fingertips.

- Interoperability – The ability to communicate and exchange data collected from multiple sources, such as medical offices, clinics, hospitals, pharmacies, laboratories, and radiology departments, allows for the direct and efficient communication of medical data.

As the health care community shifts toward greater use of electronic health records, a primary concern is creating standards for exchanging, integrating, sharing, and retrieving information accurately and safely. Private and governmental agencies have been established to set standards.

In the United States, matters of patient confidentiality and issues such as protection from patient data interception are addressed in legislation under the Health Insurance Portability and Accountability Act (HIPAA).

Whether data is recorded on paper or electronically, the complete and accurate input of information into health records is essential to providing quality patient care.

CORRECTIONS

Sometimes mistakes are made when making an entry in a medical record. Careful correction and clarification of the error are essential. The format for making corrections may vary according to specific facility or organizational guidelines. Generally, if a mistake is made in a handwritten entry, it should be identified by drawing a single line through it, then writing the correction in the margin above or immediately after the mistake. Include the date and the initials of the person making the correction (Fig. 3-10). The use of correction fluid is forbidden!

The medical record often becomes evidence in medical malpractice cases. Obliterations and signs of possible tampering can be construed as trying to withhold information

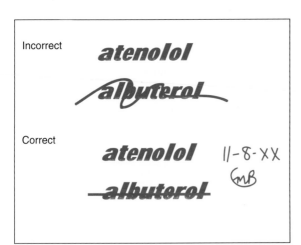

FIGURE 3-10   Proper correction of a handwritten chart entry.

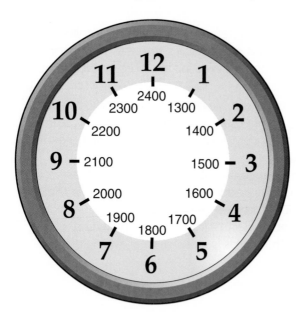

FIGURE 3-11   Military (24-hour) and standard (12-hour) time.

or covering up negligent wrongdoing. Complete and accurate record keeping is your best defense against any possible legal action.

Recording Date and Time

The date and time are usually required in entries in a medical record. Always include the month, day of the month, and year (e.g., 12/25/xx); sometimes eight digits are required (e.g., 01/08/20xx). Military time is often used to indicate the exact time of day. Military time uses a 24-hour clock, beginning with 0000 hours, which is the start of the day, and ending at 2400, which is the end of the day. For example, 1 a.m. is 0100 hours, 2 a.m. is 0200 hours, and so-on up until 11 p.m., which is 2300 hours (Fig. 3-11).

Standard (12-hour format)	Military (24-hour format)	Standard	Military
1:00 a.m.	0100 (zero one hundred hours)	1:00 p.m.	1300 (thirteen hundred hours)
2:00 a.m.	0200 (zero two hundred hours)	2:00 p.m.	1400 (fourteen hundred hours)
3:00 a.m.	0300 (zero three hundred hours)	3:00 p.m.	1500 (fifteen hundred hours)
4:00 a.m.	0400 (zero four hundred hours)	4:00 p.m.	1600 (sixteen hundred hours)
5:00 a.m.	0500 (zero five hundred hours)	5:00 p.m.	1700 (seventeen hundred hours)
6:00 a.m.	0600 (zero six hundred hours)	6:00 p.m.	1800 (eighteen hundred hours)
7:00 a.m.	0700 (zero seven hundred hours)	7:00 p.m.	1900 (nineteen hundred hours)
8:00 a.m.	0800 (zero eight hundred hours)	8:00 p.m.	2000 (twenty hundred hours)

9.00 a.m.	0900 (zero nine hundred hours)	9:00 p.m.	2100 (twenty-one hundred hours)
10:00 a.m.	1000 (ten hundred hours)	10:00 p.m.	2200 (twenty-two hundred hours)
11:00 a.m.	1100 (eleven hundred hours)	11:00 p.m.	2300 (twenty-three hundred hours)
12:00 p.m. **(noon)**	1200 (twelve hundred hours)	12:00 a.m. **(midnight)**	2400 (twenty-four hundred hours)

Rx for Success

To convert military (24-hour) time to standard (12-hour) time, subtract 1200 if the time is greater than 1200 (later than noon). For example, 1700 (seventeen hundred hours) on the 24-hour clock is converted to 5:00 p.m. standard time.

Write the abbreviation for each of the highlighted terms in the space provided on p. 133.

1.

HISTORY AND PHYSICAL

2.

HISTORY

Merrell, Ellen   June 1, 20xx

3.

CHIEF COMPLAINT: Fatigue

4.

HISTORY OF PRESENT ILLNESS: The patient is a 49-year-old female who complains of feeling very tired for more than a month. She states that she falls asleep within 30 seconds of her head hitting the pillow at night.

13.

14.

5.

PAST MEDICAL HISTORY: The patient has had the usual childhood diseases. No serious injuries or accidents. Allergies: No known drug allergies. Current Medications:

15.

6.

Estrace, 0.2 mg q.d. **FAMILY HISTORY:** Both parents, in their 80's, are living and well.

16.

SOCIAL HISTORY: Occasional alcohol consumption. She is a nonsmoker.

7.

OCCUPATIONAL HISTORY: The patient is a retail clothing manager.

REVIEW OF SYSTEMS: HEENT: Occasional sinus headache. CARDIOPULMONARY:

8.

Occasional palpitations. No chest pain, cough or shortness of breath. GASTROINTESTINAL: Some increase in weight recently. GENITOURINARY: Recent pap smear and mammogram

9.

normal. MUSCULOSKELETAL: Negative. NEUROMUSCULAR: Negative.

10.

PHYSICAL EXAMINATION

GENERAL APPEARANCE: A well-developed, obese female in no acute distress.
VITAL SIGNS: Blood pressure 110/70, pulse 80, respirations 16, temperature 97 degrees F, height 62 inches, weight 206 pounds. **HEENT:** Pupils equal, round and reactive to light and accommodation. Tympanic membranes are normal. No sinus tenderness on percussion. Oropharynx: Clear. **NECK:** Supple; no masses or tenderness. No thyromegaly.
LUNGS: Clear to percussion and auscultation. **HEART:** Rate: 80 and regular; normal sinus rhythm; no murmurs or gallops. **RECTOPELVIC:** Deferred to gynecologist.
EXTREMITIES: No clubbing, cyanosis, or edema. **NEUROLOGICAL:** Physiologic.

17.

18.

LABORATORY DATA: Chest x-ray, ECG, and pulmonary screen are unremarkable.

11.

IMPRESSION: 1. FATIGUE
                  2. HYPOTHYROIDISM
                  3. OBESITY

12.

PLAN/RECOMMENDATION/DISPOSITION: Draw blood today for CBC and thyroid panel. The patient will return to the office in one week for test results.

Reyna James, M.D.
Reyna James, M.D.

RJ:bst
D: 6/1/20xx
T: 6/2/20xx

1. _____	7. _____	13. _____
2. _____	8. _____	14. _____
3. _____	9. _____	15. _____
4. _____	10. _____	16. _____
5. _____	11. _____	17. _____
6. _____	12. _____	18. _____

Write the term or abbreviation for each of the highlighted notations in the space provided below.

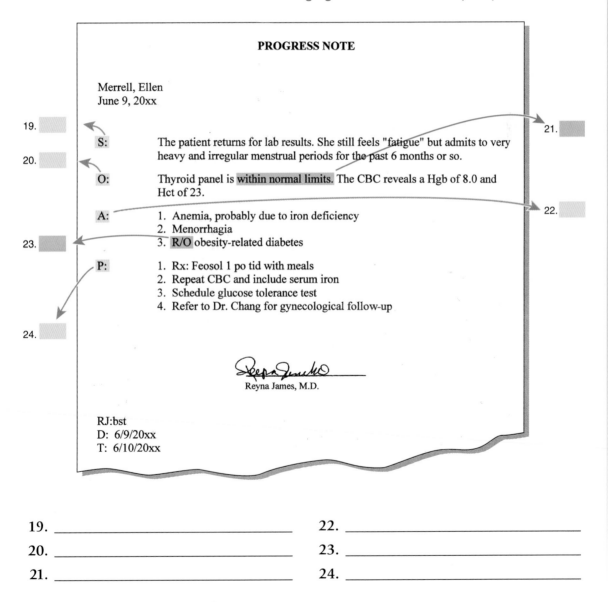

PROGRESS NOTE

Merrell, Ellen
June 9, 20xx

19.

S: The patient returns for lab results. She still feels "fatigue" but admits to very heavy and irregular menstrual periods for the past 6 months or so.

20.

O: Thyroid panel is within normal limits. The CBC reveals a Hgb of 8.0 and Hct of 23.

21.

22.

A: 1. Anemia, probably due to iron deficiency
     2. Menorrhagia
23. 3. R/O obesity-related diabetes

P: 1. Rx: Feosol 1 po tid with meals
     2. Repeat CBC and include serum iron
     3. Schedule glucose tolerance test
     4. Refer to Dr. Chang for gynecological follow-up

24.

Reyna James, M.D.

RJ:bst
D: 6/9/20xx
T: 6/10/20xx

19. _____	22. _____
20. _____	23. _____
21. _____	24. _____

Write out the expanded term or meaning for each abbreviation.

25. CC _____

26. OH _____

27. PR _____

28. BRP _____

29. PACU _____

30. PH _____

31. D/C _____

32. Sig: _____

33. ER _____

34. ICU _____

35. R/O _____

36. NPO _____

37. L&W _____

38. BP _____

39. AU _____

40. Sx _____

41. VS _____

42. ROS _____

43. pt _____

44. OD _____

45. H&P _____

46. Tx _____

47. Dx _____

48. HPI _____

Match each definition with its corresponding abbreviation or term.

49. _____ the route of oral medications   a. preop

50. _____ place for surgery   b. p.r.n.

51. _____ as desired   c. parenteral

52. _____ progress note format   d. p.o.

53. _____ after surgery   e. STAT

54. _____ pound   f. ad lib.

55. _____ as needed	g. postop
56. _____ by injection	h. OR
57. _____ before surgery	i. SOAP
58. _____ immediately	j. #

Write the meaning for the following pharmaceutical phrases.

59. VS q h ×4h, then q2h _____

60. ī p.o. q.i.d. p.c. and h.s. _____

61. aspirin (ASA) gr īī s̄s̄ _____

62. 650 mg p.o. q4h p.r.n. temp >101°F _____

63. ī suppos PR q noc p.r.n. _____

64. gt ī OU t.i.d. ×7d _____

65. cap īī p.o. STAT, then ī p.o. q6h _____

66. 15 mL p.o. q 6 h p.r.n. pain _____

Write the standard pharmaceutical abbreviations for the following.

67. one suppository in the vagina at bedtime

_____

68. two drops in left ear every 3 hours

_____

69. one capsule by mouth two times a day, morning and evening

_____

70. two by mouth immediately, then one by mouth every 6 hours

_____

71. five hundred milligrams by mouth four times a day for 10 days

_____

Give the meaning for the following error-prone abbreviations, identify why each abbreviation is commonly misinterpreted, and list the preferred term for each.

	Abbreviation	Meaning	Mistaken for	Preferred Term
72.	q.d.			
73.	q.o.d.			
74.	OS			
75.	AD			

	Abbreviation	Meaning	Mistaken for	Preferred Term
76.	AU	_____	_____	_____
77.	>	_____	_____	_____
78.	D/C	_____	_____	_____
79.	cc	_____	_____	_____

Match the following chart entries with the abbreviation for the corresponding section of the health record.

80. _____ works as a security officer   a. UCHD

81. _____ advised to lower salt intake   b. HPI

82. _____ father, age 88, L&W; mother, age 78, died, stroke   c. PE

83. _____ quit smoking 2 years ago, drinks alcohol socially   d. CC

84. _____ Diagnosis: tonsillitis   e. OH

85. _____ c/o lower back pain   f. SH

86. _____ pain in lower back for 2 weeks, worse at night   g. FH

87. _____ no reaction to any previously administered drug   h. P

88. _____ had all commonly contracted childhood diseases   i. A

89. _____ Lungs: clear. Heart: regular rate and rhythm   j. NKDA

Give the military times for the following standard times.

90. 1:00 a.m. _____

91. 2:30 p.m. _____

92. midnight _____

93. 1:00 p.m. _____

94. 7:00 p.m. _____

95. 4:50 p.m. _____

MEDICAL RECORD EXERCISES

Medical Record 3-1

Progress Note

CC: 37 y.o. ♂ c̄ diabetes c/o swelling of the Ⓡ foot and calf ×3d

S: There is no Hx of trauma, pain, SOB, or cardiac Sx, smoker ×12 yr, s̅s̅ pkg per day, denies ETOH consumption

Meds: parenteral insulin daily. NKDA

O: Pt is afebrile, BP 140/84, P 72, R 16, lungs are clear; abdomen is benign s̄ organomegaly; muscle tone and strength are WNL; there is swelling of the Ⓡ calf but s̄ erythema or tenderness

A: Edema of Ⓡ calf of unknown etiology

P: Schedule STAT vascular sonogram of lower extremities; pt is to keep the leg elevated × ī ī d, then RTC for follow-up and test results on Thursday (or sooner if ↑ edema, SOB, or CP)

Questions about Medical Record 3-1

1. What is the sex of the patient?

   a. male
   b. female

2. Where was the patient seen?

   a. emergency room
   b. outpatient office or clinic
   c. inpatient hospital
   d. not stated

3. What is the condition of the patient's abdomen?

   a. shows signs of cancer
   b. internal organs are enlarged
   c. internal organs are not enlarged
   d. muscle tone and strength are weak

4. How much does the patient smoke per day?

   a. 1 package
   b. 2 packages
   c. half a package
   d. none; patient quit smoking 12 years ago

5. How is the patient's insulin administered?

   a. orally
   b. transdermally
   c. infusion through implant
   d. by injection

6. What is the cause of the patient's complaint?

   a. unknown
   b. fever
   c. shortness of breath
   d. trauma

7. When should the sonogram be performed?

   a. immediately
   b. within 2 days
   c. at the time of follow-up
   d. only if symptoms persist

8. How long should the patient's leg be kept elevated?

   a. 1 week
   b. 2 weeks
   c. 1 day
   d. 2 days

Medical Record 3-2

Postop Orders for Medications

1. Vicodin (hydrocodone and acetaminophen), ī tab p.o. q3h p.r.n. mild pain, or īī tab p.o. q3h p.r.n. moderate pain

2. Demerol (meperidine), 100 mg IM q3h p.r.n. severe pain

3. Tylenol (acetaminophen), 650 mg p.o. q4h p.r.n. oral temp ↑ 100.4°F

4. Ambien (zolpidem), 10 mg p.o. h.s. p.r.n. sleep

5. Mylicon (simethicone), 80 mg, ī tab, chewed and swallowed q.i.d.

6. Dulcolax (bisacodyl) suppos, ī PR in a.m.

Questions about Medical Record 3-2

1. How is the Demerol to be administered?

   a. by mouth
   b. within the vein
   c. under the skin
   d. within the muscle

2. What is the Sig: on the Mylicon?

   a. one every other day
   b. one twice a day
   c. one three times a day
   d. one four times a day

3. What is the Sig: on the Dulcolax?

   a. one suppository in the rectum in the morning
   b. one suppository taken orally before noon
   c. two suppositories before breakfast
   d. one suppository as needed in the morning

4. When should the Ambien be administered?

   a. each night
   b. at bedtime
   c. as needed
   d. every hour

5. What are the instructions for administering Vicodin in the case of moderate pain?

   a. one tablet every 3 hours
   b. three tablets every hour
   c. two tablets every 3 hours
   d. three tablets every 3 hours

6. How should Tylenol be administered?

   a. one dose every 4 hours as needed
   b. one dose every 4 hours only if patient has a temperature of 100.4°F or higher
   c. one dose every 4 hours as long as the patient's temperature does not go over 100.4°F
   d. one dose every hour up to 4 per day

Medical Record 3-3

Progress Note

Mr. Michael Marsi was introduced in the Meet the Patient vignette at the beginning of the chapter. He has just seen Dr. Spaulding because he feels worse than usual today. Her Progress Note for today's visit is shown on p. 140. Review the medical record and answer the following questions.

Questions about Medical Record 3-3

1. Below are medical terms used in this record that you have not yet encountered in the text. Underline each where it appears in the record and, using a medical dictionary, define them below:

   occipital _____

   congestive heart failure (CHF) _____

   electrocardiogram (ECG) _____

PROGRESS NOTES

Patient Name: *MARSI, Michael*

DATE	FINDINGS
2-3-XX	CC: 51 y.o. ♂ c/o dizziness x 3wk and headaches 5-6 x ⊤ wk Today he woke c̄ numbness in Ⓛ leg and hand
	S Hx of ↑BP x 4yrs Smoker x 20yrs – 1pk/day ō CP & SoB occipital headaches in am moderate fat diet - 3 beers q̄ noc. NKDA
	O BP 150/100 Ⓛ arm ♀ Ht 68" Wt 198# T 98.7° P 76 R 15 Heart RRR s̄ Ⓜ Lungs Clear HEENT – WNL
	A Hypertension (HTN) R/O Congestive Heart Failure (CHF)
	P Chest x-ray (CXR) and electrocardiogram (ECG) today ↓ ETOH to ⊤ beer q̄ noc. DC Smoking Rx: Vasotec (enalapril) 5mg tab ⊤ daily ↑exercise to 3 x wk for 20-30 min stop if CP, SoB, or dizzy ↓fat and cholesterol in diet re√ BP in ⊤ wk RTO sooner if CP, SoB or dizzy JR Spaulding MD

MEDICAL RECORD 3-3   Progress Note

2. How old is Mr. Marsi? _____

3. Where was the treatment rendered? _____

4. List the three elements of the patient's complaint.

   a. _____

   b. _____

   c. _____

5. In your own words, not using medical terminology, briefly summarize Mr. Marsi's history.

   _____

   _____

   _____

6. Which of the following is not mentioned at all in this history?

   a. The prescription medication Mr. Marsi takes
   b. Mr. Marsi's smoking habit
   c. Mr. Marsi's activity level at work
   d. Mr. Marsi's consumption of alcohol

7. Dr. Spaulding and Mr. Marsi talked at length about Mr. Marsi's symptoms and how they've changed recently, and then Dr. Spaulding examined him. List three objective findings she noted in this examination.

   a. _____

   b. _____

   c. _____

8. Dr. Spaulding's assessment is that Mr. Marsi has _____

   _____

   But she also wants to make sure Mr. Marsi does not have _____

   _____

9. Dr. Spaulding's treatment plan involves four areas. List the specific plan(s) for each of these.

   a. Diagnostic tests ordered: _____

   _____

   b. Instruct the patient to change his personal habits (and how): _____

   _____

   _____

   _____

c. Drug prescribed (and how much and when): _____

_____

d. Future diagnostic check and/or action to take: _____

_____

10. When is Dr. Spaulding expecting to see Mr. Marsi again?

_____

Answers to Examine Your Understanding

1. H&P
2. Hx
3. CC
4. HPI
5. PMH
6. FH
7. SH
8. OH
9. ROS
10. PE
11. A, IMP, Dx
12. P
13. c/o
14. UCHD
15. NKDA
16. L&W
17. NAD
18. PERRLA
19. subjective
20. objective
21. WNL
22. assessment (impression, diagnosis)
23. rule out
24. plan (disposition, recommendation)
25. chief complaint
26. occupational history
27. per rectum
28. bathroom privileges
29. postanesthetic care unit
30. past history
31. discontinue or discharge
32. label; instructions to patient
33. emergency room
34. intensive care unit
35. rule out
36. nothing by mouth
37. living and well
38. blood pressure
39. both ears
40. symptom
41. vital signs
42. review of systems
43. patient
44. right eye
45. history and physical
46. treatment or traction
47. diagnosis
48. history of present illness
49. d
50. h
51. f
52. i
53. g
54. j
55. b
56. c
57. a
58. e
59. vital signs every hour for 4 hours, then every 2 hours
60. one by mouth 4 times a day, after meals and at bedtime
61. two and one-half grains of aspirin
62. 650 milligrams by mouth every 4 hours as needed for temperature greater than 101 degrees Fahrenheit
63. one suppository through the rectum every night as needed
64. one drop in both eyes 3 times a day for 7 days
65. two capsules by mouth immediately, then one by mouth every 6 hours
66. 15 milliliters by mouth every 6 hours as needed for pain
67. suppos ī PV **h.s.** *or* ī suppos PV **h.s.**
68. gtt īī **AS** q3h *or* īī gtt **AS** q3h
69. cap ī p.o. b.i.d. a.m. and p.m. *or* ī cap p.o. b.i.d. a.m. and p.m.
70. īī p.o. STAT, then ī p.o. q6h
71. 500 mg p.o. q.i.d. ×10d
72. every day; mistaken for q.i.d. (four times a day); spell out "every day" or "daily"
73. every other day; mistaken for q.d. (daily) or q.i.d. (four times a day); spell out "every other day"
74. left eye; mistaken for right eye or ear; spell out "left eye"
75. right ear; mistaken for left ear or eye; spell out "right ear"
76. both ears; mistaken for both eyes or right or left ear/eye; spell out "both ears"
77. greater than; mistaken as lesser than; spell out "greater than"

78. discharge or discontinue; mistaken for each other; spell out either "discharge" or "discontinue"
79. cubic centimeter; mistaken as "units"; use metric equivalent "ml" or "mL"

80. e	86. b	92. 2400 hours
81. h	87. j	93. 1300 hours
82. g	88. a	94. 1900 hours
83. f	89. c	95. 1650 hours
84. i	90. 0100 hours	
85. d	91. 1430 hours	

ANSWERS TO MEDICAL RECORD EXERCISES

Medical Record 3-1: Progress Note

1. a	4. c	7. a
2. b	5. d	8. d
3. c	6. a	

Medical Record 3-2: Postop Orders for Medications

1. d	3. a	5. c
2. d	4. b	6. b

Medical Record 3-3: Progress Note

1. See medical dictionary for definitions.
2. 51 years old
3. in a medical office
4. Mr. Marsi has been dizzy for 3 weeks; has had headaches 5 to 6 times in a week; and he awoke today with numbness in his left leg and hand.
5. Mr. Marsi has smoked 1 package of cigarettes a day for the past 20 years and has known high blood pressure for 4 years. He drinks 3 beers every night. His current medication is one Dyazide per day, and he has no known drug allergies.
6. c
7. Any three of the following answers are acceptable:
   • heart rate is regular
   • lungs are clear
   • blood pressure is 150/100 (abnormal finding)
   • temperature is 98.7 degrees
   • pulse is 76
   • weight is 198 pounds
   • respiratory rate is 15
   • height is 68 inches
8. hypertension (high blood pressure); congestive heart failure

9. a. Diagnostic tests ordered: chest x-ray and electrocardiogram today.
   b. Instruct the patient to change his personal habits (and how):
       • reduce alcohol intake of beer to 1 per night
       • exercise three times a week for 20 to 30 minutes (stop exercising if he experiences chest pain, shortness of breath, or dizziness)
       • stop smoking
       • reduce fat and cholesterol in his diet
   c. Drug prescribed: Vasotec (enalapril) 5 mg (milligram) strength, with instructions to take one by mouth every day
   d. Future diagnostic check: patient is to return for a blood pressure check in 1 week
10. Dr. Spaulding will see Mr. Marsi in 1 week or sooner if he experiences chest pain, shortness of breath, or dizziness.

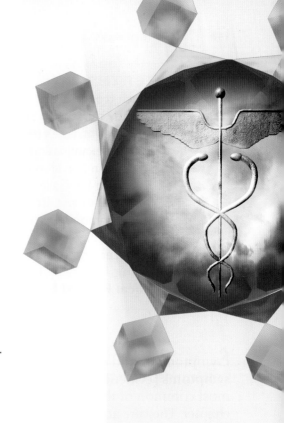

CHAPTER 4

SYMPTOMATIC AND DIAGNOSTIC TERMS

OBJECTIVES

1 Identify common symptomatic and diagnostic suffixes.

2 Define common symptomatic and diagnostic terms based on term structure analysis.

3 List common terms related to disease.

CHECKLIST

CHECKLIST	LOCATION
☐ Complete Chapter 4 Self-Instruction and Programmed Review sections	pages 148–194
☐ Review the Flash Cards related to Chapter 4	FC
☐ Complete the Chapter 4 Examine Your Understanding exercises	pages 199–204
☐ Complete Medical Record Exercises 4-1 and 4-2	pages 205–208
☐ Practice saying the Chapter 4 terms out loud with the Audio Pronunciation Glossary on the Student Resource CD-ROM	CD-ROM
☐ Complete the Chapter 4 Interactive Exercises on the Student Resource CD-ROM	CD-ROM
☐ Take the Chapter 4 Quiz on the Student Resource CD-ROM	CD-ROM
☐ When you receive 70% or higher on the Quiz, move on to Chapter 5	page 213

MEET THE PATIENT   Jane Dano seems too young to be having so much trouble. For the past three weeks, this 11-year-old girl has been constantly thirsty and seems to be urinating all of the time. She is even losing weight. Jane's mother is concerned and takes her to Dr. Spaulding for an examination. After laboratory tests showed that there was sugar in her blood and urine, Dr. Spaulding immediately referred Jane to Dr. Gallegos, an endocrinologist, who made the diagnosis of diabetes mellitus. In this chapter, you will learn the medical terms for common signs and symptoms and diagnostic terms, such as those used to identify Jane's problem. Later, you will also learn that Jane was hospitalized and cared for by several health professionals, one being a **Nursing Assistant.** Jane's hospital discharge summary is shown in **Medical Record Exercise 4-1.**

Symptomatic and diagnostic suffixes are word endings used in terms that describe **symptoms** (evidence of illness) and **diagnoses** (names of conditions or diseases). The most common of these suffixes are presented in the Self-Instruction sections of this chapter. They are accompanied by selected prefixes and combining forms to build common terms related to symptoms and diagnoses.

Core Term Components

The suffixes and prefixes used in this chapter are listed below. Pertinent combining forms will be added as you progress through programmed learning segments related to each suffix. Study these core term components first, and add those related to each of the suffixes as you work through the chapter.

SUFFIX	MEANING	FLASH CARD ID
-algia, -odynia	pain	S-2
-cele	pouching or hernia	S-3
-emia	blood condition	S-7
-genic	pertaining to origin	S-9
-ia, -ism	condition of	S-14
-iasis	formation or presence of	S-15
-ic, -tic	pertaining to	S-1
-itis	inflammation	S-18
-lepsy	seizure	S-20
-logy	study of	S-22

-malacia	softening	S-23
-mania	condition of abnormal impulse toward or frenzy	S-24
-megaly	enlargement	S-25
-oma	tumor	S-28
-osis	condition or increase	S-30
-penia	abnormal reduction	S-31
-phobia	condition of abnormal fear or sensitivity	S-34
-plegia	paralysis	S-36
-pnea	breathing	S-37
-ptosis	falling or downward displacement	S-38
-rrhage, -rrhagia	to burst forth (usually blood)	S-40
-rrhea	discharge	S-42
-spasm	involuntary contraction	S-45
-stasis	stop or stand	S-46
-y	condition or process of	S-50

PREFIX	MEANING	FLASH CARD ID
a-, an-	without	P-1
auto-	self	P-8
bi-	two or both	P-27
brady-	slow	P-9
de-	from, down, or not	P-10
dia-	across or through	P-11
dys-	painful, difficult, or faulty	P-12
endo-	within	P-14
epi-	upon	P-15
eu-	normal	P-16
hyper-	above or excessive	P-21
hypo-	below or deficient	P-22
macro-	large	P-24
meta-	beyond, after, or change	P-25
micro-	small	P-26

(continued)

PREFIX	MEANING	FLASH CARD ID
neo-	new	P-28
ortho-	straight, normal, or correct	P-29
poly-	many	P-34
tachy-	fast	P-38

SELF-INSTRUCTION: -algia and -odynia (pain)

Add the following combining forms to your study of -algia and -odynia before starting the Programmed Review below.

COMBINING FORM	MEANING	FLASH CARD ID
arthr/o	joint	CF-6
cephal/o	head	CF-12
gastr/o	stomach	CF-26
my/o	muscle	CF-40
oste/o	bone	
ot/o	ear	

PROGRAMMED REVIEW: -algia and -odynia (pain)

ANSWERS	REVIEW
ending -algia, -odynia	**4.1** A symptomatic suffix is a term _____ used to describe evidence of illness. Pain is one of the most common symptoms of illness. The two suffixes that refer to pain are _____ and _____.
joint suffix, pain arthralgia	**4.2** Using the combining form *arthr/o*, meaning _____, combined with *-algia*, the _____ meaning _____, the term for joint pain is _____.
bone ostealgia osteodynia	**4.3** Using *oste/o*, the combining form for _____, two terms for bone pain are _____ and _____.

muscle myalgia myodynia	**4.4** Using *my/o*, the combining form meaning _____, two terms for muscle pain are _____ and _____.
head cephalalgia, cephalodynia	**4.5** *cephal/o* is a combining form referring to the _____. Using the suffixes meaning pain, two terms for headache are _____ and _____.
pain, stomach epi- upon, pain stomach	**4.6** Gastralgia is a symptomatic term that describes a condition of _____ in the _____. In epigastralgia, the addition of _____, the prefix meaning _____, modifies this term to indicate that the _____ is in the epigastrium, which is the area of the abdomen overlying the _____.
ot/o otalgia, otodynia	**4.7** The combining form for ear is _____. When a patient describes an earache, the medical term noted will either be _____ or _____.

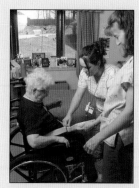

Health Care Professionals   MEET THE NURSING ASSISTANT

Nursing assistants are well-trained members of the health care team who assist nurses in providing basic nursing care to help meet the needs of patients, clients, and residents in a variety of health care settings. These needs include hygiene, safety, comfort, nutrition, exercise, and elimination, as well as basic emotional needs. Nursing assistants ensure that humanistic care, or care that places the emphasis on each person's unique needs, is given.

A more detailed description of nursing assistant as a health care career can be found on the Student Resource CD-ROM and at the companion website at www.thePoint.lww.com/WillisQC.

SELF-INSTRUCTION: -cele (pouching or hernia)

Add the following combining forms to your study of -cele before starting the Programmed Review below.

COMBINING FORM	MEANING	FLASH CARD ID
cyst/o	bladder or sac	CF-18
hydr/o	water	CF-31
rect/o	rectum	
varic/o	swollen, twisted vein	

PROGRAMMED REVIEW: -cele (pouching or hernia)

ANSWERS	REVIEW
	4.8 Hernia is a term used to explain the pouching of a part from its normal location. Common types include inguinal hernia (pouching of the intestine through layers of the abdominal wall in the groin area) and hiatal hernia (protrusion of part of the stomach upward through the hiatus, an opening in the diaphragm). The diagnostic suffix -cele is
pouching	also used in several terms describing a/an _____
hernia	or _____.
water	**4.9** In the male testicle, two terms using -cele name common afflictions. hydr/o is the combining form meaning _____. Combined with -cele, it forms the
hernia	term that describes a pouching or _____ of
hydrocele	fluid in the testicle: _____ (Fig. 4-1). When varic/o, a combining form referring to a swollen, twisted vein, is linked to -cele, it forms the term for swollen,
varicocele	twisted veins near the testicle, called _____. Notice that there is no direct reference to the testicle in either term.

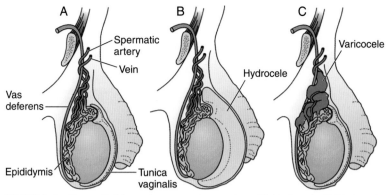

FIGURE 4-1 Testes. **A.** Normal testes and appendages. **B.** Hydrocele. **C.** Varicocele

4.10 Related to females, *-cele* is used in terms that describe a sagging or _____ of pelvic organs into the vagina as a result of weakening of the muscles and ligaments that provide support, a condition known as pelvic floor relaxation (Fig. 4-2). Interestingly, there is no direct reference to the vagina in these terms, only the link of *-cele* to the combining form naming the structure that is _____ into it. Knowing this, the term that describes a sagging or pouching of the bladder into the vagina links *cyst/o*, the combining form meaning sac or _____, with *-cele*, in the term _____. Likewise, *rect/o*, a combining form meaning _____, is used in the term describing the pouching of the rectum into the vagina, or _____.

pouching

pouching

bladder
cystocele
rectum
rectocele

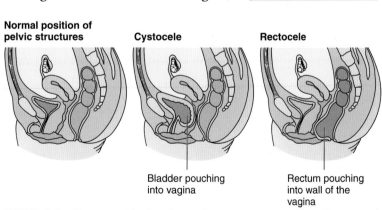

FIGURE 4-2 Two types of pelvic floor relaxation, causing pouching (protrusion) into the vagina.

SELF-INSTRUCTION: -ia (condition of)

Add the following combining forms to your study of -ia before starting the Programmed Review below.

COMBINING FORM	MEANING	FLASH CARD ID
cardi/o	heart	CF-11
dips/o	thirst	
phag/o	eat or swallow	CF-47
phas/o	speech	CF-48
phren/o	diaphragm, mind	
pneumon/o	air or lung	CF-51
psych/o	mind	CF-53
schiz/o	split	
thym/o	thymus gland or mind	
ur/o	urine	CF-67

PROGRAMMED REVIEW: -ia (condition of)

ANSWERS	REVIEW
condition of	4.11 The simple suffix -ia is used in various symptomatic and diagnostic terms to indicate a/an _____ ____. The root that it modifies is key to the definition of the term.
slow heart condition of bradycardia tachycardia dysrhythmia without faulty	4.12 brady- is a prefix meaning _____. Combined with cardi, the root meaning _____, and -ia, meaning _____ ____, the term for the condition of a slow heart rate is _____. In comparison, the condition of a fast heart rate is _____. Both bradycardia and tachycardia are considered arrhythmias (loss or abnormality of rhythm, especially irregularity of the heartbeat). The synonym for arrhythmia is _____ (formed by substituting the prefix a-, meaning _____, with the prefix dys-, meaning painful, difficult, or _____).

lung -ia	**4.13** Pneumonia, the term for a condition of lung infection, is formed by the link of *pneumon/o*, meaning _____, with _____, the suffix indicating a condition of.
condition of speech, without aphasia difficult dysphasia	**4.14** The term describing the inability to speak is formed by combining *-ia*, the suffix meaning _____ ____, with *phas/o*, the combining form meaning _____, and *a-*, the prefix meaning _____. The term is _____. A change of the prefix in aphasia from *a-*, meaning without, to *dys-*, meaning painful, faulty, or _____, forms the term for the condition of difficulty speaking: _____.
mind mind split condition of mind painful, difficult faulty, mind condition of	**4.15** *psych/o* is a combining form meaning _____. *phren/o*, meaning diaphragm, and *thym/o*, meaning thymus gland, are combining forms that also mean _____. For example, in the term schizophrenia, *schiz/o*, a combining form meaning _____, is linked to *phren/o* and *-ia*, the suffix meaning _____ ____, to name the mental illness in which the _____ is said to be split from reality, as evidenced by disorganized thinking, delusions, hallucinations, and other psychotic symptoms. Dysthymia, a term for mild depression, was formed by a link of *dys-*, the prefix meaning _____, _____, or _____, to *thym/o*, meaning _____, and *-ia*, the suffix meaning _____ ____.
swallow without condition of	**4.16** *phag/o* means to eat or _____. Modified by *a-*, the prefix meaning _____, and *-ia*, the suffix meaning _____ ____, the term that describes the condition in which one is unable to

aphagia dysphagia	swallow is _____. The condition of difficulty eating or swallowing is therefore termed _____.
prefix many urine polyuria thirst polydipsia	**4.17** When *-ia* is combined with *poly-*, a/an _____ meaning _____, to modify *ur/o*, the combining form meaning _____, it forms the term for the condition of excessive urination: _____. When *-ia* is linked to *poly-* and *dips/o*, a combining form meaning _____, it forms the term for excessive thirst, or _____. Both of these conditions are common symptoms of diabetes mellitus (see ⊘ Vital Statistics: Diabetes Mellitus).

🩺 Vital Statistics ▸ DIABETES MELLITUS (*dī-ă-bē′tēz mel-i-tus*)

Origin: Diabetes is a Greek word for siphon (which includes *dia-*, meaning across or through, and *bain/o*, to pass or go); mellitus is a Latin word for sweetened honey. From earliest accounts, patients with diabetes mellitus were said to pass large amounts of sweet-tasting urine that often attracted ants and other insects.

Diabetes mellitus (DM) is a metabolic disorder caused by the absence or insufficient production of insulin (a hormone secreted by the pancreas), which results in the inability of tissue cells to absorb sugar (glucose) in the blood. Insulin (*in′sŭ-lin*), originating from the Latin word for island, is a hormone secreted by the beta cells of the islets of Langerhans of the pancreas that regulates the metabolism of glucose by allowing it to move from the blood into cells to produce energy. Due to the absence of or insufficient function of insulin, glucose levels rise in the blood (hyperglycemia) and pass into the urine (glucosuria), and cells are starved of energy.

There are three main forms of diabetes mellitus: type 1, type 2, and gestational diabetes. These forms have similar signs and symptoms but different causes. In type 1 diabetes mellitus (*tīp 1 dī-ă-bēt′z mel-i-tŭs*), no beta cell production of insulin occurs, and the patient is dependent on insulin for survival. In type 2 diabetes mellitus (*tīp 2 dī-ă-bē′tēz mel-i-tŭs*), either the body produces insufficient insulin or insulin resistance (a defective use of the insulin that is produced) occurs; the patient usually is not dependent on insulin for survival. Gestational diabetes occurs during pregnancy but typically resolves after the baby is delivered.

Recalling our patient, Jane Dano, at the beginning of the chapter, polyuria (excessive urination) and polydipsia (excessive thirst) are common symptoms of diabetes mellitus.

Screening for diabetes mellitus includes testing for the presence of sugar in urine, such as part of a urinalysis. The diagnosis is confirmed by measure of glucose in the blood. Treatment is centered on maintenance of a normal level of glucose in the blood to alleviate symptoms and reduce the risk of complications. This includes a healthy diet and exercise regimen, medications that boost the efficiency of insulin in type 2 diabetics, and insulin injections for patients with type 1 diabetes mellitus (and some patients with type 2 diabetes mellitus).

SELF-INSTRUCTION: *-emia* (blood condition)

Add the following combining forms to your study of *-emia* before starting the Programmed Review below.

COMBINING FORM	MEANING	FLASH CARD ID
glyc/o	sugar (glucose)	
isch/o	to hold back	
leuk/o	white	CF-35
lip/o	fat	CF-4
ox/o	oxygen	

PROGRAMMED REVIEW: *-emia* (blood condition)

ANSWERS	REVIEW
blood condition	**4.18** Evolved from the Greek word haima, *-emia* is the suffix that means _____ _____. There are various terms ending in *-emia*. You'll recall it was presented in Chapter 1 in the term hyperlipemia, which refers to a blood
excessive fat	condition of _____ _____.
	4.19 Glycemia, the term for the presence of sugar in the blood, is formed by linking *-emia* to *glyc/o*, a combining form

sugar (glucose)	meaning _____. Further modification of this term by
hyper-	the addition of _____, the prefix meaning above or
	excessive, forms the term that describes an excessive level of
hyperglycemia	blood sugar, or _____. When modified
below	by *hypo-*, the prefix meaning _____ or
deficient	_____, the term for a condition of low blood
hypoglycemia	sugar is _____.

	4.20 *ox/o* is a combining form meaning oxygen. Combined
deficient	with *hypo-*, the prefix meaning below or _____,
	and the suffix *-emia*, it forms the term that describes a
	deficient level of oxygen in the blood, known as
hypoxemia	_____. (Apply the rule explained in Chapter 1,
	noting that occasionally, when a prefix ends in a vowel and
	the root begins with a vowel, the final vowel is dropped
	from the prefix.)

	4.21 Anemia is a diagnostic term formed by the link of
blood condition	*-emia*, meaning _____ _____, to *an-*, the
without	prefix meaning _____. The components in this term
	give a hint to the name of this condition of reduced numbers
	of red blood cells and their diminished ability to transport
	oxygen to the tissues.

combining	**4.22** In leukemia, the link of *leuk/o*, a/an _____
form, white, -emia	_____ meaning _____, with _____,
	the suffix meaning blood condition, forms the term that
	identifies malignant (cancerous) disease of the
	blood-forming organs, marked by abnormal leukocytes (or
white	_____ blood cells).

	4.23 Ischemia is a medical term describing the loss of blood flow or supply of blood to tissue, as caused by narrowing or occlusion of a vessel. It is formed by linking *isch/o*, a
back	combining form meaning to hold _____, with *-emia*, the
blood condition	suffix meaning _____ _____. Ischemic, the adjective form of the term, was formed by replacing *-ia*
pertaining to	with *-ic*, the suffix meaning _____ ____.

SELF-INSTRUCTION: *-genic* (pertaining to origin)

Add the following combining forms to your study of *-genic* before starting the Programmed Review below.

COMBINING FORM	MEANING	FLASH CARD ID
bronch/o	bronchus (airway)	
iatr/o	treatment	CF-33

PROGRAMMED REVIEW: *-genic* (pertaining to origin)

ANSWERS	REVIEW
origin	**4.24** *-genic* is a suffix meaning pertaining to _____. Combined with *bronch/o*, a combining form referring to the
bronchus (airway)	_____, that which originates in the bronchus is
bronchogenic	called _____. When *iatr/o*, a combining
treatment	form meaning _____, is linked to *-genic*, it forms the term that pertains to that which is produced as a
iatrogenic	result of treatment: _____.

SELF-INSTRUCTION: *-itis* (inflammation)

Add the following combining forms to your study of *-itis* before starting the Programmed Review.

COMBINING FORM	MEANING	FLASH CARD ID
appendic/o	appendix	
dermat/o	skin	CF-21
hepat/o	liver	CF-29
metr/o, metri/o, uter/o	uterus	
nas/o, rhin/o	nose	CF-43
oophor/o	ovary	
pharyng/o	pharynx or throat	
phleb/o, ven/o	vein	CF-68
salping/o	uterine or fallopian tube	CF-56
thromb/o	clot	CF-64
tonsill/o	tonsil	
vagin/o	vagina	

PROGRAMMED REVIEW: -itis (inflammation)

ANSWERS	REVIEW
inflammation	**4.25** -itis, meaning _____, is one of the most common suffixes used in symptomatic and diagnostic terms. When attached to a root, it indicates that the given
inflamed	structure or tissue is _____. Note that there are
two, one	_____ "m"s in inflammation and only _____ in inflamed. Characteristics of inflammation include redness, swelling, and pain. In dermatitis, the inflammation is of the _____
skin	(Fig. 4-3).

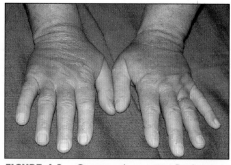

FIGURE 4-3   Contact dermatitis. Redness, swelling, and various lesions on the skin occur as a result of exposure to lanolin.

rhin/o	**4.26** -*nas/o* and _____ are combining forms referring to the nose. Using this second combining form, the term for
rhinitis	inflammation of the nose is _____. Using
throat	*pharyng/o*, the combining form for _____, the term for
pharyngitis	inflammation of the throat is _____.
inflammation	Tonsillitis describes _____ of the
tonsil(s)	_____. When -*itis* is linked to *ot/o*, the combining
ear	form meaning _____, it forms the term for inflammation of
otitis	the ear, or _____. Otitis externa specifically indicates that the inflammation is in the outer ear canal, whereas
inflammation	otitis media indicates that the _____ is
middle	in the _____ ear. (*medi/o*, you'll recall from Chapter 2, is a combining form meaning middle.)
	4.27 You'll recall that pneumonia is a term describing a/an
condition of, lung	_____ ____ the _____ from infection. This condition of infection, typically from bacteria or viruses, causes inflammation; however, the specific term describing inflammation of the lung, as commonly caused by hypersensitivity to chemicals or dust, is formed by a link of
lung	*pneumon/o*, the combining form meaning air or _____,
pneumonitis	with the suffix meaning inflammation: _____.
inflammation	Bronchitis refers to _____ of the bronchi, which are the airways in the lungs. The singular form of
bronchus	bronchi is _____.
	4.28 Arthritis is a general term that describes inflammation
joint(s)	of the _____. The additional combining form in the
inflammation	term osteoarthritis indicates that the _____
bone, joint(s)	includes the _____ and _____.

liver	**4.29** *hepat/o* is the combining form meaning _____.
hepatitis	The term for inflammation of the liver is _____.
	Hepatitis A, B, and C are the most common types.
	4.30 *appendic/o* is the combining form meaning
appendix	_____. Inflammation of the appendix is
appendicitis	_____.
	4.31 You'll recall that the combining forms for vein are *ven/o*
phleb/o	and _____. Using this second combining form, the
phlebitis	term for inflammation of a vein is _____. In
	thrombophlebitis, the additional link to *thromb/o*, meaning
clot	_____, modifies the term to describe the
inflammation, vein	_____ of a/an _____ with
	formation of a clot.
inflammation	**4.32** The suffix *-itis* is used to name _____
	of female reproductive organs. Inflammation of the vagina, the
vaginitis	canal that leads to the uterus, is called _____.
uterine (or fallopian)	*salping/o*, the combining form meaning _____
tube	_____, is used to name an inflammation of the uterine
salpingitis	tube or tubes: _____. *oophor/o*, a combining
ovary	form meaning _____, is used in the term for inflammation
oophoritis	of the ovary or ovaries: _____ . *endo-* is a
within	prefix meaning _____. When combined with *metr/o*, a
uterus	combining form meaning _____, and modified by *-itis*,
endometritis	it forms _____, the term describing an
	inflammation of the endometrium (the tissue lining the uterus).
	Pelvic inflammatory disease (PID) describes inflammation of
	multiple organs in the pelvic cavity; this condition usually
	involves the fallopian tubes, ovaries, and endometrium and is
	most often caused by bacteria.

SELF-INSTRUCTION: -malacia (softening)

Add the following combining forms to your study of -malacia before starting the
Programmed Review below.

COMBINING FORM	MEANING	FLASH CARD ID
chondr/o	cartilage	
laryng/o	larynx (voice box)	
trache/o	trachea (windpipe)	

PROGRAMMED REVIEW: -malacia (softening)

ANSWERS	REVIEW
-malacia softening bone	**4.33** The suffix meaning softening is _____. One of the most common terms in which -malacia is used is osteomalacia, the term for _____ of _____. This condition, known as rickets in children, is caused by calcium and vitamin D deficiency.
cartilage chondromalacia	**4.34** chondr/o is a combining form meaning _____. The term for softened cartilage is _____.
trachea (windpipe) tracheomalacia laryngomalacia	**4.35** trache/o is the combining form for the _____. The disorder of the trachea that causes it to be abnormally collapsible (softened) due to the lack of a structural framework is called _____. A similar term relating to a softened (collapsible) larynx is _____.

SELF-INSTRUCTION: -mania (condition of abnormal impulse toward or frenzy)

Add the following combining forms to your study of -mania before starting the Programmed Review.

COMBINING FORM	MEANING	FLASH CARD ID
necr/o	death	CF-44

PROGRAMMED REVIEW: *-mania* (condition of abnormal impulse toward or frenzy)

ANSWERS	REVIEW
abnormal impulse toward death necromania	**4.36** *-mania* appears as a word or suffix related to a condition of _____ _____ _____ or frenzy. When linked to *necr/o*, a combining form meaning _____, it forms the term referring to a condition of abnormal impulse toward death, or _____.
frenzy condition of pertaining to two, both mania	**4.37** Mania, as a stand-alone term, refers to a state of abnormal elation and increased activity or _____. The adjective for mania is formed by replacing *-ia*, the suffix meaning _____ ____, with *-ic*, the suffix meaning _____ ____. Manic depression is a mental illness also known as bipolar disorder. The prefix *bi-*, meaning _____ or _____, gives hints to the two mood swings that are characteristic of the disorder: the "up" of abnormal elation and increased activity in _____ and the extreme "down" state of depression (see ⬤ Vital Statistics: Mental Illness).

MEET THE PATIENT   Steve Sanchez is a 45-year-old patient who suffers from bipolar disorder, which is a mental illness. Also known as manic depression, bipolar disorder is an affective disorder that is characterized by mood swings of mania and depression (extreme up and down states). Dr. Spaulding has referred him to several health care practitioners for care, including a psychologist for psychotherapy, a psychiatrist for drug therapy, and an Occupational Therapist. His occupational therapist works with an occupational therapy assistant (OTA); together, they help Steve secure a comfortable, affordable living situation and a low-stress job, as well as membership in a peer support group, all in an effort to help him lead a meaningful life.

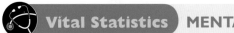 **MENTAL ILLNESS**

Mental illness refers to any disorder of the brain or mind that alters thought, mood, or behavior. Common classifications of mental illness include:

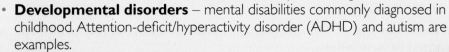

- **Mood disorders** – conditions that affect how a person feels, also called **affective disorders.** Major depression and bipolar disorder are examples of mood disorders.
- **Anxiety disorders** – conditions of emotional distress. Generalized anxiety disorder (GAD) is the most common anxiety disorder. Other types include obsessive-compulsive disorder, panic disorder, phobia, and posttraumatic stress disorder (PTSD).
- **Cognitive disorders** – conditions impairing one's ability to think and reason. Alzheimer disease is an example of a cognitive disorder.
- **Developmental disorders** – mental disabilities commonly diagnosed in childhood. Attention-deficit/hyperactivity disorder (ADHD) and autism are examples.
- **Eating disorders** – disturbances in eating behavior. Anorexia nervosa and bulimia nervosa are common eating disorders.
- **Substance abuse disorders** – mental disorders resulting from abuse of substances such as drugs, alcohol, and other toxins that result in personal and social dysfunction. Substance abuse disorders are identified by the abused substance, such as alcohol abuse, amphetamine abuse, opioid (narcotic) abuse, and polysubstance abuse.
- **Psychotic disorders** – mental disorders that impair one's ability to recognize reality. Schizophrenia is an example of a psychotic disorder.

 ON CLOSER INSPECTION **Anorexia vs. Anorexia Nervosa**

Anorexia is a common symptomatic term indicating that one is *without an appetite.* It is not to be confused with anorexia nervosa, the term for an eating disorder in which the individual has abnormal perceptions about his or her body weight, evidenced by an overwhelming fear of becoming fat that results in a refusal to eat and body weight well below normal.

Health Care Professionals   MEET THE OCCUPATIONAL THERAPIST

Occupational therapists (OTs) work with individuals who suffer from mentally, physically, developmentally, or emotionally disabling conditions. OTs use treatments to develop, recover, or maintain the daily living and work skills of their patients. The therapist's goal is to help clients have independent, productive, and satisfying lives. OTs provide services in a wide variety of settings to individuals of all ages so that they can engage in their daily occupations of work, productive activity, self-care, and leisure/play. They 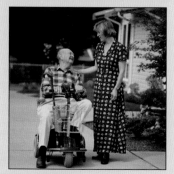 serve individuals, groups, and populations with illnesses and disabilities. In addition, OTs provide wellness and prevention services to improve health and overall quality of life.

◉ A more detailed description of occupational therapy as a health care career can be found on the Student Resource CD-ROM and at the companion website at www.thePoint.lww.com/WillisQC.

SELF-INSTRUCTION: *-megaly* (enlargement)

Add the following combining forms to your study of *-megaly* before starting the Programmed Review below.

COMBINING FORM	MEANING	FLASH CARD ID
acr/o	extremity or topmost	CF-2
megal/o	large	
splen/o	spleen	

PROGRAMMED REVIEW: *-megaly* (enlargement)

ANSWERS	REVIEW
	4.38 *-megaly*, the compound suffix (formed by a link of *-y*, meaning condition or process of, to *megal/o*, meaning large)

enlargement	describes _____. Linked to *hepat/o*, the
liver	combining form meaning _____, the term for an
hepatomegaly	enlargement of the liver is _____. *splen/o*
spleen	is the combining form for _____. An enlargement of
splenomegaly	the spleen is called _____.

enlargement	**4.39** Cardiomegaly refers to _____ of the
heart	_____ (also termed megalocardia). *megal/o* is a
large	combining form meaning _____.

	4.40 The condition of enlarged extremities due to
	hypersecretion of the pituitary growth hormone after puberty
	was coined by linking *acr/o*, the combining form meaning
extremity	topmost or _____, with *-megaly*, meaning
enlargement	_____, to form the term
acromegaly	_____ (Fig. 4-4). Acromegalic is the
adjective	_____ form of the term.

FIGURE 4-4   Enlarged hands and facial features in a patient with acromegaly.

SELF-INSTRUCTION: -osis (condition or increase)

Add the following combining forms to your study of -osis before starting the Programmed Review below.

COMBINING FORM	MEANING	FLASH CARD ID
ather/o	fatty, or lipid, paste	CF-7
arteri/o	artery	
cyt/o	cell	CF-19
isch/o	to hold back	
kyph/o	humpbacked	
lord/o	bent	
nephr/o	kidney	CF-45
neur/o	nerve	
scoli/o	twisted	
scler/o	hard	CF-58
sten/o	narrow	CF-60
vertebr/o, spondyl/o	vertebra	CF-69

PROGRAMMED REVIEW: -osis (condition or increase)

ANSWERS	REVIEW
	4.41 Many symptomatic and diagnostic terms use the suffix
condition, increase	-osis to indicate a/an _____ or _____.
	4.42 -osis is used in several terms to name conditions of abnormal curvature of the spine. The combining form
kyph/o	meaning humpback is _____. Combined with -osis, it forms the term for the abnormal posterior curvature of the thoracic spine, known as a humpback condition:
kyphosis	_____. lord/o, a combining form meaning
bent	_____, is used in the term to identify an anterior bend or sway back condition of the lumbar spine called
lordosis	_____. Lordotic is a term meaning
pertaining to	_____ ____ lordosis. Scoliosis, the term

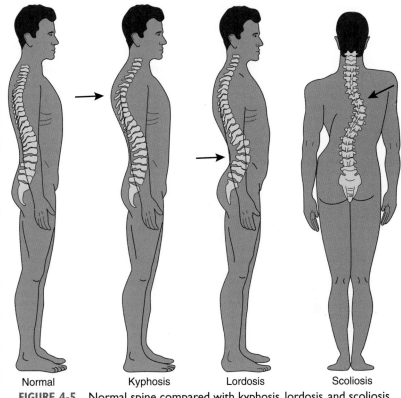

Normal   Kyphosis   Lordosis   Scoliosis

FIGURE 4-5   Normal spine compared with kyphosis, lordosis, and scoliosis.

describing the condition of a lateral S-shaped curve of the spine, is formed by linking -*osis* to *scoli/o*, the combining form

twisted

meaning _____ (Fig. 4-5).

---

condition, increase

nerve

mind

4.43   Neurosis, a general term formed by a link of -*osis*, meaning _____ or _____, to *neur/o*, a combining form meaning _____, describes any mental condition in which anxiety is a prominent feature. Psychosis is a condition of the _____ that is characterized by a distortion of reality and the inability to communicate or function within one's environment (see 🜨 Vital Statistics: Mental Illness).

kidney	**4.44** Some conditions involve degeneration (deterioration) of tissues. *nephr/o*, a combining form for _____, combined with *-osis*, forms the term that defines the condition
nephrosis	of degeneration of the renal tubules: _____. The combining forms for vertebra are *vertebr/o* and
spondyl/o	_____. Use of the latter combining form linked to *-osis* forms the term describing a condition of the
spondylosis	vertebrae (due to joint degeneration): _____.

inflammation	**4.45** Recall from earlier study that endometritis is the term for _____ of the endometrium (tissue lining the uterus). Replacing *-itis* with *-osis* changes the term
endometriosis	to _____, indicating a condition or
increase	_____ of the endometrium. The precise definition describes the migration of portions of the endometrium outside the uterine cavity. Once again, the suffix is a key component that modifies and gives essential meaning to the term.

	4.46 *-osis* refers to an increase in the following terms:
increase, large	macrocytosis: _____ of _____ (red) cells;
increase, small	microcytosis: _____ of _____ (red) cells;
increase, white	leukocytosis: _____ of _____ cells.

hard	**4.47** When *-osis* is combined with *scler/o*, the combining form meaning _____, it forms the general term for a
sclerosis	condition or increase of hardened tissue: _____.
condition	In arteriosclerosis, the _____ or
increase, arteries	_____ is of hardened _____. *ather/o*,
fatty (lipid) paste	a combining form meaning _____ _____, is used in atherosclerosis, a term specifically referring to the

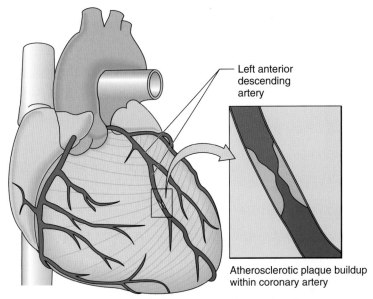

Atherosclerotic plaque buildup
within coronary artery

Left anterior
descending
artery

FIGURE 4-6   Coronary artery disease (CAD).

hardening of fatty (lipid) paste within the walls of arteries.

pertaining to

Using *-ic*, the suffix meaning _____ ____,
the adjective form of atherosclerosis is

atherosclerotic

_____. When hardened fatty paste
(atherosclerotic plaque) builds up within the wall of a blood
vessel, it can have many cumulative ill effects. Atherosclerosis
within the coronary arteries causes coronary artery disease
(CAD) (Fig. 4-6).

narrow

4.48   *sten/o*, a combining form meaning _____,
combined with *-osis* forms the term to describe a/an

condition

_____ or increase of narrowing:

stenosis

_____. Stenosis is a general term used in
reference to any abnormal narrowing of a structure, such as

adjective

an artery or heart valve. Stenotic is the _____
form of the term. Atherosclerotic plaque buildup within the
walls of blood vessels causes stenosis.

condition, increase

clot

4.49 Thrombosis, a term formed by a link of *-osis*, meaning _____ or _____, to *thromb/o*, a combining form meaning _____, describes a condition of stationery clot formation within the heart or a blood vessel. Often when a thrombus (clot) forms, it causes a

stenosis

condition of narrowing, or _____. It can also cause a plug, known as an occlusion (Fig. 4-7).

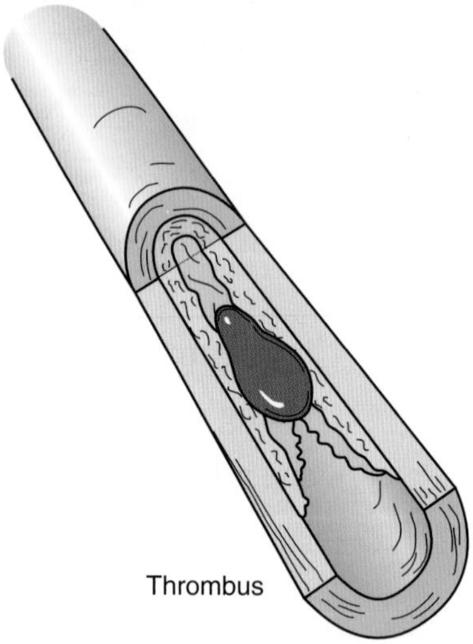

Thrombus

FIGURE 4-7   Thrombus within a blood vessel, causing occlusion.

back

4.50 You'll recall from earlier study of *-emia* that ischemia is a condition in which blood is held _____. This occurs in a blood vessel when there is a loss of blood flow for any reason but commonly because of stenosis (a condition of

narrowing

clot

_____) or thrombosis (a condition of _____ formation). Prolonged ischemia, caused by the occlusion of a blood vessel, results in the loss of oxygenated blood to tissue cells. *necr/o*, the combining form

death

necrosis

meaning _____, is used to describe a condition of tissue death known as _____. The scar left by

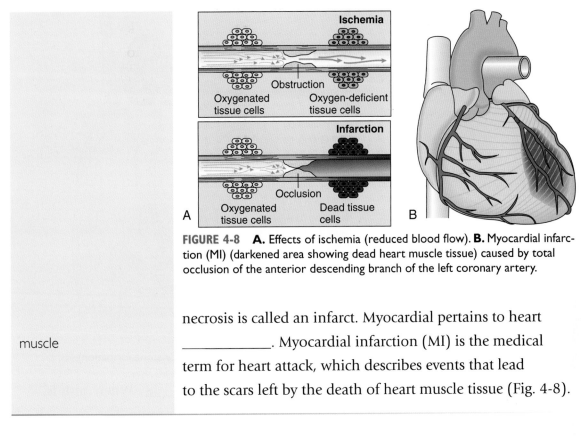

FIGURE 4-8   A. Effects of ischemia (reduced blood flow). **B.** Myocardial infarction (MI) (darkened area showing dead heart muscle tissue) caused by total occlusion of the anterior descending branch of the left coronary artery.

muscle	necrosis is called an infarct. Myocardial pertains to heart _____. Myocardial infarction (MI) is the medical term for heart attack, which describes events that lead to the scars left by the death of heart muscle tissue (Fig. 4-8).

SELF-INSTRUCTION: -iasis (formation or presence of)

Add the following combining forms to your study of -iasis before starting the Programmed Review below.

COMBINING FORM	MEANING	FLASH CARD ID
chol/e	bile	CF-14
lith/o	stone	

PROGRAMMED REVIEW: -iasis (formation or presence of)

ANSWERS	REVIEW
condition, increase	**4.51** You have just studied terms modified by *-osis*, the suffix meaning _____ or _____. A similar suffix that refers to a condition characterized by a

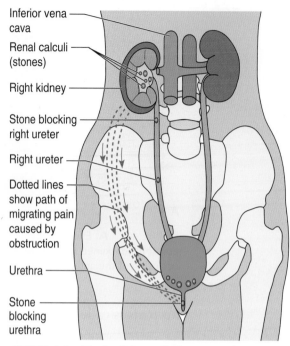

Inferior vena cava

Renal calculi (stones)

Right kidney

Stone blocking right ureter

Right ureter

Dotted lines show path of migrating pain caused by obstruction

Urethra

Stone blocking urethra

FIGURE 4-9   Nephrolithiasis (kidney stone formation).

-iasis	formation or presence of is _____. When *-iasis* is
stone	linked to *lith/o,* a combining form meaning _____, it
	forms the term referring to the formation or presence of a
lithiasis	stone or stones: _____. Microlithiasis refers
formation, presence	to the _____ or _____ of a stone
small	that is _____ in size. Another term for stone is calculus.
	Recall that the combining forms meaning kidney are *nephr/o*
ren/o, kidney	and _____. Renal calculi are _____ stones.
	Nephrolithiasis indicates the presence of one or more
kidney	_____ stones (Fig. 4-9).
bile	**4.52** *chol/e* is a combining from meaning _____. Bile is
	produced in the liver and stored in the cholecyst, or gallbladder.
	(Gall, a synonym for bile, refers to its bitterness.)
formation	Cholelithiasis refers to the _____ or
presence, stones	_____ of one or more bile or gall _____.

SELF-INSTRUCTION: *-lepsy* (seizure)

Add the following combining form to your study of *-lepsy* before starting the Programmed Review below.

COMBINING FORM	MEANING	FLASH CARD ID
narc/o	stupor or sleep	CF-42

PROGRAMMED REVIEW: *-lepsy* (seizure)

ANSWERS	REVIEW
-lepsy prefix upon seizure	**4.53** A seizure is a sudden, transient disturbance in brain function resulting from the abnormal firing of nerve impulses. The suffix meaning seizure is _____. The term epilepsy, a condition characterized by recurrent seizures, was formed by the combination of *epi-*, the _____ meaning _____, with *-lepsy*, the suffix meaning _____.
sleep narcolepsy	**4.54** When *narc/o*, a combining form meaning stupor or _____, is combined with *-lepsy*, it forms the term describing the sleep disorder characterized by a sudden, uncontrollable need to sleep: _____.

SELF-INSTRUCTION: *-oma* (tumor)

Add the following combining forms to your study of *-oma* before starting the Programmed Review.

COMBINING FORM	MEANING	FLASH CARD ID
aden/o	gland	CF-3
carcin/o	cancer	CF-10
fibr/o	fiber	
melan/o	black	CF-39
onc/o	tumor	
plas/o	formation	CF-50
sarc/o	flesh	CF-57

PROGRAMMED REVIEW: -oma (tumor)

ANSWERS	REVIEW
tumor	**4.55** -oma is a diagnostic suffix meaning _____. Tumors form as the result of an abnormal and uncontrolled growth of cells. Cells change from normal (typical) into atypical forms, including tumor formation (neoplasm). plas/o is a
formation	combining form meaning _____, and dys- is a
faulty	prefix meaning bad, difficult, or _____. Dysplasia is the term used to describe abnormal cell and tissue
new	development, and neoplasia, a condition of _____ formation, is the term used to describe the formation of cells and tissue into tumor. Cancerous tumors are called malignant neoplasia, and noncancerous tumors are called
neoplasia	benign _____.
-oma	**4.56** Again, the suffix for tumor is _____. Linked to carcin/o, a combining form meaning cancer, the common term for a cancerous (malignant) epithelial tumor is
carcinoma	_____. Squamous cell carcinoma (SCC) and basal cell carcinoma (BCC), therefore, are skin cancer
tumor(s)	_____ (Fig. 4-10).

FIGURE 4-10   The lesion on this patient's forehead was diagnosed as a basal cell carcinoma (BCC), the most common and easily treatable type of skin cancer.

black	**4.57** *melan/o* is a combining form meaning _____, and melanocytes are the cells that give color to the skin. Combined with *-oma*, the term for a malignant tumor of the
melanoma	skin composed of melanocytes is _____ (Fig. 4-11).

Signs of melanoma

A **Asymmetry:** One half does not match the other half.

B **Border irregularity:** The edges are ragged, notched, or blurred.

C **Color:** The pigmentation is not uniform. Shades of tan, brown, and black are present. Red, white, and blue may add to the mottled appearance.

D **Diameter greater than 6 millimeters:** Any sudden or continuing increase in size should be of special concern.

FIGURE 4-11   Malignant melanoma. The characteristic ABCD warning signs are present in this photo of a nevus (mole) that has developed into a malignant melanoma.

bone	**4.58** You'll recall that *oste/o* means _____. Linked to *-oma*, the term for a benign (noncancerous) tumor of the
osteoma	bone is _____. *sarc/o*, a combining form meaning
flesh	_____, is used in terms indicating the presence of malignant connective tissue. Therefore, an osteosarcoma
tumor	describes a malignant bone _____.

muscle	**4.59** *my/o* is a combining form meaning _____. A
tumor	myoma is a muscle _____. *fibr/o* is the combining form
fiber	used to describe _____. A fibromyoma is a benign tumor in the uterus composed of smooth muscle and fibrous connective tissue. (It is also called simply a fibroma.)

gland	**4.60** *aden/o* is a combining form meaning _____.
cancer	Combined with *carcin/o*, meaning _____, and *-oma*,

tumor	meaning _____, the term describing a cancerous tumor of glandular (secretory) tissue is
adenocarcinoma	_____.

	4.61 Cancerous tumors invade and destroy surrounding tissue and spread through blood and lymph to other parts of the body. Benign tumors do not. The term for the spread of cancer to distant organs or tissue is metastasis, a term formed
stop, stand	by the link of *-stasis*, meaning _____ or _____, with
beyond, after	*meta-*, a prefix meaning _____, _____, or
change	_____.

tumor	**4.62** *onc/o* is the combining form meaning _____.
study of	Combined with *-logy*, the suffix meaning _____ ____, the term describing the specialty concerned with the study of
oncology	tumors and cancers is _____.

Rx for Success

Keeping watch on the pronunciation, spelling, and context in which a term is used will help you avoid errors in understanding those terms that sound similar but are spelled differently and have different meanings. Examples include:
- *hepatoma (tumor of liver)*
  hematoma (tumor of blood)
- *aphagia (inability to swallow)*
  aphasia (inability to speak)

SELF-INSTRUCTION: -penia (abnormal reduction)

Add the following combining form to your study of *-penia* before starting the Programmed Review.

COMBINING FORM	MEANING	FLASH CARD ID
erythr/o	red	CF-24

PROGRAMMED REVIEW: *-penia* (abnormal reduction)

ANSWERS	REVIEW
abnormal reduction white red erythrocytopenia	**4.63** *-penia* is a suffix meaning _____ _____. This term component is often seen in terms describing symptoms related to an abnormal reduction of blood cells. For example, in leukocytopenia, the abnormal reduction is of _____ blood cells. (The more commonly used term is simply leukopenia.) Similarly formed, but using *erythr/o*, the combining form meaning _____, the term describing an abnormal reduction of red blood cells is _____. (This term is also more commonly known as erythropenia.)
clot cell thrombocytopenia all	**4.64** The combination of *thromb/o*, a combining form meaning _____, with *cyt/o*, the combining form meaning _____, and the suffix *-penia* forms the term for the abnormal reduction of thrombocytes, the cells responsible for blood clotting: _____. Pancytopenia indicates an abnormal reduction of _____ cellular components in the blood.
bone pertaining to	**4.65** Another use of *-penia* is in osteopenia, the term describing an abnormal reduction of _____. Osteopenic is the adjective form using the suffix *-ic*, meaning _____ ____. Both terms relate to early warning signs of osteoporosis, a condition of decreased bone density and increased porosity, causing bones to become brittle and liable to break (fracture) (Fig. 4-12).

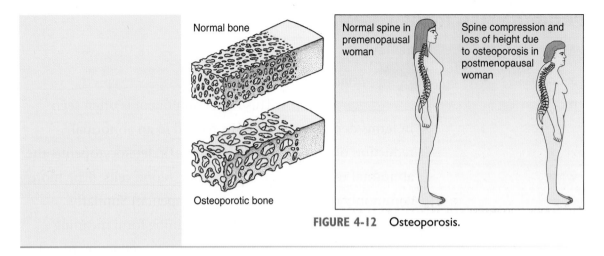

Normal bone

Osteoporotic bone

Normal spine in premenopausal woman

Spine compression and loss of height due to osteoporosis in postmenopausal woman

FIGURE 4-12   Osteoporosis.

SELF-INSTRUCTION: -*phobia* (condition of exaggerated fear or sensitivity)

Add the following combining form to your study of -*phobia* before starting the Programmed Review below.

COMBINING FORM	MEANING	FLASH CARD ID
phot/o	light	CF-49

PROGRAMMED REVIEW: -*phobia* (condition of exaggerated fear or sensitivity)

ANSWERS	REVIEW
exaggerated fear, sensitivity light photophobia	**6.66** Phobia is a stand-alone term, and -*phobia* is a suffix, both describing the condition of _____ _____ or _____. When linked to *phot/o*, a combining form meaning _____, the term referring to a condition of exaggerated sensitivity to light is _____.
condition of	**6.67** Phobia refers to the _____ ____ exaggerated fear. As a suffix, it is used in many terms related to anxiety disorders (see ⬤ Vital Statistics: Mental

topmost	Illness). You'll recall that *acr/o* is a combining form meaning extremity or _____. A person with acrophobia has
high	a fear of _____ places (heights). *necr/o*, a combining
death	form meaning _____, is used to name the condition of
necrophobia	an exaggerated fear of death: _____.

SELF-INSTRUCTION: *-pnea* (breathing)

Terms related to breathing are formed by a link of *-pnea* to a descriptive prefix. Add a review of the prefixes presented at the beginning of this chapter to your study of *-pnea* before starting the Programmed Review below.

PROGRAMMED REVIEW: *-pnea* (breathing)

ANSWERS	REVIEW
	4.68 The symptomatic suffix indicating breathing is *-pnea*.
breathing	The link of *-pnea*, meaning _____, to *eu-*,
normal	a prefix meaning good or _____, forms the term for
eupnea	normal breathing, or _____. *dys-* is a prefix meaning
painful, difficult, faulty	_____, _____, or _____. The
dyspnea	term for difficult breathing is therefore _____.
breathe	Apnea describes the inability to _____. *tachy-* is a
fast	prefix meaning _____. The term for fast breathing is
tachypnea	_____. Bradypnea is a term indicating
slow	_____ breathing. In some conditions, such as during an asthma attack, the patient is unable to breathe except in an upright position. The term, derived from the
straight	combination of the prefix *ortho-*, meaning _____,
normal, correct	_____, or _____, with *-pnea*, is
orthopnea, adjective	_____. Orthopneic is the _____ used to describe orthopnea.

SELF-INSTRUCTION: -ptosis (falling or downward displacement)

Add the following combining form to your study of -ptosis before starting the Programmed Review below.

COMBINING FORM	MEANING	FLASH CARD ID
blephar/o	eyelid	CF-9

PROGRAMMED REVIEW: -ptosis (falling or downward displacement)

ANSWERS	REVIEW
	4.69 Ptosis is used as a stand-alone term as well
downward	as a suffix, meaning falling or _____
displacement	_____. The adjective form is ptotic. Using
kidney	*nephr/o*, the combining form meaning _____, the
	term describing a downward displacement of a kidney is
nephroptosis	_____. Using *gastr/o*, the combining
stomach	form meaning _____, the downward displacement
gastroptosis	of the stomach is termed _____. *blephar/o*,
eyelid	a combining form meaning _____, combined with
	-ptosis forms the specific term for drooping of the eyelid:
blepharoptosis	_____. Most ophthalmologists,
eye	physicians who treat the _____, simply use the term ptosis
	(Fig. 4-13).

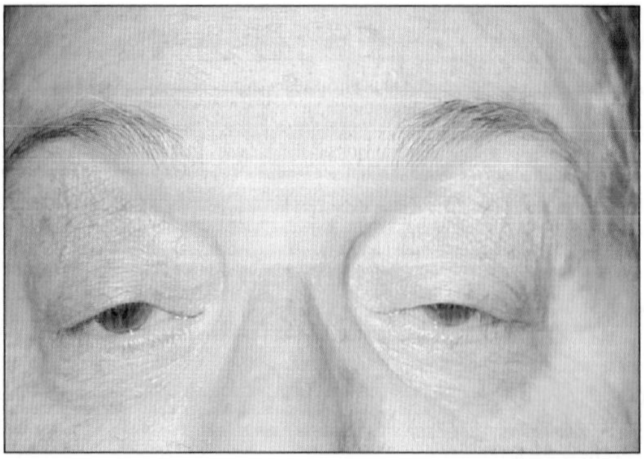

FIGURE 4-13   Blepharoptosis (ptosis). Marked bilateral blepharoptosis caused by paralysis.

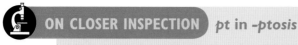

ON CLOSER INSPECTION *pt* in *-ptosis*

You'll remember from the rules of pronunciation covered in Chapter 1 that "pt" has a "t" sound, such as in ptosis (*tō'sis*); however, it is acceptable to pronounce both the "p" and the "t" when "pt" is found within a term, e.g., nephroptosis (*nef-rop-tō'sis*).

SELF-INSTRUCTION: *-plegia* (paralysis)

Terms related to paralysis are formed by a link of *-plegia* to a descriptive prefix. Add the following prefixes to your study of *-plegia* before starting the Programmed Review below.

PREFIX	MEANING	FLASH CARD ID
hemi-	half	P-18
para-	alongside of or abnormal	P-31
quadri-	four	P-27

PROGRAMMED REVIEW: *-plegia* (paralysis)

ANSWERS	REVIEW
suffix	**4.70** *-plegia* is a/an _____ meaning
paralysis	_____. It is combined in medical terms with prefixes that indicate the type of paralysis. Linked
half	to *hemi-*, it forms the term for paralysis of _____ of
hemiplegia	the body (right or left): _____. *quadri-*
prefix, four	is the _____ meaning _____. Paralysis of
quadriplegia	all four limbs is therefore termed _____.
alongside	*para-*, the prefix meaning abnormal or _____
of	____, is used to name paralysis of the lower extremities:
paraplegia	_____.

SELF-INSTRUCTION: -rrhage and -rrhagia (to burst forth, usually blood)

Add the following combining form to your study of -rrhage and -rrhagia before starting the Programmed Review below.

COMBINING FORM	MEANING	FLASH CARD ID
men/o	month (menstruation)	

PROGRAMMED REVIEW: -rrhage and -rrhagia (to burst forth, usually blood)

ANSWERS	REVIEW
burst	**4.71** -rrhage and -rrhagia are suffixes meaning to _____
forth	_____, usually blood. In hemorrhage, the burst
blood	forth is specifically of _____. Menorrhagia indicates
burst forth	an excessive _____ _____ of blood at the
	time of the month during female menstruation (a heavy
	period). *men/o* is a combining form referring to
month	_____, and *metr/o* is a combining form referring to the
uterus	_____. Combined with -rrhagia, it forms the term for
	bleeding from the uterus at any time other than menstruation
	(bleeding from the uterus between periods):
metrorrhagia	_____.

SELF-INSTRUCTION: -rrhea (discharge)

Add the following combining forms to your study of -rrhea before starting the Programmed Review.

COMBINING FORM	MEANING	FLASH CARD ID
nas/o, rhin/o	nose	CF-43

PROGRAMMED REVIEW: -rrhea (discharge)

ANSWERS	REVIEW
discharge rhin/o rhinorrhea	**4.72** The Greek word rhoia, meaning flow, is the origin of -rrhea, the symptomatic suffix used to describe a/an _____. Recall that there are two combining forms meaning nose: *nas/o* and _____. Using the second combining form, a runny discharge from the nose is called _____.
without amenorrhea painful difficult, faulty dysmenorrhea	**4.73** Menorrhea describes menstrual discharge (menstruation). The addition of the prefix *a-*, meaning _____, forms the term for the absence of menstrual discharge (a sign of pregnancy): _____. Using the prefix *dys-*, meaning _____, _____, or _____, the term for painful menstrual discharge is _____.
ear otorrhea	**4.74** *ot/o* is the combining form for _____. The discharge (-rrhea) of purulent (infectious) matter from the ear as a result of infection is simply termed _____.
through discharge diarrhea	**4.75** Formed from the prefix *dia-*, meaning across or _____, and the suffix -rrhea, meaning _____, the term describing frequent loose or liquid stool is _____.
discharge	**4.76** In ancient times, the term for the purulent urethral discharge in males, now known as a characteristic of infection, was thought to be a leakage of semen. *gon/o*, meaning seed (as in sperm), was combined with -rrhea, meaning _____, to form the term that today describes the contagious invasion of bacteria known as

| gonorrhea | _____ (a contagious, sexually transmitted inflammation of the genital mucous membranes caused by invasion of the gonococcus, *Neisseria gonorrhea*). |

Rx for Success

Don't be rolled over by the

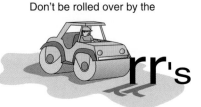

*We have the Greeks to thank for the suffixes with **double rr's**. Take a careful look at these symptomatic and diagnostic ones so that you will spell them correctly in terms! Also, keep in mind that "rrh" has an "r" sound.*

Suffix	Meaning	Example
-rrhea	discharge	rhinorrhea (runny discharge from the nose)
-rrhage or -rrhagia	to burst forth (usually blood)	hemorrhage (a burst forth of blood) menorrhagia (a burst forth of blood during menstruation)

SELF-INSTRUCTION: *-spasm* (involuntary contraction)

Add the following combining form to your study of *-spasm* before starting the Programmed Review below.

COMBINING FORM	MEANING	FLASH CARD ID
enter/o	small intestine	CF-23

PROGRAMMED REVIEW: *-spasm* (involuntary contraction)

ANSWERS	REVIEW
suffix, involuntary	**4.77** The word spasm is used as a stand-alone term or at the end of a term as a symptomatic or diagnostic _____ that describes a/an _____

contraction	_____. -*spasm* is used as a suffix in several terms. Using the combining form meaning vessel,
involuntary	vasospasm is defined as a/an _____
contraction, vessel	_____ of a blood _____. Linked to
bronchus (airway)	*bronch/o*, meaning _____, the term for involuntary
bronchospasm	spasm of the bronchi is _____. The combining form referring to the small intestine is
enter/o	_____. The term for involuntary contraction of the
enterospasm	small intestine is therefore _____. Using the combining form for eyelid, blepharospasm describes a/an
involuntary contraction	_____ _____ of the
eyelid	_____.

SELF-INSTRUCTION: -ism (condition of)

Add the following combining forms to your study of *-ism* before starting the Programmed Review below.

COMBINING FORM	MEANING	FLASH CARD ID
cerebr/o	largest part of the brain	
pulmon/o	lung	CF-54
thyroid/o	thyroid gland (shield)	

PROGRAMMED REVIEW: -ism (condition of)

ANSWERS	REVIEW
condition of	**4.78** The suffix *-ism*, meaning _____ ____, is part of many diagnostic terms. *hyper-*, the prefix meaning
excessive	above or _____, and its counterpart, *hypo-*,
deficient	meaning below or _____, are used in terms for conditions of thyroid gland secretion. An excessive thyroid
hyper	gland secretion is termed _____thyroidism, whereas the
hypo	condition of deficient thyroid secretion is _____thyroidism.

self, condition of	**4.79** Autism, a term formed by a link of *auto-*, the prefix meaning _____, with *-ism*, meaning _____ ____, is the name for the developmental disability that renders the individual unable to communicate or relate to anything beyond one's self (see ⊚ Vital Statistics: Mental Illness).
clot condition of emboli lung brain	**4.80** You'll recall that thrombus is the name for a stationary _____. Embolus is the name given a detached thrombus that travels within a blood vessel and obstructs where it lodges (Fig. 4-14). Embolism describes the _____ ____ an embolus. The plural of embolus is _____. A pulmonary embolism (PE) is a clot that has lodged in a blood vessel in the _____. A cerebral embolism is a clot that has lodged in a blood vessel in the _____. The damage to brain tissue that occurs as a result of a cerebral embolism is known as a stroke or cerebrovascular accident (CVA) (Fig. 4-15).

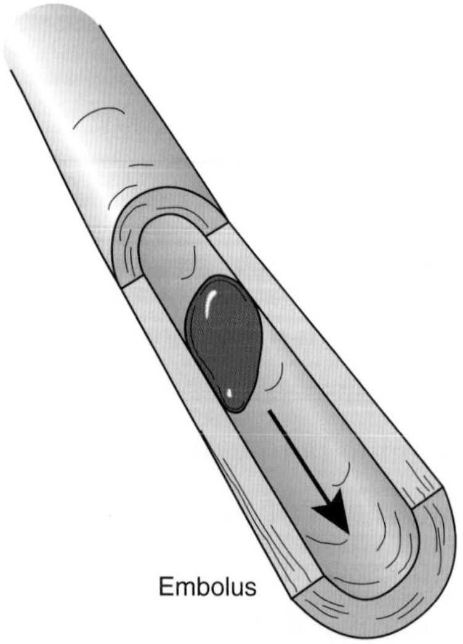

Embolus

FIGURE 4-14   Embolism.

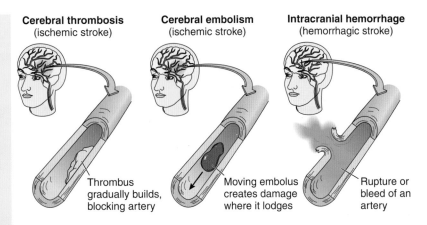

Cerebral thrombosis
(ischemic stroke)

Cerebral embolism
(ischemic stroke)

Intracranial hemorrhage
(hemorrhagic stroke)

Thrombus
gradually builds,
blocking artery

Moving embolus
creates damage
where it lodges

Rupture or
bleed of an
artery

FIGURE 4-15   Types of stroke (cerebrovascular accident [CVA]).

4.81 In a few terms, the "i" in *-ism* is replaced with a "y" to show Greek origin. Paroxysm, the term referring to a condition marked by the sudden onset of symptoms, is an example. The combination of *aneury/o*, a combining form referring to a widening, with *-ysm*, forms _____, the Greek term that refers to a condition of widening in the wall of the heart, aorta, or artery caused by a congenital defect or acquired weakness (Fig. 4-16). The bleed or rupture of an aneurysm in a blood vessel in the brain causes an event known as a hemorrhagic stroke, which is another type of cerebrovascular accident (CVA).

aneurysm

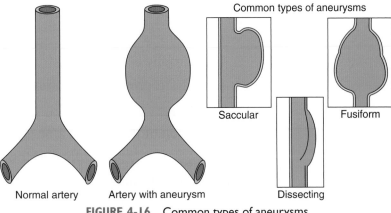

Common types of aneurysms

Saccular

Fusiform

Normal artery

Artery with aneurysm

Dissecting

FIGURE 4-16   Common types of aneurysms.

SELF-INSTRUCTION: -y (condition or process of)

Add the following combining forms to your study of -y before starting the Programmed Review below.

COMBINING FORM	MEANING	FLASH CARD ID
lymph/o	clear fluid	
path/o	disease	CF-46
troph/o	nourishment or development	CF-65

PROGRAMMED REVIEW: -y (condition or process of)

ANSWERS	REVIEW
condition	**4.82** The suffix -y, meaning _____ or
process	_____, is a common simple suffix that is seen in many symptomatic and diagnostic terms. You'll recall that
without	the prefix a- means _____. Combined with troph/o, a combining form meaning nourishment or
development	_____, and -y, the suffix meaning
condition	_____ or process, the term describing shrinking or wasting of tissue, such as muscle, is
atrophy	_____. On the other hand, hypertrophy is a term
excessive	that indicates the above normal or _____ increase in size of an organ or tissue. The adjective form
atrophic	of atrophy is _____; the adjective form of
hypertrophic	hypertrophy is _____. Analyzing the
painful	term dystrophy, the prefix meaning _____,
difficult, faulty	_____, or _____ gives a clue to the
condition	definition of the term as a/an _____ or
process	_____ of faulty development of a tissue or organ. The adjective form of dystrophy is
dystrophic	_____.

condition process, heart	**4.83** Cardiomyopathy is a term linking -*y* to several components in order to describe a/an _____ or _____ of diseased _____ muscle.
fluid gland, disease condition or process	**4.84** Lymphadenopathy, the term describing a condition of enlarged (diseased) lymph nodes, was formed by linking lymph, meaning clear _____, with *aden/o*, meaning _____, *path/o*, meaning _____, and -*y*, meaning _____ or _____ (Fig. 4-17).

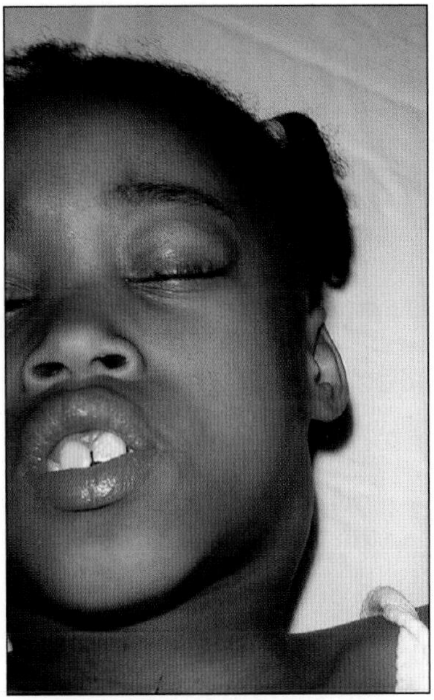

FIGURE 4-17   Enlarged lymph glands below the jaw (submandibular lymphadenopathy) in child with mumps (parotiditis).

SELF-INSTRUCTION: Common Terms Related to Disease

The following is a list of terms related to disease that commonly accompany symptomatic and diagnostic terms and are important to learn. Add the following to your study before starting the Programmed Review that follows.

TERM	MEANING
acute	sharp; a condition that has intense, often severe symptoms and a short course
benign	mild or noncancerous
chronic	a condition that develops slowly and persists over a period of time
degeneration	gradual deterioration of normal cells and body functions
degenerative disease	any disease in which deterioration of the structure or function of tissue occurs
diagnosis	determination of the presence of a disease based on an evaluation of symptoms, signs, and test findings (results) (*dia* = through; *gnosis* = knowing)
etiology	the cause of a disease (*etio* = cause)
exacerbation	an aggravation, or "flare-up," of symptoms (*ex* = out; *acerbo* = harsh)
febrile	relating to a fever, or elevated temperature
localized	limited to a definite area or part
malignant	harmful or cancerous
prognosis	foreknowledge; prediction of the likely outcome of a disease based on the general health status of the patient and knowledge of the usual course of the disease; often noted in one word (e.g., prognosis: good)
progressive	pertaining to the advance of a condition as the signs and symptoms increase in severity
remission	a period in which symptoms and signs stop or abate
sign	a mark; objective evidence of disease that can be seen or verified by an examiner
symptom	subjective evidence of disease that is perceived by the patient and often noted in his or her own words
syndrome	a running together; combination of symptoms and signs that give a distinct clinical picture indicating a particular condition or disease (e.g., menopausal syndrome)

PROGRAMMED REVIEW: Common Terms Related to Disease

ANSWERS	REVIEW
sign symptom objective febrile a pain or ache subjective symptom	**4.85** Originating from the Latin word for a mark, the term describing objective evidence of disease that can be seen or verified by an examiner is called a/an _____. The term used to describe subjective evidence of disease that is perceived by the patient is a/an _____. Many different signs and symptoms manifest disease in the body. For example, fever in the body can be verified by taking the patient's temperature, _____ evidence that may be a sign of disease. A patient is considered to be _____ if he or she has an increase in body temperature and to be __febrile if he or she is without a fever. Cephalalgia, or head _____, is an example of _____ evidence that is a/an _____ of disease.
across, through knowing diagnosis prognosis etiology	**4.86** The prefix *dia-* means _____ or _____, and *gnos/o* means _____. Through knowledge gained by education and training, a doctor makes a/an _____ when naming a disease and gives a/an _____ when predicting its likely outcome. The cause or _____ of a disease is often unknown.
acute, chronic	**4.87** Some conditions have an intense, often severe or _____ onset, whereas others that are _____ develop slowly and persist over time.
localized systemic	**4.88** Conditions limited to a definite body area or part are considered to be _____, whereas those that are _____ affect the whole body.

malignant, benign	**4.89** If a condition is cancerous, it is termed _____; if it is noncancerous, it is _____.
exacerbation remission	**4.90** An aggravation, or "flare-up," of symptoms is referred to as a/an _____. A condition is said to be in _____ during the period in which signs and symptoms have stopped.
not degeneration	**4.91** Degenerative disease occurs as a result of gradual deterioration of tissue with loss of function. The prefix *de-*, meaning from, down, or _____, is used in the term for this process: _____.
progressive	**4.92** A condition is considered to be _____ when the symptoms and signs advance with increased severity. The progression ranges from slow to rapid.
syndrome	**4.93** The term describing a combination of symptoms and signs that give a distinct clinical picture is called a syndrome. For example, hot flashes, weight gain, mood swings, and irregular menstruation are signs and symptoms that indicate a woman is going through menopause, a condition known as menopausal _____.

Pronunciation Summary

Following you will find a list of medical terms that you have learned to build and spell in this chapter, followed by the page number on which each term can be found and its written pronunciation. ◉ Take a minute to listen to the audio pronunciations of these terms on the Student Resource CD-ROM, and then practice pronouncing them out loud. For additional practice and reinforcement, write the definition of each term on a separate piece of paper.

acromegaly/167
ak-rō-meg'ă-lē

acrophobia/181
ak-rō-fō'bē-ă

acute/192
ă-kyūt'

adenocarcinoma/177
ad'ĕ-nō-kar-si-nō'mă

amenorrhea/185
ă-men-ō-rē'ă

anemia/158
ă-nē'mē-ă

aneurysm/189
an'yū-rizm

aphagia/156
ă-fā'jē-ă

aphasia/155
ă-fā'zē-ă

apnea/181
ap'nē-ă

appendicitis/162
ă-pen-di-sī'tis

arteriosclerosis/170
ar-tēr'ē-ō-skler-ō'sis

arthralgia/150
ar-thral'jē-ă

atherosclerosis/170
ath'er-ō-skler-ō'sis

atrophy/190
at'rō-fē

autism/188
aw'tizm

benign/192
bē-nīn'

bipolar disorder/164
bī-pō'lăr dis-ōr'děr

blepharoptosis/182
blef'ă-rop'tō-sis

blepharospasm/187
blef'ă-rō-spazm

bradycardia/154
brad-ē-kar'dē-ă

bradypnea/181
brad-ip-nē'ă

bronchogenic/159
brong-kō-jen'ik

bronchospasm/187
brong'kō-spazm

carcinoma/176
kar-si-nō'mă

cardiomegaly/167
kar-dē-ō-meg'ă-lē

cardiomyopathy/191
kar'dē-ō-mī-op'ă-thē

cephalalgia/151
sef'al-al'jē-ă

cephalodynia/151
sef'a-lō-din'ē-ă

cerebrovascular accident (CVA)/188,189
ser'ĕ-brō-vas'kyū-lăr ak'si-dent

cholelithiasis/174
kō'lē-li-thī'ă-sis

chondromalacia/163
kon'drō-mă-lā'shē-ă

chronic/192
kron'ik

coronary artery disease (CAD)/171
kōr'ŏ-nār-ē ar'těr-ē di-zēz'

cystocele/153
sis'tō-sēl

degeneration/192
dē-jen-ĕr-ā'shŭn

dermatitis/160
děr-mă-tī'tis

diagnosis/148
dī-ag-nō'sis

diarrhea/185
dī-ă-rē'ă

dysmenorrhea/185
dis-men-ō-rē'ă

dysphagia/156
dis-fā′jē-ă

dysphasia/155
dis-fā′zē-ă

dysplasia/176
disp-nē′ă

dyspnea/181
disp-nē′ă

dysrhythmia/154
dis-rith′mē-ă

dysthymia/155
dis-thī′mē-ă

dystrophy/190
dis′trō-fē

endometriosis/170
en′dō-mē-trē-ō′sis

enterospasm/187
en′tĕr-ō-spazm

epigastralgia/151
ep′i-gas-tral′jē-ă

epilepsy/175
ep′i-lep′sē

erythrocytopenia/179
ĕ-rith′rō-sī′tō-pē′nē-ă

etiology/192
ē-tē-ol′ŏ-jē

eupnea/181
yūp-nē′ă

exacerbation/192
ek-zas-ĕr-bā′shŭn

febrile/192
feb′ril

fibroma/177
fi-brō′mă

fibromyoma/177
fi′brō-mī-ō′mă

gastroptosis/182
gas′trōp-tō′sis

hemiplegia/183
hem-ē-plē′jē-ă

hemorrhage/186
hem′ŏ-răj

hepatitis/162
hep-ă-tī′tis

hepatomegaly/167
hep′ă-tō-meg′ă-lē

hydrocele/152
hī′drō-sēl

hyperglycemia/158
hī′pĕr-glī-sē′mē-ă

hyperlipemia/157
hī′pĕr-li-pē′mē-ă

hyperthyroidism/187
hī-pĕr-thī′royd-izm

hypertrophy/190
hī-pĕr′trō-fē

hypoglycemia/158
hī′pō-glī-sē′mē-ă

hypothyroidism/187
hī′pō-thī′royd-izm

hypoxemia/158
hī-pok-sē′mē-ă

iatrogenic/159
ī-at′rō-jen′ik

ischemia/159
is-kē′mē-ă

ischemic/159
is-kē′mik

kyphosis/168
kī-fō′sis

laryngomalacia/163
lă-ring′gō-mă-lā′shē-ă

leukemia/158
lū-kē′mē-ă

leukocytosis/170
lū′kō-sī-tō′sis

leukocytopenia/179
lū′kō-sī′tō-pē′nē-ă

leukopenia/179
lū′kō-pē′nē-ă

lithiasis/174
lith-ī′ă-sis

localized/192
lō9kăl-ı̄zd

lordosis/168
lōr-dō′sis

lymphadenopathy/191
lim-fad′ĕ-nop′ă-thē

macrocytosis/170
mak′rō-sī-tō′sis

malignant/192
mă-līg′nănt

mania/164
mā′nē-ă

manic depression/164
man′ik dē-presh′ŭn

melanoma/177
mel′ă-nō′mă

menorrhagia/184
men-ō-rā′jē-ă

metastasis/178
mĕ-tas′tă-sis

metrorrhagia/184
mē-trō-rā′jē-ă

microcytosis/170
mī′krō-sī-tō′sis

microlithiasis/174
mī′krō-li-thī′ă-sis

myalgia/151
mī-al′jē-ă

myocardial infarction (MI)/173
mī-ō-kar′dē-ăl in-fark′shŭn

myodynia/151
mī′ō-din′ē-ă

myoma/177
mī-ō′mă

narcolepsy/175
nar′kō-lep-sē

necromania/164
nek′rō-mā′nē-ă

necrophobia/181
nek′rō-fō′bē-ă

necrosis/172
nĕ-krō′sis

neoplasia/176
nē′ō-plā′zē-ă

nephrolithiasis/174
nef′rō-li-thī′ă-sis

nephroptosis/182
nef′rop-tō′sis

nephrosis/170
ne-frō′sis

neurosis/169
nū-rō′sis

oncology/178
ong-kol′ŏ-jē

orthopnea/181
ōr-thop-nē′ă

ostealgia/150
os-tē-al′jē-ă

osteoarthritis/161
os′tē-ō-ar-thrī′tis

osteodynia/150
os-tē-ō-din′ē-ă

osteomalacia/163
os′tē-ō-mă-lā′shē-ă

osteopenia/179
os′tē-ō-pē′nē-ă

osteosarcoma/177
os′tē-ō-sar-kō′mă

otalgia/151
ō-tal′jē-ă

otitis media/161
ō-tī′tis mē′dē-ă

otodynia/151
ō-tō-din′ē-ă

otorrhea/185
ō-tō-rē′ă

paraplegia/183
par-ă-plē′jē-ă

pharyngitis/161
fă-rin-jī'tis

phlebitis/162
fle-bī'tis

photophobia/180
fō-tō-fō'bē-ă

pneumonia/155
nū-mō'nē-ă

pneumonitis/161
nū-mō-nī'tis

polydipsia/156
pol-ē-dip'sē-ă

polyuria/156
pol-ē-yū'rē-ă

prognosis/192
prog-nō'sis

progressive/192
prō-gres'iv

psychosis/169
sī-kō'sis

quadriplegia/183
kwah'dri-plē'jē-ă

rectocele/153
rek'tō-sēl

rhinitis/161
ñ-nī'tis

rhinorrhea/185
ñ-nō-rē'ă

remission/192
rē-mish'ŭn

salpingitis/162
sal-pin-jī'tis

schizophrenia/155
skiz-ō-frē'nē-ă

sclerosis/170
sklĕ-rō'sis

scoliosis/168
skō-lē-ō'sis

sign/192
sīn

splenomegaly/167
splē-nō-meg'ă-lē

spondylosis/170
spon-di-lō'sis

stenosis/171
ste-nō'sis

symptom/148, 192
simp'tŏm

syndrome/192
sin'drōm

tachycardia/154
tak-i-kar'dē-ă

tachypnea/181
tak-ip-nē'ă

thrombocytopenia/179
throm'bō-sī-tō-pē'nē-ă

thrombophlebitis/162
throm'bō-fle-bī'tis

tonsillitis/161
ton-si-lī'tis

tracheomalacia/163
trā'kē-ō-mă-lā'shē-ă

vaginitis/162
vaj-i-nī'tis

varicocele/152
var'i-kō-sēl

vasospasm/187
vā'sō-spazm

Examine Your Understanding

For the following terms, draw a line or lines to separate the prefixes (P), combining forms (CF), roots (R), and suffixes (S). Then, write the meaning of each component on the corresponding blank to define the term.

EXAMPLE

hyperlipemia

hyper/lip/emia

above or excessive / *fat* / *blood condition*

         P   R   S

1. anemia

_____ / _____
       P   S

2. arthralgia

_____ / _____
       R   S

3. hydrocele

_____ / _____
       CF   S

4. erythrocytopenia

_____ / _____ / _____
       CF   CF   S

5. hepatitis

_____ / _____
       R   S

6. endometriosis

_____ / _____ / _____
       P   R   S

7. dysplasia

_____ / _____ / _____
       P   R   S

8. melanoma

_____ / _____
       R   S

9. orthopnea

_____ / _____
       P   S

10. thrombophlebitis

_____ / _____ / _____
CF   R   S

11. schizophrenia

_____ / _____ / _____
CF   R   S

12. iatrogenic

_____ / _____
CF   S

13. chondromalacia

_____ / _____
CF   S

14. bronchospasm

_____ / _____
CF   S

15. metastasis

_____ / _____
P   S

16. gastralgia

_____ / _____
R   S

17. splenomegaly

_____ / _____
CF   S

18. lymphadenopathy

_____ / _____ / _____ / _____
R   CF   R   S

19. cephalodynia

_____ / _____
R   S

20. osteosarcoma

_____ / _____ / _____
CF   R   S

21. hyperthyroidism

_____ / _____ / _____
P   R   S

22. oncology

_____ / _____
CF   S

23. blepharoptosis

_____ / _____
      CF   S

24. adenocarcinoma

_____ / _____ / _____
      CF   R   S

25. varicocele

_____ / _____
      CF   S

26. amenorrhea

_____ / _____ / _____
      P   CF   S

27. atrophic

_____ / _____ / _____
      P   R   S

28. cystocele

_____ / _____
      CF   S

29. bradypnea

_____ / _____
      P   S

30. hypothyroidism

_____ / _____ / _____
      P   R   S

Match the following conditions.

31. _____ bradycardia

32. _____ aphasia

33. _____ nephrosis

34. _____ tachycardia

35. _____ kyphosis

36. _____ atrophy

37. _____ hypertrophy

38. _____ dysphasia

39. _____ dystrophy

40. _____ lordosis

41. _____ necrosis

a. diseased muscle

b. loss of blood flow

c. difficulty swallowing

d. sway back

e. difficult speech

f. excessive development

g. deficient thyroid

h. dead tissue

i. humpback

j. without development

k. inability to speak

42. _____ dysphagia   l. slow heart

43. _____ myopathy   m. degenerative kidney

44. _____ hypothyroidism   n. fast heart

45. _____ ischemia   o. faulty development

Circle the correct meaning for the following term components.

46. *-malacia*

   a. discharge   b. enlargement   c. hernia   d. softening

47. *-ia*

   a. condition of   b. increase   c. pertaining to   d. abnormal
                                                                      reduction

48. *-cele*

   a. enlargement   b. involuntary   c. hernia   d. stop or stand
                            contraction

49. *-rrhea*

   a. discharge   b. blood   c. tumor   d. to burst forth
                            condition   blood

50. *-ic*

   a. condition of   b. increase   c. tumor   d. pertaining to

51. *-odynia*

   a. resembling   b. pain   c. pouching   d. abnormal
                                                                      reduction

52. *-ptosis*

   a. falling down   b. involuntary   c. tumor   d. discharge
                            contraction

53. *-itis*

   a. hard   b. straight   c. inflammation   d. left

54. *-osis*

   a. discharge   b. condition   c. tumor   d. pertaining to

Identify the synonym for the following term components.

55. *nas/o* _____

56. *-odynia* _____

57. *vertebr/o* _____

58. *ven/o* _____

Give the medical term for the following conditions.

59. inflammation of the ear _____

60. inflammation of the nose _____

61. inflammation of the throat _____

62. inflammation of a joint _____

63. enlargement of the liver _____

64. discharge from the nose _____

65. painful menstrual discharge _____

66. downward displacement of the eyelid _____

67. downward displacement of the kidney _____

68. pain in the joint _____

69. pain in the head _____

70. pain in the stomach _____

71. bleeding from the uterus _____

72. bleeding from the ear _____

73. presence or formation of stone or stones _____

Match the features of the following psychiatric terms.

74. _____ acrophobia
75. _____ necromania
76. _____ mania
77. _____ psychosis
78. _____ neurosis
79. _____ dysthymia
80. _____ autism

a. anxiety
b. distorted reality
c. mild depression
d. abnormal elation and increased activity
e. only relates to one's self
f. abnormal impulse toward death
g. fear of heights

Identify the meaning of the following suffixes.

81. -malacia _____

82. -spasm _____

83. -lepsy _____

84. -iasis _____

85. -tic _____

Match the following terms with their meanings.

86. _____ febrile   a. period in which symptoms stop

87. _____ syndrome   b. probable outcome of a disease

88. _____ chronic   c. name of a disease based on history, exam, and
                                        testing

89. _____ remission   d. elevated temperature

90. _____ etiology   e. set of symptoms characteristic of a particular
                                        disease or condition

91. _____ malignant   f. an aggravation of symptoms

92. _____ prognosis   g. developing slowly over time

93. _____ diagnosis   h. limited to a definite area or part

94. _____ exacerbation   i. cancerous

95. _____ localized   j. the study of the cause of a disease

96. _____ acute   k. objective evidence of disease

97. _____ benign   l. subjective evidence of disease

98. _____ degenerative   m. mild or noncancerous

99. _____ symptom   n. deterioration of the structure or function of tissue

100. _____ sign   o. having intense, often severe symptoms

MEDICAL RECORD EXERCISES

Medical Record 4-1

You first read about Jane Dano in the Meet the Patient vignette at the beginning of the chapter. She was referred by Dr. Spaulding to an endocrinologist, who decided to admit her to Central Medical Center. One week later, she was discharged, and her Discharge Summary is shown in Medical Record 4-1 (page 206). Review the medical record and answer the following questions.

Questions about Medical Record 4-1

1. Below are medical terms used in this record that you have not yet encountered in the text. Underline each term where it appears in the record and, using a medical dictionary, define them below.

    nocturia _____

    urinalysis _____

    ketones _____

    dietitian _____

    human insulin _____

    NPH insulin _____

    Use an online resource to define and learn about the following:

    USDA Dietary Guidelines _____

2. What was significant in Jane's history?

    a. she had lost weight
    b. she was excessively thirsty
    c. she needed to urinate frequently
    d. all of the above

3. Which of the following describes Jane's condition?

    a. metabolic disorder caused by absence or insufficient production of insulin
    b. condition of hypersecretion of the thyroid gland
    c. condition of hyposecretion of the thyroid gland
    d. condition resulting in an excessive amount of insulin in the bloodstream

4. During Jane's hospital course, what was the condition that required "spot dosing" at lunch?

    a. low blood sugar
    b. high blood sugar
    c. glucose in her urine
    d. presence of ketones

CENTRAL MEDICAL CENTER

211 Medical Center Drive • Central City, US 90000-1234 • PHONE: (012) 125-6784 • FAX: (012) 125-9999

DISCHARGE SUMMARY

ADMITTING DIAGNOSIS: New onset Type 1 diabetes mellitus.

FINAL DIAGNOSIS: New onset Type 1 diabetes mellitus.

HISTORY OF PRESENT ILLNESS: The patient is an 11-year-old white female who presented with a 3-week history of polyuria and polydipsia. She has also had nocturia for the past 2 months and associated weight loss. She was seen by J. Spaulding, M.D., her private physician, on the day of admission. A urinalysis was positive for glucose. The patient was then referred to this examiner for further evaluation and management of new onset Type 1 diabetes mellitus.

HOSPITAL COURSE: The patient was admitted to the third floor. She was initially treated with regular insulin and then progressed to a 2-shot regimen with regular insulin and NPH before breakfast and regular insulin and NPH before dinner. She also required some spot dosing at lunch for hyperglycemia. Prior to discharge, her blood sugars had stabilized. She did not have any overnight hypoglycemia. Her ketones were clear, and she had spilled 10 gm of glucose in her urine. Also, during the course of hospitalization, the parents and the patient underwent extensive education with nursing staff and the dietitian including how to give insulin injections and do home blood glucose monitoring.

DISCHARGE PROGRAM: The patient is to be seen in the Diabetic Clinic in approximately 2 weeks. **DIET:** She is on a 2000-calorie diet based on USDA Dietary Guidelines with three meals and two snacks. Physical activity is ad lib. The patient may return to school at the end of the week. **SPECIAL INSTRUCTIONS:** The parents are to check blood sugar at 2 a.m. for the first two nights at home. They are also to call for insulin dose adjustments daily for the first week after discharge.

DISCHARGE MEDICATIONS: Novolin Human Insulin, 12 units of regular and 12 units of NPH, to be given 20 minutes before breakfast; 10 units of regular and 6 units of NPH to be given 20 minutes before dinner.

R Gallegos M.D.

R. Gallegos, M.D.

RG:ti
D:11/19/20xx
T:11/20/20xx

DISCHARGE SUMMARY		
	PT. NAME:	DANO, JANE
	ID NO:	IP-403831
	ROOM NO:	310
	ADM. DATE:	November 11, 20xx
	DIS. DATE:	November 18, 20xx
	ATT. PHYS:	R. GALLEGOS, M.D.

MEDICAL RECORD 4-1 Discharge Summary

5. What was noted in the discharge instructions about Jane's physical activity?

   a. She should only be as active as necessary.
   b. She may be as active as she desires.
   c. She is limited to bedrest.
   d. She must exercise 20 minutes before breakfast.

6. Which test will Jane and her family be performing at home?

   a. vital signs
   b. body weight
   c. insulin injections
   d. blood sugar monitoring

Medical Record 4-2

S 45 y.o. ♂ with long history of asthma presents with SOB and severe wheezing. The pt has felt poorly for the past 3 days but significantly worse in the last hour. The pt is orthopneic and has had a nonproductive cough for the last few days but denies fever or chills.

   PMH: Singulair, 10 mg tab po q noc, Proventil inhaler qid prn. NKDA

O VS: T 98°F, P 128, R 36, BP 180/90
   Pertinent PE Findings: Skin – diaphoretic. Chest – bilateral expiratory wheezes. Heart – rapid rate s̄ murmur. The electrocardiogram (ECG) demonstrates sinus tachycardia

A Asthma exacerbation
   R/O myocardial infarction

P Admit to ICU for treatment and cardiac assessment

Questions about Medical Record 4-2

1. 📖 Below are medical terms used in this record that you have not yet encountered in the text. Underline each term where it appears in the record and, using a medical dictionary, define them below.

   asthma _____

   diaphoretic _____

   expiratory _____

   wheezes _____

   (sinus) tachycardia _____

2. What is the sex of this patient?

    a. male
    b. female

3. How often may the patient inhale the Proventil?

    a. as desired
    b. twice a day
    c. three times a day
    d. four times a day

4. How is the Singulair taken?

    a. one tablet by mouth every night
    b. 10 milligrams inhaled once a day
    c. one tablet by mouth at bedtime if needed
    d. one tablet every other night

5. What is noted about the patient's skin?

    a. it is dry
    b. it is cold
    c. it is sweaty
    d. it is itching

6. What did the electrocardiogram (ECG) of the heart reveal?

    a. high blood pressure
    b. wheezes
    c. rapid contractions of the heart
    d. a heart murmur

7. Why is the patient being admitted to the hospital?

    a. to treat the asthma and the heart attack
    b. to treat the asthma and find out if the patient has had a heart attack
    c. to treat the asthma, tachycardia, and heart attack
    d. to treat the asthma and heart murmur

8. What is noted about the patient's breathing?

    a. normal
    b. slow
    c. shallow
    d. only able to breathe in an upright position

9. What does "exacerbation" refer to in this record?

    a. a period in which symptoms and signs stop
    b. gradual deterioration of normal cells and body functions
    c. a condition that develops slowly and persists over a period of time
    d. an aggravation of symptoms

Answers to Examine Your Understanding

1. an/emia
   <u>without</u> / <u>blood condition</u>
       P   S

2. arthr/algia
   <u>joint</u> / <u>pain</u>
      R   S

3. hydro/cele
   <u>water</u> / <u>pouching or hernia</u>
      CF   S

4. erythro/cyto/penia
   <u>red</u> / <u>cell</u> / <u>abnormal reduction</u>
   CF   CF   S

5. hepat/itis
   <u>liver</u> / <u>inflammation</u>
      R   S

6. endo/metri/osis
   <u>within</u> / <u>uterus</u> / <u>condition or increase</u>
       P   R   S

7. dys/plas/ia
   <u>painful, difficult, or faulty</u> / <u>formation</u> / <u>condition of</u>
                P   R   S

8. melan/oma
   <u>black</u> / <u>tumor</u>
      R   S

9. ortho/pnea
   <u>straight, normal, or correct</u> / <u>breathing</u>
                P   S

10. thrombo/phleb/itis
    <u>clot</u> / <u>vein</u> / <u>inflammation</u>
      CF   R   S

11. schizo/phren/ia
    <u>split</u> / <u>mind (or diaphragm)</u> / <u>condition of</u>
       CF   R   S

12. iatro/genic
    <u>treatment</u> / <u>pertaining to origin</u>
        CF   S

13. chondro/malacia
    <u>cartilage</u> / <u>softening</u>
        CF   S

14. broncho/spasm
    <u>bronchus (airway)</u> / <u>involuntary contraction</u>
           CF   S

15. meta/stasis
    <u>beyond, after, or change</u> / <u>stop or stand</u>
                 P   S

16. gastr/algia
    <u>stomach</u> / <u>pain</u>
       R   S

17. spleno/megaly
    <u>spleen</u> / <u>enlargement</u>
       CF   S

18. lymph/adeno/path/y
    <u>clear fluid</u> / <u>gland</u> / <u>disease</u> / <u>condition or process of</u>
       R   CF   R   S

19. cephal/odynia
    <u>head</u> / <u>pain</u>
      R   S

20. osteo/sarc/oma
    <u>bone</u> / <u>flesh</u> / <u>tumor</u>
      CF   R   S

21. hyper/thyroid/ism
    <u>above or excessive</u> / <u>thyroid gland (shield)</u> / <u>condition of</u>
         P   R   S

22. onco/logy
    <u>tumor</u> / <u>study of</u>
      CF   S

23. blepharo/ptosis
    <u>eyelid</u> / <u>falling or downward displacement</u>
      CF   S

24. adeno/carcin/oma
    <u>gland</u> / <u>cancer</u> / <u>tumor</u>
      CF   R   S

25. varico/cele
    <u>swollen, twisted vein</u> / <u>pouching or hernia</u>
        CF   S

26. a/meno/rrhea
    <u>without</u> / <u>month (menstruation)</u> / <u>discharge</u>
       P   CF   S

27. a/troph/ic
    <u>without</u> / <u>nourishment or development</u> / <u>pertaining to</u>
       P   R   S

28. cysto/cele
    <u>bladder or sac</u> / <u>pouching or hernia</u>
       CF   S

29. brady/pnea
    <u>slow</u> / <u>breathing</u>
      P   S

30. hypo/thyroid/ism
    <u>below or deficient</u> / <u>thyroid gland (shield)</u> / <u>condition of</u>
        P   R   S

31. l
32. k
33. m
34. n
35. i
36. j
37. f
38. e
39. o
40. d
41. h
42. c
43. a
44. g
45. b
46. d
47. a
48. c
49. a
50. d
51. b
52. a
53. c
54. b
55. rhin/o
56. -algia
57. spondyl/o
58. phleb/o
59. otitis
60. rhinitis
61. pharyngitis
62. arthritis
63. hepatomegaly
64. rhinorrhea
65. dysmenorrhea
66. blepharoptosis
67. nephroptosis
68. arthralgia or arthrodynia
69. cephalalgia or cephalodynia
70. gastralgia or gastrodynia
71. metrorrhagia
72. otorrhagia
73. lithiasis
74. g
75. f
76. d
77. b
78. a
79. c
80. e
81. softening
82. involuntary contraction
83. seizure
84. formation or presence of
85. pertaining to
86. d
87. e
88. g
89. a
90. j
91. i
92. b
93. c
94. f
95. h
96. o
97. m
98. n
99. l
100. k

ANSWERS TO MEDICAL RECORD EXERCISE 4-1

1. See medical dictionary/resources.
2. d
3. a
4. b
5. b
6. d

ANSWERS TO MEDICAL RECORD EXERCISE 4-2

1. See medical dictionary.
2. a
3. d
4. a
5. c
6. c
7. b
8. d
9. d

CHAPTER **5**

DIAGNOSTIC TESTS AND PROCEDURES

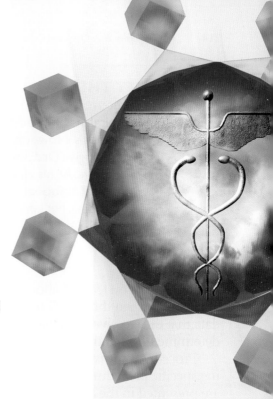

OBJECTIVES

☐ Identify common suffixes related to diagnostic tests and procedures.

☐ Define common terms related to diagnostic tests and procedures using term structure analysis.

☐ Recognize the types of diagnostic imaging modalities.

☐ Identify common clinical laboratory tests.

CHECKLIST   LOCATION

CHECKLIST	LOCATION
☐ Complete Chapter 5 Self-Instruction and Programmed Review sections	pages 214–251
☐ Review the Flash Cards related to Chapter 5	FC
☐ Complete the Chapter 5 Examine Your Understanding exercises	pages 254–257
☐ Complete Medical Record Exercises 5-1, 5-2, and 5-3	pages 258–265
☐ Practice saying the Chapter 5 terms out loud with the Audio Pronunciation Glossary on the Student Resource CD-ROM	CD-ROM
☐ Complete the Chapter 5 Interactive Exercises on the Student Resource CD-ROM	CD-ROM
☐ Take the Chapter 5 Quiz on the Student Resource CD-ROM	CD-ROM
☐ When you receive 70% or higher on the Quiz, move on to Chapter 6	page 269

MEET THE PATIENT   Henry Lin is a 69-year-old male who has been recovering at home after hospitalization for leukemia. During his hospital stay, he had a bone marrow biopsy, which confirmed the diagnosis. Now, it is important for Mr. Lin to regularly see an oncologist, Dr. Ellison, to ensure that his transfusion therapy is effective. At his appointments, he typically has his blood tested by a **Clinical Laboratory Technologist**, and the results are copied to Dr. Spaulding, Mr. Lin's primary care physician (see **Medical Record Exercise 5-3**).

In Chapter 4, you learned about subjective symptoms and objective signs that patients report and exhibit when they are ill or injured. Physicians supplement that information with the data that they receive from diagnostic tests and procedures in order to make diagnoses and determine how treatment is progressing. This chapter focuses on those tests and procedures.

Procedural suffixes are word endings used in terms that describe methods of performing specific procedures or studies, such as medical tests. The most common of these suffixes are presented in the Self-Instruction sections of this chapter. They are joined by selected prefixes and combining forms to build terms related to diagnostic tests and procedures.

Core Term Components

The suffixes and prefixes used in this chapter are listed below. Pertinent combining forms will be added as you progress through programmed learning segments related to each suffix. Study these core components first, and add those related to each of the suffixes as you work through the chapter.

SUFFIX	MEANING	FLASH CARD ID
-al, -eal	pertaining to	S-1
-gram	record	S-11
-graph	instrument for recording	S-12
-graphy	process of recording	S-13
-ist	one who specializes in	S-17
-logy	study of	S-22
-logist	one who specializes in the study or treatment of	S-21
-meter	instrument for measuring	S-26
-metry	process of measuring	S-27
-opsy	process of viewing	S-29
-scope	instrument for examination	S-43
-scopy	process of examination	S-44

PREFIX	MEANING	FLASH CARD ID
auto-	self	P-8
bi-	two or both	P-27
endo-	within	P-14
ex-	out or away	P-13
poly-	many	P-34
trans-	across or through	P-11
ultra-	beyond or excessive	P-39

SELF-INSTRUCTION: -gram (record)

Add the following combining forms to your study of -gram before starting the Programmed Review below.

COMBINING FORM	MEANING	FLASH CARD ID
abdomin/o	abdomen	CF-1
angi/o	vessel	CF-5
arteri/o	artery	
cardi/o	heart	CF-11
electr/o	electricity	
encephal/o	entire brain	CF-22
esophag/o	esophagus	
mamm/o	breast	CF-38
my/o	muscle	CF-40
rect/o	rectum	
son/o	sound	
vagin/o	vagina	
ven/o	vein	CF-68

PROGRAMMED REVIEW: -gram (record)

ANSWERS	REVIEW
record	**5.1** The suffix -gram, meaning _____, is commonly used in terms referring to a document that displays or provides the details of a diagnostic test or procedure. Linked to electr/o, the combining form
electricity	meaning _____, and cardi/o, the

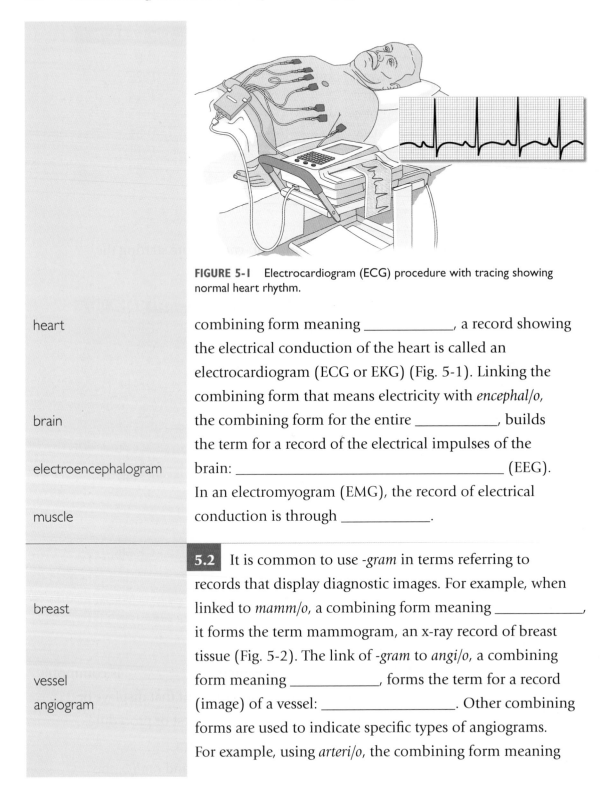

FIGURE 5-1   Electrocardiogram (ECG) procedure with tracing showing normal heart rhythm.

heart

combining form meaning _____, a record showing the electrical conduction of the heart is called an electrocardiogram (ECG or EKG) (Fig. 5-1). Linking the combining form that means electricity with *encephal/o*,

brain

the combining form for the entire _____, builds the term for a record of the electrical impulses of the

electroencephalogram

brain: _____ (EEG). In an electromyogram (EMG), the record of electrical

muscle

conduction is through _____.

5.2   It is common to use *-gram* in terms referring to records that display diagnostic images. For example, when

breast

linked to *mamm/o*, a combining form meaning _____, it forms the term mammogram, an x-ray record of breast tissue (Fig. 5-2). The link of *-gram* to *angi/o*, a combining

vessel

form meaning _____, forms the term for a record

angiogram

(image) of a vessel: _____. Other combining forms are used to indicate specific types of angiograms. For example, using *arteri/o*, the combining form meaning

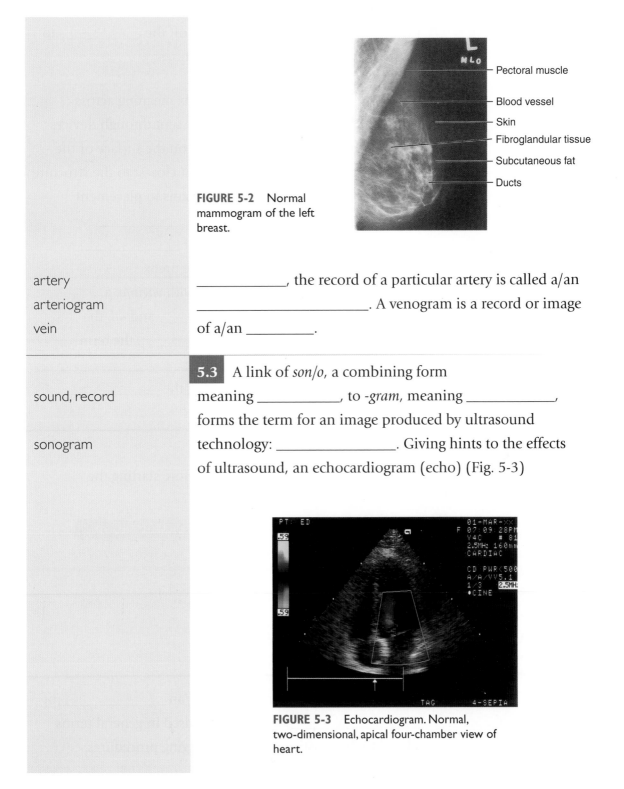

- Pectoral muscle
- Blood vessel
- Skin
- Fibroglandular tissue
- Subcutaneous fat
- Ducts

FIGURE 5-2   Normal mammogram of the left breast.

artery

arteriogram

vein

_____ , the record of a particular artery is called a/an _____. A venogram is a record or image of a/an _____ .

sound, record

sonogram

5.3   A link of *son/o*, a combining form meaning _____ , to -*gram*, meaning _____ , forms the term for an image produced by ultrasound technology: _____. Giving hints to the effects of ultrasound, an echocardiogram (echo) (Fig. 5-3)

FIGURE 5-3   Echocardiogram. Normal, two-dimensional, apical four-chamber view of heart.

heart	provides images of sound bouncing off the _____ to provide a motion picture of its structures.
through	**5.4** You'll recall that *trans-* is a prefix meaning across or _____. Sound waves are sent through devices called transducers, which are placed on the surface of the body or within a cavity for placement closest to the structure to be scanned. Transesophageal pertains to placement
through, esophagus	across or _____ the _____.
through	Transabdominal pertains to across or _____
abdomen	the _____. Using *endo-*, the prefix
within	meaning _____, combined with *vagin/o*, a
vagina	combining form meaning _____, and *-al*, the
pertaining to	suffix meaning _____ ____, the term
endovaginal	that describes within the vagina is _____.
within, rectum	Endorectal pertains to _____ the _____.

SELF-INSTRUCTION: *-graphy* (process of recording)

Add the following combining forms to your study of *-graphy* before starting the Programmed Review below.

COMBINING FORM	MEANING	FLASH CARD ID
radi/o	ray or radiation	
somn/o	sleep	
tom/o	to cut	

PROGRAMMED REVIEW: *-graphy* (process of recording)

ANSWERS	REVIEW
process	**5.5** *-graphy*, the suffix referring to a/an _____ of
recording	_____, is commonly used in general terms related to diagnostic testing and imaging procedures.

ray	Linked to *radi/o*, meaning _____ or radiation, the term to describe the process of recording x-ray images
radiography	is _____. A link of *tom/o*, a combining
cut	form meaning to _____, with *-graphy*, forms
tomography	_____, the term used to describe the x-ray process of making cross-sectional images of the body. Computed tomography (CT) describes the process of converting the tomographic x-ray slices into a three-dimensional image. Later in the chapter, you will see examples of these types of diagnostic images.

vessel	**5.6** By linking *angi/o*, the combining form meaning _____, to *-graphy*, we form the general term referring to the process of recording images of
angiography	blood vessels: _____.

sound	**5.7** When *-graphy* is linked to *son/o*, the combining form meaning _____, it forms the term describing the
recording	process of _____ sound wave
sonography	images: _____. The addition of *ultra-*,
prefix, beyond	the _____ meaning _____
excessive	or _____, forms the synonym for
ultrasonography	sonography: _____.

many	**5.8** *poly-*, the prefix meaning _____, is linked to
sleep	*somn/o*, the combining form meaning _____, in the term for the process of recording and evaluating
polysomnography	sleep: _____ (Fig. 5-4).

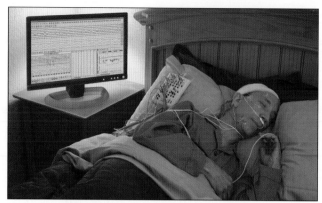

FIGURE 5-4   Polysomnography (PSG).

SELF-INSTRUCTION: -graph (instrument for recording)

Review the combining forms introduced earlier in the chapter, which also relate to the suffix -*graph*, before starting the Programmed Review below.

PROGRAMMED REVIEW: -graph (instrument for recording)

ANSWERS	REVIEW
	5.9 You'll recall that an electrocardiogram (ECG or EKG)
record	is a/an _____ of the electrical conduction
heart	of the _____. Replacing the suffix -*gram* in this term
instrument	with -*graph*, the suffix meaning _____
recording	for _____, forms the name of the
	instrument (or machine) used to produce an
electrocardiograph	ECG: _____.
	The instrument used to produce an electromyogram
electromyograph	is therefore called a/an _____,
	and the instrument that records electric currents
	generated by the brain is called
electroencephalograph	a/an _____.
record	**5.10** A sonogram is a/an _____ of
sound	_____ (ultrasound). The instrument for recording
sonograph	sound (ultrasound) is called a/an _____.

ON CLOSER INSPECTION   Radiograph

As you have learned, the suffix *-graph* is used in terms that refer to an instrument for recording. However, an exception to this rule occurs in radiology: *-graph* is the preferred suffix used to refer to the x-ray image itself, or the radiograph. A radiograph is taken by a radiologic technologist (also known as radiographer) and interpreted or read by a radiologist, a physician specializing in the study of radiology. (See ✚ Meet the Radiologic Technologist in Chapter 3.)

 Vital Statistics   METHODS OF PHYSICAL EXAMINATION

A physician's physical examination is a critical aspect of the recognition, diagnosis, and treatment of injury and illness. The physical examination is performed using the following methods:

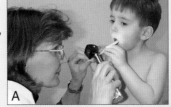
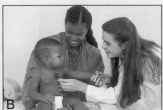
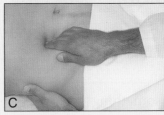
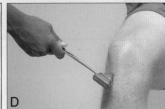
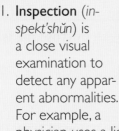

1. **Inspection** (*in-spekt'shŭn*) is a close visual examination to detect any apparent abnormalities. For example, a physician uses a light source to inspect a patient's mouth and throat (photo A).

2. **Auscultation** (*aws-kŭl-tā'shŭn*), a Greek word meaning "to listen," involves listening to the sounds within the body, typically with the aid of a stethoscope (photo B). Physicians commonly auscultate the chest for heart and lung sounds.

3. **Palpation** (*pal-pā'shŭn*) stems from a Latin word meaning "to touch" and refers to an examination with the hands to feel tissues and organs of the body (photo C).

4. **Percussion** (*pĕr-kŭsh'ŭn*) is a method of tapping over the body to elicit vibrations and sounds in order to estimate the size, border, or fluid content of a cavity, such as the chest, or using a percussion hammer to elicit deep tendon reflexes (DTRs) (photo D).

Rx for Success

*Don't confuse the term **palpation** (a method of physical examination using the hands to feel tissues and organs of the body) with **palpitation** (the subjective feeling of pounding, skipping, or racing heartbeats).*

SELF-INSTRUCTION: -scope (instrument for examination)

Add the following combining forms to your study of -*scope* before starting the Programmed Review below.

COMBINING FORM	MEANING	FLASH CARD ID
colon/o	colon (large intestine)	
ophthalm/o	eye	
ot/o	ear	CF-8
steth/o	chest	CF-63

PROGRAMMED REVIEW: -scope (instrument for examination)

ANSWERS	REVIEW
-scope instrument, examination small	**5.11** The suffix used to name an instrument for examination is _____. A microscope is a/an _____ for _____ of something _____.
eye ophthalmoscope ear chest stethoscope	**5.12** -*scope* is included in the name of several instruments used in performing physical examination (see 🔵 Vital Statistics: Methods of Physical Examination). When linked to *ophthalm/o,* a combining form meaning _____, the instrument used to examine the interior of the eye is called a/an _____. An otoscope is used to examine the _____. Using *steth/o,* a combining form for _____, the instrument for examination of the chest is called a/an _____. The stethoscope is placed on the chest in order to hear heart and lung sounds.

prefix, within	**5.13** *endo-*, the _____ meaning _____, combined with *-scope*, forms the term for any instrument used to examine within the body, particularly the interior
endoscope	of a tubular or hollow organ: _____. Endoscopes are named for the body part or cavity they examine and are rigid or flexible depending on the extent of the examination and the need to maneuver within a cavity. Ophthalmoscopes and otoscopes are examples of rigid endoscopes. A colonoscope is an example of a flexible endoscope used to examine the
colon	interior of the _____.

Rx for Success

You'll recall from Chapter 1 that the consonants "ph" have an "f" sound. This holds true for the pronunciation of ophthalmoscope (of-thal'mŏ-skōp). Make a note so you will pronounce and spell this term with confidence.

SELF-INSTRUCTION: -scopy (process of examination)

Add the following combining forms to your study of *-scopy* before starting the Programmed Review.

COMBINING FORM	MEANING	FLASH CARD ID
an/o	anus	
arthr/o	joint	CF-6
bronch/o	bronchus (airway)	
cyst/o, vesic/o	bladder or sac	CF-18
duoden/o	duodenum	
gastr/o	stomach	CF-26
lapar/o	abdomen	CF-1
nas/o	nose	CF-43
pharyng/o	pharynx or throat	
proct/o	rectum and anus	CF-52
sigmoid/o	sigmoid colon	

MEET THE PATIENT   Mr. Antonio Villata is an accountant whose employer, The Hospital Corporation, values preventive medicine and recognizes its cost savings to individuals and the company itself. So each year, Mr. Villata sees Dr. Spaulding for a comprehensive physical examination as part of his wellness program. This year, while performing a routine sigmoidoscopic exam, she found a polyp in Mr. Villata's intestine, which necessitated a referral to Dr. Roger Blain, a gastro-enterologist, for further evaluation. Mr. Villata subsequently underwent a colonoscopy with biopsy. This procedure was performed by Dr. Blain, who dictated a report describing each step. This report was later typed by a **Medical Transcriptionist** into the format of an Endoscopy Laboratory Report, which became part of Mr. Villata's health care record. You will see this report later in the chapter as **Medical Record Exercise 5-2**.

PROGRAMMED REVIEW: -scopy (process of examination)

ANSWERS	REVIEW
	5.14 You'll recall that an endoscope is any instrument
within	used to examine _____ the body, particularly the
	interior of a tubular or hollow organ. Using -scopy, the
process, examination	suffix meaning _____ of _____,
	the general term that describes the process of examination
endoscopy	within the body is _____. The name for
	each endoscopic procedure corresponds to the part of the
	body that is examined. For example, an ophthalmoscope is
eye	an instrument used to examine the interior of the _____,
	and the process of examination of the interior of the eye is
ophthalmoscopy	called _____. ot/o is a combining
ear	form meaning _____, and the process of examination of
otoscopy	the ear canal is therefore called _____.
	Nasopharyngoscopy describes the process of examining

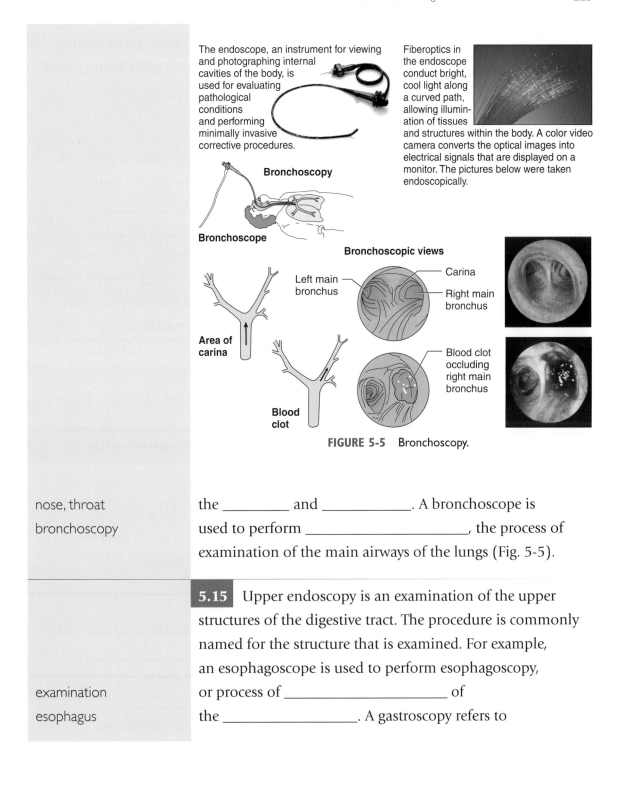

The endoscope, an instrument for viewing and photographing internal cavities of the body, is used for evaluating pathological conditions and performing minimally invasive corrective procedures.

Fiberoptics in the endoscope conduct bright, cool light along a curved path, allowing illumination of tissues and structures within the body. A color video camera converts the optical images into electrical signals that are displayed on a monitor. The pictures below were taken endoscopically.

Bronchoscopy

Bronchoscope

Bronchoscopic views

Carina

Left main bronchus

Right main bronchus

Area of carina

Blood clot occluding right main bronchus

Blood clot

FIGURE 5-5   Bronchoscopy.

nose, throat	the _____ and _____. A bronchoscope is
bronchoscopy	used to perform _____, the process of examination of the main airways of the lungs (Fig. 5-5).

5.15 Upper endoscopy is an examination of the upper structures of the digestive tract. The procedure is commonly named for the structure that is examined. For example, an esophagoscope is used to perform esophagoscopy,

examination

esophagus

or process of _____ of the _____. A gastroscopy refers to

stomach	examination of the _____. An esophagogastro-duodenoscopy (EGD) describes the process of examination
esophagus, stomach	of the _____, _____, and
duodenum	_____.
	5.16 Lower endoscopy is the process of examination of the anus, rectum, and colon. Anoscopy involves using
anoscope, anus	a/an _____ to examine the _____.
rectum	A proctoscope is used to examine the _____
anus	and _____. The process of examination of the rectum
proctoscopy	and anus is called _____. The "S"-shaped curve of the lower part of the colon is the sigmoid colon. Using *sigmoid/o*, the combining form meaning
sigmoid colon	_____ _____, the instrument used to examine the sigmoid colon is called a/an
sigmoidoscope	_____. The process of examination
sigmoidoscopy	of the sigmoid colon is called _____. Colonoscopy describes the process of examining the
colon	entire _____.
	5.17 *cyst/o* and *vesic/o* are combining forms
bladder	meaning _____ or sac. Using *cyst/o*, the term for the process of examination of the bladder
cystoscopy	is _____.
	5.18 Some examinations require surgical incisions, such
examination	as laparoscopy, or the process of _____ of
abdomen, process	the _____, and arthroscopy, the _____
examination, joint	of _____ of a/an _____. (Laparoscopic and arthroscopic surgery are covered in Chapter 6.)

Health Care Professionals MEET THE MEDICAL TRANSCRIPTIONIST

You have been exposed to many medical records in this text. Who creates these records? By definition, a medical transcriptionist (MT) is a person who converts dictated medical information into a written text document that can be printed or retained as an electronic record of a patient's medical care. Medical transcriptionists must comply with specific standards that apply to the style of medical records and to the legal and ethical requirements for keeping patient information confidential. Transcriptionists work in settings such as hospitals and outpatient clinics, as well as for private transcription services or as independent contractors out of their homes.

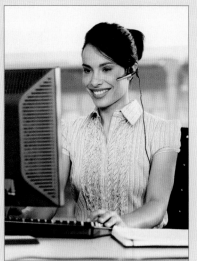

A more detailed description of medical transcription as a health care career can be found on the Student Resource CD-ROM and at the companion website at www.thePoint.lww.com/WillisQC.

SELF-INSTRUCTION: *-meter* (instrument for measuring)

Add the following combining forms to your study of *-meter* before starting the Programmed Review below.

COMBINING FORM	MEANING	FLASH CARD ID
audi/o	hearing	
spir/o	breathing	CF-59
therm/o	heat	CF-62

PROGRAMMED REVIEW: *-meter* (instrument for measuring)

ANSWERS	REVIEW
	5.19 The suffix referring to an instrument for measuring
-meter	is _____. You'll recall that *therm/o* is a combining
heat	form meaning _____. Combined with *-meter*, the
instrument	suffix meaning _____

measuring thermometer	for _____, the instrument used to measure heat (temperature) is a/an _____.
hearing audiometer	**5.20** Using *audi/o*, a combining form meaning _____, the instrument for measuring hearing is called a/an _____.
breathing spirometer	**5.21** You'll remember that *-pnea* is the suffix meaning breathing. *spir/o*, the combining form meaning _____, is linked to *-meter* in the term used to name an instrument for measuring breathing: _____.

SELF-INSTRUCTION: *-metry* (process of measuring)

Add the following combining forms to your study of *-metry* before starting the Programmed Review below.

COMBINING FORM	MEANING	FLASH CARD ID
opt/o	eye	
pulmon/o	lung	CF-54

PROGRAMMED REVIEW: *-metry* (process of measuring)

ANSWERS	REVIEW
instrument, measuring process of -metry	**5.22** You'll recall that *-meter* is the suffix meaning _____ for _____. The link of *-y*, a simple suffix meaning _____ ____, with *-meter* forms the compound suffix referring to the process of measuring: _____.
eye	**5.23** *opt/o* is a combining form meaning _____. A doctor of optometry is therefore a specialist in

process, measuring	the _____ of _____ the eye. Optometrists measure the eye and prescribe lenses to correct vision, as well as treat eye conditions. *ophthalm/o,*
eye	another combining form meaning _____, is used to name the medical doctor (MD) who performs optometric procedures as well as medical and surgical treatment of
ophthalmo	the eye: _____logist.

	5.24 Using *audi/o,* a combining form meaning
hearing	_____, the process of measuring hearing is
audiometry	_____. The specialist who performs
audio	audiometry is called a/an _____logist.

	5.25 You'll recall that a spirometer is an instrument to
breathing	measure _____. The process of measuring
spirometry	breathing is therefore called _____ (Fig. 5-6). Spirometry is part of pulmonary function testing
lung	(*pulmon/o* is the combining form meaning _____, and
pertaining	-*ary* is an adjective ending that means _____
to	____). The combining form meaning lung is used to name

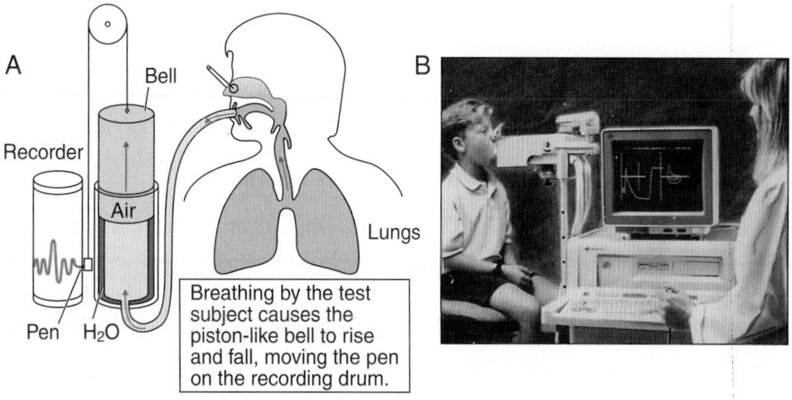

A
Bell
Recorder
Air
Pen   H₂O

Breathing by the test subject causes the piston-like bell to rise and fall, moving the pen on the recording drum.

Lungs

B

FIGURE 5-6   **A.** Principles of spirometry. **B.** Spirometry procedure.

| pulmono | the physician who analyzes pulmonary function studies in the diagnosis and treatment of lung conditions: _____logist. |

SELF-INSTRUCTION: -opsy (process of viewing)

Add the following combining forms to your study of -opsy before starting the Programmed Review below.

COMBINING FORM	MEANING	FLASH CARD ID
bi/o	life	
cis/o	to cut	
nephr/o, ren/o	kidney	CF-45
path/o	disease	CF-46

PROGRAMMED REVIEW: -opsy (process of viewing)

ANSWERS	REVIEW
	5.26 Formed by a link of *op/o*, a combining form meaning eye, with *-y*, the simple suffix meaning condition
process of	or _____ ____, the compound suffix that means
-opsy	process of viewing is _____. You'll recall that *bi/o* is
life	the combining form meaning _____. When *bi/o* is
biopsy	combined with *-opsy*, it forms the term _____, referring to the process of viewing life by removal of suspicious tissue from living patients for pathological
disease	analysis. *path/o* is a combining form meaning _____
	and *-logist* is a suffix referring to one who specializes in
study of	the _____ ____. A pathologist is a physician who
	performs biopsy and other procedures in the study of
disease	_____.

cut

out

ex

5.27 There are several types of biopsy (Bx) (Fig. 5-7). You'll recall that *cis/o* means to _____. An incisional biopsy is one in which a cut is made into an area of suspicious tissue to remove a small portion for examination. *ex-*, the prefix meaning _____, is used to name the type of biopsy in which the entire lesion (such as a polyp) is removed intact: ____cisional Bx. An endoscopic biopsy

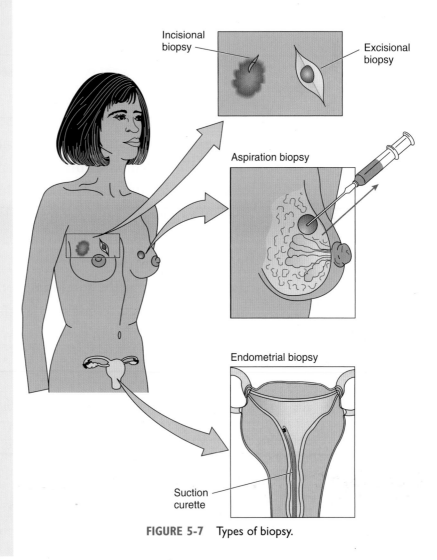

Incisional biopsy

Excisional biopsy

Aspiration biopsy

Endometrial biopsy

Suction curette

FIGURE 5-7   Types of biopsy.

within biopsy	is one that is performed during an examination _____ a body cavity. Some biopsies are obtained using a needle to draw out or aspirate tissue. This type is simply called a needle _____.
kidney kidney biopsy	**5.28** Additional terms are used to identify the tissue that is removed for biopsy (Bx). For example, *nephr/o* and *ren/o* are combining forms meaning _____. Renal Bx is commonly used to refer to a/an _____ _____.
self, -opsy pathologist	**5.29** Autopsy, a term referring to "seeing with one's own eyes," is formed by the combination of *auto-*, a prefix meaning _____, with _____, the suffix meaning process of viewing. Autopsy is the examination of a body after death to determine the condition of tissues and organs and identify the disease or injury that may have been the cause of death. Autopsy, as well as biopsy, is performed by a physician who specializes in the study of disease, known as a/an _____ (formed by linking the combining form for disease with the suffix that refers to one who specializes in the study of).

Rx for Success

How do you keep bi- *and* bi/o *straight? Memorize the fact that* bi- *is a prefix meaning two or both, and* bi/o *is a combining form meaning life. Biopsy refers to viewing life or living tissue, and bilateral refers to both sides.*

Common Diagnostic Tests and Procedures

Diagnostic tests and procedures are an integral part of patient care, so it is essential for health care professionals to be familiar with those that are most common, as well as the types of technology used to produce them.

SELF-INSTRUCTION: Diagnostic Imaging

Methods of diagnostic imaging have rapidly expanded since Wilhelm Roentgen discovered x-rays in 1895. By using x-rays, physicians and scientists could see through the body to produce images of the skeleton and other body structures. However, the radiation used to produce the x-rays was found to be "ionizing," that is, a process that changes the electrical charge of atoms and may affect body cells. Overexposure to ionizing radiation was found to have harmful side effects, such as cancer. However, over the years, researchers and scientists have found new ways to produce images that require significantly lower doses of radiation and minimize the risk to the patient.

Further advancement has led to the discovery and use of other imaging modalities (or techniques) that fall under the umbrella of the medical specialty known as radiology. Common ionizing modalities include: radiography (x-ray), computed tomography (CT), and nuclear medicine. Common nonionizing modalities that present no apparent risk include magnetic resonance imaging (MRI) and sonography, or ultrasound (U/S or US).

Radiography

Radiography (x-ray) is an imaging modality that uses x-rays (ionizing radiation) to produce images of the body's anatomy for the diagnosis of a condition or impairment. An image is created when a small amount of radiation is passed through the body to expose a sensitive film. The image is called a radiograph (Fig. 5-8).

Computed Tomography

Computed tomography (CT), also known as computed axial tomography (CAT), is a radiologic procedure that uses a machine, called a scanner, to examine a body site by taking a series of cross-sectional (tomographic) x-ray films in a full circle rotation. A computer then calculates and converts the rates of absorption and density of the x-rays into a three-dimensional picture on a screen (Fig. 5-9).

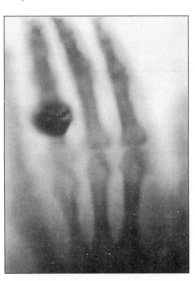

FIGURE 5-8   First published x-ray record, showing the hand and signet ring of Professor Roentgen's wife, produced on December 22, 1895.

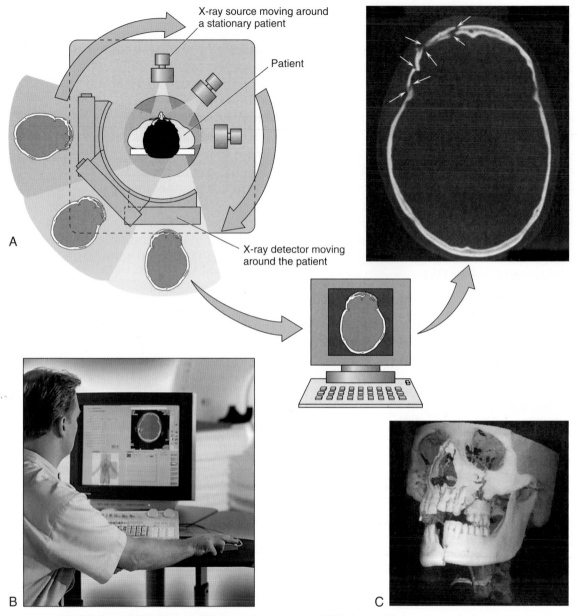

FIGURE 5-9   **A.** Principles of computed tomography (CT). *Inset,* CT showing multiple open fractures (arrows) of skull. **B.** CT imaging process. **C.** Ninety-nine tomographic images were compiled in this three-dimensional CT reconstruction of a skull showing traumatic injury to facial bones suffered as the result of a motor vehicle accident (MVA).

Nuclear Medicine Imaging

Nuclear medicine imaging, or radionuclide organ imaging, uses an injected or ingested radioactive isotope (also called radionuclide), which is a chemical that has been "tagged" with radioactive compounds that emit gamma rays. A gamma camera detects and produces an image of the distribution of the gamma rays in the body. This technique is useful in determining the size, shape, location, and function of body organs, such as the brain, lungs, bones, and heart. The most common techniques used to produce radionuclide organ images are SPECT (single photon emission computed tomography) and PET (positron emission tomography) (Fig. 5-10).

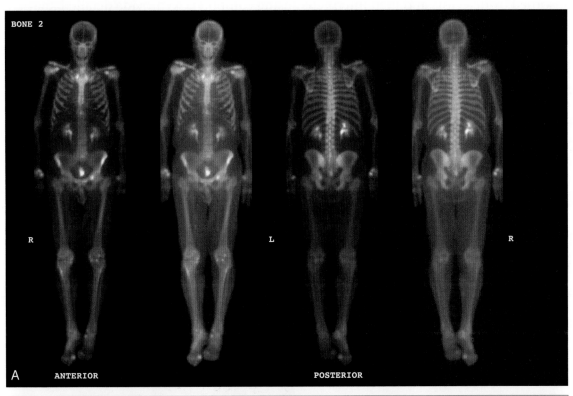

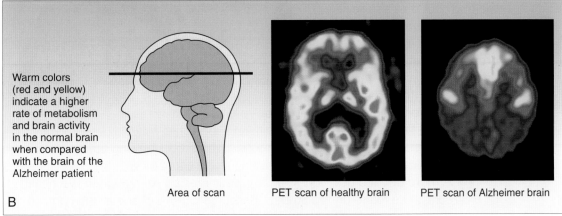

Warm colors (red and yellow) indicate a higher rate of metabolism and brain activity in the normal brain when compared with the brain of the Alzheimer patient

Area of scan   PET scan of healthy brain   PET scan of Alzheimer brain

FIGURE 5-10   Nuclear medicine imaging (radionuclide organ imaging). **A.** SPECT whole-body bone scan. **B.** Positron emission tomography (PET) scans of brain.

Magnetic Resonance Imaging

Magnetic resonance imaging (MRI) is a nonionizing imaging technique that uses magnetic fields and radiofrequency waves to visualize anatomic structures within the body. A large magnet surrounds the patient as a scanner subjects the body to a radio signal that temporarily alters the alignment of the hydrogen atoms in the patient's tissue. As the radio wave signal is turned off, the atoms realign, and the energy produced is absorbed by detectors and then interpreted using computers to provide detailed anatomic images of the body part. This modality is particularly useful in examining soft tissues, joints, and the brain and spinal cord (Fig. 5-11).

Sonography

Sonography, which is also known as diagnostic ultrasound (U/S or US), uses high-frequency sound waves (ultrasound) to visualize body tissues. Ultrasound waves sent through a scanning device, called a transducer, are reflected off structures within the body and then analyzed by a computer to produce moving images on a monitor. Sonography is used to examine many parts of the body, including the abdomen, male and female reproductive organs, thyroid and parathyroid glands, and the cardiovascular system (Fig. 5-12).

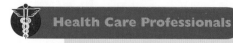 **Health Care Professionals**   MEET THE DIAGNOSTIC MEDICAL SONOGRAPHER

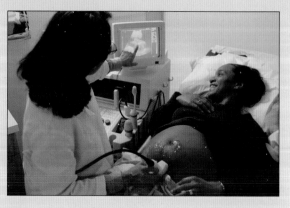

Diagnostic medical sonographers are imaging professionals who use ultrasound waves, which are nonradiating and noninvasive, to see into the human body. Sonographers not only scan parts of the body, but they also review the patient's medical record, perform a patient assessment, prepare the patient for the exam, provide a preliminary technical report to the interpreting physician, surgeon, or radiologist, and follow up to ensure quality results. Sonography is an umbrella field that covers several different specialties, including general, OB/GYN, and cardiac sonographers, and vascular technologists, among others. Each area of specialization requires specific training and credentialing.

A more detailed description of diagnostic medical sonographer as a health care career can be found on the Student Resource CD-ROM and at the companion website at www.thePoint.lww.com/WillisQC.

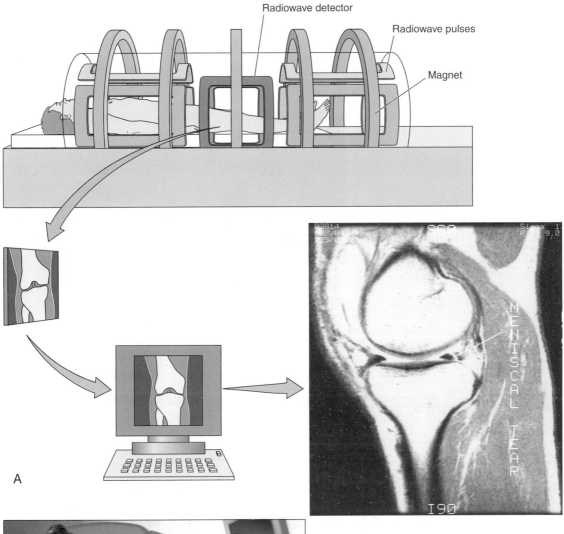

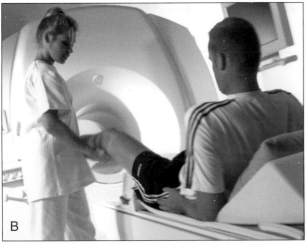

FIGURE 5-11   A. Principles of magnetic resonance imagine (MRI). Patient is positioned within a magnetic field as radiowave signals are conducted through the selected body part. Energy is absorbed by tissues and then released. A computer processes the released energy and formulates the image. *Inset,* MRI of knee (lateral view) identifying a torn meniscus. **B.** MRI unit.

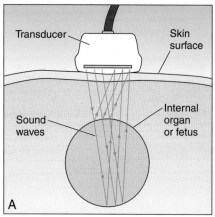

Transducer — Skin surface
Sound waves — Internal organ or fetus
A

Energy in the form of sound waves is reflected off internal organs, or off the fetus during pregnancy, and transformed into an image on a TV-type monitor.

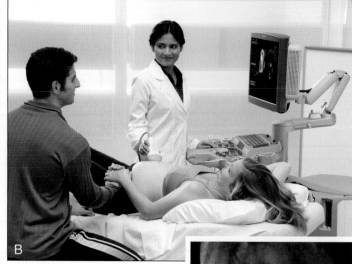

B

C

FIGURE 5-12   **A.** Principles of sonography. **B.** Obstetrical sonography. **C.** Three-dimensional sonogram of fetus "waking up."

Use of Contrast

Some imaging procedures require the internal administration of a contrast medium to enhance the visualization of anatomic structures. There are many different kinds of contrast media, including barium, iodinated compounds, gasses (such as air or carbon dioxide), and other chemicals known to increase visual clarity. Depending on the medium, it may be injected, swallowed, or introduced through an enema or catheter (Fig. 5-13).

PROGRAMMED REVIEW: Diagnostic Imaging

ANSWERS	REVIEW
ionizing	**5.30** The diagnostic modality using _____ radiation (x-rays) to produce images of the body's
radiology	anatomy is called _____. This term is

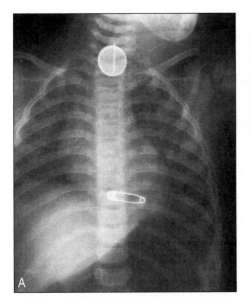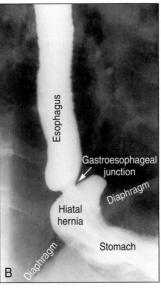

FIGURE 5-13 Examples of x-ray images taken with and without contrast. **A.** Plain radiograph (without contrast) showing two impacted foreign bodies in a child, aged 2.5 years. This child ingested a safety pin and an ornamental pin. Endoscopic removal was required. **B.** Upper gastrointestinal radiograph showing hiatal hernia visualized by contrast.

study of radiograph radiologic technologist radiologist cancer	derived from the combining form *radi/o*, meaning x-ray (radiation), and the suffix *-logy*, meaning _____ ____. The x-ray image is called a/an _____. It is taken by a radiographer or _____ _____ and interpreted by a physician who specializes in the study of radiology, who is called a/an _____. Ionizing radiation has an effect on body tissue, and overexposure can have harmful side effects such as _____.
CT cut, process of	**5.31** Computer technology was first applied to medical imaging with the development of computed tomography, abbreviated ____. *tom/o*, a combining form meaning to _____, and *-graphy*, meaning _____ ____

recording	_____, give clues to how the CT scanner operates. The scanner is used to take a series of
tomo	cross-sectional, or _____graphic, x-ray films that are
computer	converted by a/an _____ into a three-dimensional picture on a screen.

	5.32 Nuclear medicine imaging, or
radionuclide	_____ organ imaging, is another
ionizing	modality using _____ radiation. The technique involves the injection or ingestion of a
isotope	radioactive _____, which emits gamma rays.
gamma	An image is produced using a/an _____ camera to detect the distribution of the gamma rays. Radionuclide organ images are useful in determining the size, shape,
function	location, and _____ of body organs. SPECT (single photon emission computed tomography)
positron emission	and PET (_____ _____
tomography	_____) are common techniques used to produce radionuclide organ images.

	5.33 There are two major nonionizing imaging
risk	modalities that have shown no apparent _____ to
magnetic resonance	patients: MRI, or _____ _____
imaging	_____, and ultrasound (U/S or US) or
sonography, magnet	_____. MRI uses a large _____
radio	and _____ waves to visualize anatomical structures
soft	within the body, especially _____ tissues. Sonography,
sound	from the combining form *son/o*, meaning _____,
recording	and *-graphy*, meaning a process of _____, uses high-frequency sound waves to produce body images.

	5.34 In order to enhance visualization of anatomic structures, some imaging procedures require the internal
contrast	administration of a/an _____ medium.
media	The plural of medium is _____. There are many different types of contrast media that are known to
visual	increase _____ clarity.

COMMON CLINICAL LABORATORY TESTS

Analyses of urine, stool, and blood specimens are recorded among the earliest efforts to understand conditions of disease. The advance of technology has led to the development of many highly sophisticated laboratory tests. It is valuable for health care professionals to recognize the most common of these and the manner in which specimens are obtained.

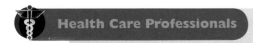 **Health Care Professionals**

MEET THE CLINICAL LABORATORY TECHNOLOGIST

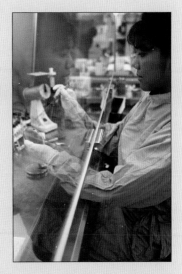

As you learned in the opening vignette concerning Dr. Spaulding's patient, Henry Lin, clinical laboratory testing plays a crucial role in the detection, diagnosis, and treatment of disease. Clinical laboratory technologists, also referred to as clinical laboratory scientists or medical technologists, perform most of these tests.

Clinical laboratory technologists perform complex chemical, biological, hematological, immunologic, microscopic, and bacteriological tests. They make cultures of body fluid and tissue samples to determine the presence of bacteria, fungi, parasites, or other microorganisms. Most clinical laboratory technologists work in hospitals, but there are also jobs in physician offices and in medical and diagnostic laboratories.

✿ A more detailed description of clinical laboratory technologist as a health care career can be found on the Student Resource CD-ROM and at the companion website at www.thePoint.lww.com/WillisQC.

SELF-INSTRUCTION: Blood Tests

Add the following terms to your study before starting the Programmed Review.

TERM	MEANING
phlebotomy, *syn.* venipuncture	incision into or puncture of a vein to withdraw blood for testing (*phleb/o* and *ven/o* are combining forms meaning vein)
blood chemistry	a test of the fluid portion of blood to measure the amounts of its chemical constituents (e.g., glucose and cholesterol)
blood sugar (BS), *syn.* blood glucose	measurement of the level of sugar, or glucose, in the blood
blood chemistry panels	specialized combinations of automated blood chemistry tests performed on a single sample of blood; used as a general screen for disease or to target specific organs or conditions (e.g., metabolic panel and lipid panel)
basic metabolic panel (BMP)	combination of tests used as a general screen for disease; includes calcium, carbon dioxide (CO_2), chloride, creatinine, glucose, potassium, sodium, and blood urea nitrogen (BUN)
comprehensive metabolic panel (CMP)	tests in addition to the basic metabolic panel for expanded screening; includes albumin, bilirubin, alkaline phosphatase, protein, alanine aminotransferase (ALT), and aspartate aminotransferase (AST) (Fig. 5-14)
lipid panel	a measure of fat in the blood, including the level of total cholesterol, low-density lipoprotein (LDL) cholesterol, high-density lipoprotein (HDL) cholesterol, and triglycerides
blood culture	a test to determine if infection is present in the blood-stream by isolating a specimen of blood in an environment that encourages the growth of microorganisms; the specimen is observed, and the organisms that grow in the culture are identified
complete blood count (CBC)	a common test performed as a screen of general health or for diagnostic purposes; the following is a listing of the component tests included in a CBC (Fig. 5-15)
white blood count (WBC)	a count of the number of white blood cells in a given volume of blood, obtained using manual or automated laboratory methods
red blood count (RBC)	a count of the number of red blood cells in a given volume of blood, obtained using manual or automated laboratory methods
hemoglobin (HGB or Hgb)	a test to determine the blood level of hemoglobin (expressed in grams)
hematocrit (HCT or Hct)	a measurement of the percentage of packed red blood cells in a given volume of blood

---

CENTRAL MEDICAL CENTER
211 Medical Center Drive • Central City, US 90000-1234 • PHONE: (012) 125-6784 • FAX: (012) 125-9999

11/02/20xx
14:27

NAME   : TEST, PATIENT   LOC: TEST   DOB: 02/03/xx   AGE: 38Y
MR#   : TEST-221   SEX: M
ACCT#   : H111111111

M63561 COLL: 11/02/20xx 13:24   REC: 11/02/20xx 13:25

COMPREHENSIVE METABOLIC PANEL

Blood Urea Nitrogen	*30	[5 - 25]	mg/dl
(BUN)			
Sodium	139	[135 - 153]	mEq/L
Potassium	4.2	[3.5 - 5.3]	mEq/L
Chloride	105	[101 - 111]	mEq/L
Carbon Dioxide (CO$_2$)	27	[24 - 31]	mmol/L
Glucose, Random	*148	[70 - 110]	mg/dl
Creatinine	*1.5	[< 1.5]	mg/dl
SGOT (AST)	18	[10 - 42]	U/L
SGPT (ALT)	*8	[10 - 60]	U/L
Alkaline Phosphatase	58	[42 - 121]	U/L
Total Protein	6.5	[6.0 - 8.0]	G/dl
Albumin	3.7	[3.5 - 5.0]	G/dl
Amylase	33	[< 129]	U/L
Bilirubin, Total	0.7	[< 1.5]	mg/dl
Calcium, Total	9.7	[8.6 - 10.6]	mg/dl

TEST, PATIENT   TEST-221   END OF REPORT   PAGE 1
11/02/20xx 14:27

INTERIM REPORT COMPLETED

FIGURE 5-14   Comprehensive metabolic panel (CMP) report. Normal ranges are in brackets [ ].

blood indices	calculations based on the RBC, HGB, and HCT results to determine the average size, hemoglobin concentration, and content of red blood cells for classification of anemia; reported as mean cell volume (MCV), mean cell hemoglobin (MCH), and mean cell hemoglobin concentration (MCHC)
differential count	a determination of the number of each type of white blood cell (leukocyte) seen on a stained blood smear; each type is counted and reported as a percentage of the total examined

Type of Leukocyte	Normal Range
lymphocytes	25–33%
monocytes	3–7%
neutrophils	54–75%

CENTRAL MEDICAL CENTER
211 Medical Center Drive • Central City, US 90000-1234 • PHONE: (012) 125-6784 • FAX: (012) 125-9999

11/02/20xx
14:27

NAME   : TEST, PATIENT   LOC: TEST   DOB: 2/2/xx   AGE: 27Y
MR#   : TEST-221   SEX: M
ACCT#   : H111111111

M63558 COLL: 11/2/20xx 13:23   REC: 11/2/20xx 13:24

HEMOGRAM
CBC

WBC	*11.5	[4.5 - 10.5]	K/UL
RBC	5.84	[4.6 - 6.2]	M/UL
HGB	17.2	[14.0 - 18.0]	G/DL
HCT	50.8	[42.0 - 52.0]	%
MCV	87	[82 - 92]	FL
MCH	29.5	[27 - 31]	PG
MCHC	33.9	[32 - 36]	G/DL
PLT	202	[150 - 450]	K/UL
Auto Lymph %	15	[20 - 40]	%
Auto Mono %	2	[1 - 11]	%
Auto Neutro %	82	[50 - 75]	%
Auto Eos %	1	[0 - 6]	%
Auto Baso %	0	[0 - 2]	%
Auto Lymph #	1.7	[1.5 - 4.0]	K/UL
Auto Mono #	0.2	[0.2 - 0.9]	K/UL
Auto Neutro #	9.4	[1.0 - 7.0]	K/UL
Auto Eos #	0.1	[0 - 0.7]	K/UL
Auto Baso #	0.0	[0 - 0.2]	K/UL

TEST, PATIENT   TEST-221   END OF REPORT   PAGE 1
11/02/20xx   14:27   INTERIM REPORT

INTERIM REPORT COMPLETE

FIGURE 5-15 Complete blood count (CBC) report. Normal ranges are in brackets [ ].

	eosinophils	1–3%
	basophils	0–1%
platelet count (PLT)	a calculation of the number of thrombocytes in the blood; the normal adult range is 150,000–450,000 platelets in a given volume of blood	

 ON CLOSER INSPECTION **RBC and WBC**

RBC and WBC are common abbreviations for red blood cell and white blood cell, respectively. However, in a complete blood count (CBC) report, RBC and WBC refer to the actual count of these blood cells. Since the word "count" is not used in the reporting, the context will be your guide as to whether the reference of RBC or WBC is to the cells or to the count of the cells.

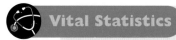 **Vital Statistics**   **BLOOD CHEMISTRY TESTS**

Blood chemistry tests are commonly ordered either separately or as part of a panel to evaluate abnormal conditions that cause disease. The following is a list of several individual tests and reasons for their use.

Chemistry Test	Used to Evaluate Conditions Related to:
albumin	liver, kidney
alkaline phosphatase	liver, bone, gallbladder
alanine aminotransferase (ALT)	liver, heart muscle
aspartate aminotransferase (AST)	liver, heart muscle
bilirubin	liver
blood urea nitrogen (BUN)	kidney function
calcium	bones, heart, nerves, kidneys, and teeth
creatinine	kidney
electrolytes (e.g., bicarbonate, chloride, potassium, and sodium)	metabolic balance (homeostasis)
glucose	diagnosis and monitoring of diabetes mellitus
lipids (e.g., cholesterol, LDL, and HDL)	evaluating risk for coronary artery disease
protein	liver, kidney

PROGRAMMED REVIEW: Blood Tests

ANSWERS	REVIEW
	5.35 Blood tests are studies performed with samples of blood. The blood sample, often drawn by a phlebotomist, is obtained through a needle puncture of a vein called a
phlebotomy	venipuncture or _____ (a term formed by a link of *phleb/o*, a Greek combining form
vein	meaning _____, with *-tomy*, the suffix
incision	meaning _____.
	5.36 Blood tests generally examine the chemical constituents of the blood or the physical properties of different kinds of blood cells. A test of the fluid portion of

chemistry, panel	blood for presence of chemical constituents is called blood _____. A blood chemistry _____ includes a combination of chemistry tests using a single sample of blood. Some panels target specific organs or conditions, such as a lipid or arthritis panel. There are two panels of chemistry tests that are used as a general or
metabolic	expanded screen for disease: basic _____
comprehensive	panel (BMP) and _____
metabolic panel	_____ _____ (CMP).
culture	**5.37** To determine the presence and type of an infection in the blood, a blood sample may be put in an environment that encourages the growth of microorganisms in order for them to be identified. This test is called a blood _____.
blood count	**5.38** A complete _____ _____ (CBC) is a diagnostic test with several components that is often performed as a general screen. The RBC is a count of the
red blood	number of erythrocytes, or _____ _____ cells in a given volume of blood. A WBC is a count of the number
white, cells	of leukocytes, or _____ blood _____. The test of the blood level of hemoglobin is often called simply a
HGB, Hgb	hemoglobin, abbreviated _____ or _____. The measurement of the percentage of packed red blood cells in a given volume of blood is called
hematocrit	the _____ (HCT or Hct).
	5.39 Calculations based on the RBC count, HGB determination, and HCT results are used to determine the size, make-up, and content of red blood cells in order to

indices	classify an anemia. These calculations are called the blood _____.
platelet platelet count	**5.40** Thrombocytes are also counted as part of a CBC. Remember that another term for thrombocyte is _____. Thus, this measure is simply called a/an _____ _____ (PLT).
white cyte, phil differential count	**5.41** Recall that there are five kinds of leukocytes, or _____ blood cells (WBCs): lymphocyte, mono_____, neutrophil, eosino_____, and basophil. The determination of the percentage of each type in the total of all types is called a/an _____ _____.

SELF-INSTRUCTION: Urine Tests

Add the following terms to your study before starting the Programmed Review.

TERM	MEANING
urinalysis (UA) (Fig. 5-16)	physical, chemical, and microscopic examination of urine (*urin/o* is a combining form meaning urine)
specific gravity (SpGr)	measure of the concentration or dilution of urine
pH	measure of the acidity or alkalinity of urine
glucose, *syn.* sugar	chemical test used to detect sugar in the urine; most often used to screen for diabetes mellitus
albumin (alb), *syn.* protein	chemical test used to detect the presence of albumin (protein) in the urine; high levels are a sign of kidney disease
ketones	chemical test used to detect the presence of ketone bodies in the urine; a positive test indicates that fats are being used by the body instead of carbohydrates, which occurs during starvation or an uncontrolled diabetic state

CENTRAL MEDICAL CENTER

211 Medical Center Drive • Central City, US 90000-1234 • PHONE: (012) 125-6784 • FAX: (012) 125-9999

11//02/20xx
13:49

NAME : TEST, PATIENT   LOC: TEST   DOB: 2/2/XX   AGE: 38Y
MR#   :   TEST-221   SEX: M
ACCT # :   H111111111

M63560 COLL: 11/2/20xx 13:24   REC: 11/2/20xx   13:25

URINE BASIC			
Color	STRAW		
Appearance	CLEAR		
Specific Gravity	1.010	[1.003 - 1.035]	
pH	5.5	[5.0 - 9.0]	
Protein	NEG	[0 - 10]	MG/DL
Glucose	NEG	[NEG]	
Ketones	NEG	[NEG]	
Bilirubin	NEG	[NEG]	
Urine Occult Blood	NEG	[NEG]	
Nitrites	NEG		

URINE MICROSCOPIC		
Epithelial Cells	3 to 4	/HPF
WBCs	0 to 1	/HPF
RBCs	0	/HPF
Bacteria	0	
Mucous Threads	0	

TEST, PATIENT   TEST-221   END OF REPORT   PAGE 1
11/02/20xx   13:49   INTERIM REPORT
INTERIM REPORT COMPLETED

FIGURE 5-16   Sample urinalysis (UA) report.

occult blood, urine	chemical test for the presence of hidden blood in the urine as a result of red blood cell hemolysis; indicates bleeding in the kidneys (occult = hidden)

bilirubin	chemical test used to detect bilirubin in the urine; seen in gallbladder and liver disease
urobilinogen	chemical test used to detect bile pigment in the urine; increased amounts are seen in gallbladder and liver disease
nitrite	chemical test to determine the presence of bacteria in the urine by measuring the amount of nitrite, a waste product that bacteria produce
microscopic findings	microscopic identification of abnormal constituents in the urine (e.g., red blood cells and white blood cells); reported per high power field (hpf) or low power field (lpf)
urine culture and sensitivity (C&S)	isolation of a urine specimen in a culture medium to encourage the growth of microorganisms; the organisms that grow in the culture are identified, as are drugs to which they are sensitive

PROGRAMMED REVIEW: Urine Tests

ANSWERS	REVIEW
	5.42 Urinalysis, abbreviated UA, is a term formed by the combination of *urin/o*, the combining form
urine	meaning _____, with -*al*, a simple suffix
pertaining to	meaning _____ ____, and -*lysis*, the suffix
breakdown, dissolution	meaning _____ or _____. Urinalysis includes physical, chemical, and microscopic testing of urine. It is typically done as a general screen for health.
	5.43 The measurement of the concentration of urine, showing the kidney's ability to concentrate or dilute urine,
specific gravity	is _____ _____ (SpGr).

pH	**5.44** The measurement of the acidity or alkalinity of any fluid is called its _____. The urinalysis includes urine pH.
glucose diabetes	**5.45** Sugar in the urine is called _____. A test for glucose in urine is a common screen for _____ mellitus.
protein albumin	**5.46** The chemical test that detects the presence of albumin or _____ in the urine is called a urine _____ or protein test.
ketones	**5.47** The test to detect the presence of ketone bodies in the urine is simply called _____.
breaking down urine occult blood	**5.48** You'll recall that the suffix -*lysis* means dissolution or _____ _____. Hemolysis occurs when the intact membranes of red blood cells break down. The cells, once intact, are now hidden. The presence of free flowing hemoglobin, the pigment normally contained within red blood cells, is a clue to their hidden state. The chemical test of urine to determine the presence of these once intact and now hidden blood cells is _____ _____ _____.
bilirubin	**5.49** Bilirubin is a component of bile, which is secreted by the liver and is not normally present in urine. The test for its presence in urine is simply called _____.
urobilinogen liver	**5.50** The chemical test for the presence of a bile pigment in the urine is _____. Increased amounts of urobilinogen are seen in gallbladder and _____ disease.

bacteriuria nitrite	**5.51** The presence of bacteria in the urine is termed _____ (formed by a link of *bacteri/o* and *-uria*). Nitrite is a waste product produced by bacteria. The chemical test to determine the presence of this waste product in urine, thereby indicating bacteriuria, is simply called _____.
microscopic findings	**5.52** Urine is examined under a microscope to identify abnormal constituents such as blood cells. The results of this examination are called _____ _____.
urine culture, sensitivity	**5.53** The isolation of a urine specimen in a culture medium to grow microorganisms and identify drugs to which they are sensitive is called a/an _____ _____ and _____ (C&S).

Pronunciation Summary

Following you will find a list of medical terms that you have learned to build and spell in this chapter, followed by the page number on which each term can be found and its written pronunciation. ⬤ Take a minute to listen to the audio pronunciations of these terms on the Student Resource CD-ROM, and then practice pronouncing them out loud. For additional practice and reinforcement, write the definition of each term on a separate piece of paper.

albumin (alb)/247
al-bū′min

angiogram/216
an′jē-ō-gram

angiography/219
an′jē-og′rǎ-fē

anoscope/226
ā′nō-skōp

anoscopy/226
ā-nos′kŏ-pē

arteriogram/217
ahr-tēr′ē-ō-gram

arthroscopy/226
ahr-thros′kŏ-pē

audiologist/229
aw′dē-ol′ŏ-jist

audiometer/228
aw′dē-om′ě-těr

audiometry/229
aw′dē-om′ě-trē

autopsy/232
aw′top-sē

basic metabolic panel (BMP)/242
bā′sik met-ă-bol′ik păn′l

bilirubin/249
bil-i-rū′bin

biopsy/230
bī′op-sē

blood chemistry/242
blŭd kem′is-trē

blood chemistry panels/242
blŭd kem′is-trē păn′lz

blood culture/242
blŭd kŭl′chŭr

blood glucose/242
blŭd glŭ′kōs

blood indices/243
blŭd in′di-sēz

blood sugar (BS)/242
blŭd shu-găr

bronchoscope/225
brong′kō-skōp

bronchoscopy/225
brong-kos′kŏ-pē

colonoscopy/226
kō′lŏn-os′kŏ-pē

complete blood count (CBC)/242
kom-plēt′ blŭd kownt

comprehensive metabolic panel (CMP)/242
kom-pre-hen′siv met-ă-bol′ik păn′l

computed tomography (CT)/219,233
kŏm-pyū′tĕd tŏ-mog′ră-fē

cystoscopy/226
sis-tos′kŏ-pē

differential count/243
dif-ĕr-en′shăl kownt

echocardiogram (echo)/217
ek′ō-kahr′dē-ō-gram

electrocardiogram (ECG or EKG)/216
ĕ-lek′trō-kahr′dē-ō-gram

electrocardiograph/220
ĕ-lek′trō-kahr′dē-ō-graf

electroencephalogram/216
ĕ-lek′trō-en-sef′ă-lō-gram

electroencephalograph/220
ĕ-lek′trō-en-sef′ă-lō-graf

electromyogram (EMG)/216
ĕ-lek′trō-mī′ō-gram

electromyograph/220
ĕ-lek′trō-mī′ō-graf

endoscope/223
en′dō-skōp

endoscopy/224
en-dos′kŏ-pē

esophagogastroduodenoscopy (EGD)/226
ĕ-sof′ă-gō-gas′trō-dū′ō-den-os′kŏ-pē

esophagoscope/225
ĕ-sof′ă-gō-skōp

esophagoscopy/225
ĕ-sof′ă-gos′kŏ-pē

gastroscopy/225
gas-tros′kŏ-pē

hematocrit (HCT or Hct)/242
hē-mat′ō-krit

hemoglobin (HGB or Hgb)/242
hē′mō-glō′bin

ketones/247
kē′tōnz

laparoscopy/226
lap′ă-ros′kŏ-pē

magnetic resonance imaging (MRI)/236
mag-net′ik rez′ō-năns im′ăj-ing

mammogram/216
mam′ō-gram

microscope/222
mī′krŏ-skōp

microscopic findings/249
mī′krŏ-skop′ik find′ingz

nasopharyngoscopy/224
nā′zō-far-in-gos′kŏ-pē

nitrite/249
nī′trīt

nuclear medicine imaging/234
nū′klē-ăr med′i-sin im′ăj-ing

occult blood, urine/248
ŏ-kŭlt blŭd, yūr′in

ophthalmologist/229
of′thăl-mol′ŏ-jist

ophthalmoscope/222
of-thal′mŏ-skōp

ophthalmoscopy/224
of′thăl-mos′kŏ-pē

optometrist/229
op-tom′ě-trist

optometry/228
op-tom′ě-trē

otoscope/222
ō′tō-skōp

otoscopy/224
ō-tos′kŏ-pē

pathologist/230,232
pa-thol′ŏ-jist

phlebotomy/242
fle-bot′ŏ-mē

platelet count (PLT)/244
plāt′let kownt

polysomnography/219
pol′ē-som-nog′ră-fē

proctoscope/226
prok′tō-skōp

proctoscopy/226
prok-tos′kŏ-pē

protein/247
prō′tēn

pulmonary/229
pul′mŏ-nār-ē

pulmonologist/230
pul′mŏ-nol′ŏ-jist

radiography/219,233
rā′dē-og′ră-fē

radionuclide organ imaging/234
rā′dē-ō-nū′klīd ōr′găn im′ăj-ing

red blood count (RBC)/242
rěd blŭd kownt

sigmoidoscope/226
sig-moy′dō-skōp

sigmoidoscopy/226
sig′moy-dos′kŏ-pē

sonogram/217
sŏn′ō-gram

sonograph/220
son′ō-graf

sonography/219,236
sŏ-nog′ră-fē

specific gravity (SpGr)/247
spě-sif′ik grav′i-tē

spirometer/228
spī-rom′ě-těr

spirometry/229
spī-rom′ě-trē

stethoscope/222
steth′ŏ-skōp

thermometer/228
thěr-mom′ě-těr

tomography/219
tŏ-mog′ră-fē

ultrasonography/219
ŭl′tră-sŏ-nog′ră-fē

ultrasound (U/S or US)/236
ŭl′tră-sownd

urinalysis (UA)/247
yūr′in-al′i-sis

urine culture and sensitivity (C&S)/249
yūr′in kŭl′chŭr and sen′si-tiv′i-tē

urobilinogen/249
yūr′ō-bi-lin′ō-jen

venipuncture/242
ven′i-pŭngk′shŭr

venogram/217
vē′nō-gram

white blood count (WBC)/242
wīt blŭd kownt

Examine Your Understanding

For the following terms, draw a line or lines to separate the prefixes (P), combining forms (CF), roots (R), and suffixes (S). Then, write the meaning of each component on the corresponding blank to define the term.

EXAMPLE

hyperlipemia

hyper/lip/emia

above or excessive / *fat* / *blood condition*

P   R   S

1. sonograph

_____ / _____
       CF   S

2. cystoscopy

_____ / _____
       CF   S

3. mammography

_____ / _____
       CF   S

4. spirometry

_____ / _____
       CF   S

5. pathology

_____ / _____
       CF   S

6. stethoscope

_____ / _____
       CF   S

7. polysomnography

_____ / _____ / _____
       P   CF   S

8. audiometry

_____ / _____
       CF   S

9. electroencephalogram

_____ / _____ / _____
       CF   CF   S

10. transesophageal

_____ / _____ / _____
       P   R   S

Circle the meaning of the following term components.

11. *auto-*

 a. across   b. out   c. both   d. self

12. *angi/o*

 a. artery   b. vessel   c. heart   d. vein

13. *bi-*

 a. both   b. many   c. life   d. away

14. *gastr/o*

 a. liver   b. stomach   c. abdomen   d. intestine

15. *somn/o*

 a. sound   b. sleep   c. breathing   d. chest

16. *cyst/o*

 a. airway   b. breathing   c. chest   d. bladder or sac

Briefly describe the difference between the following term components.

17. *angi/o* vs. *arteri/o*

 _____

18. *spir/o* vs. *-pnea*

 _____

19. *endo-* vs. *trans-*

 _____

20. *ot/o* vs. *opt/o*

 _____

Match the following suffixes with their meanings.

21. _____ *-gram*   a. instrument for measuring
22. _____ *-opsy*   b. one who specializes in the study or treatment of
23. _____ *-metry*   c. instrument for examination
24. _____ *-graphy*   d. process of measuring
25. _____ *-logy*   e. process of recording
26. _____ *-logist*   f. record
27. _____ *-meter*   g. study of
28. _____ *-scope*   h. process of viewing

Write out the expanded term for each abbreviation.

29. EEG _____

30. MRI _____

31. echo _____

32. Bx _____

33. CT _____

34. EMG _____

35. U/S _____

36. C&S _____

37. CBC _____

38. ECG _____

39. UA _____

Match the following.

40. _____ computed tomography

41. _____ magnetic resonance imaging

42. _____ radiology

43. _____ radionuclide organ imaging

44. _____ sonography

a. standard x-rays

b. gamma rays

c. ultrasound waves

d. radio waves

e. 3-D x-rays

Name the endoscope used to perform each of the following procedures.

45. bronchoscopy _____

46. colonoscopy _____

47. ophthalmoscopy _____

48. laparoscopy _____

49. otoscopy _____

50. cystoscopy _____

For each of the following, circle the term component that corresponds to the meaning given.

51. kidney	ren/o	cyst/o	hepat/o
52. rectum	rect/o	proct/o	col/o
53. life	bi-	-opsy	bi/o
54. eye	ot/o	ox/o	ophthalm/o

55. hearing   *ot/o*   *ophthalm/o*   *audi/o*

56. throat   *pharyng/o*   *bronch/o*   *nas/o*

57. vein   *angi/o*   *ven/o*   *arteri/o*

58. ear   *ot/o*   *audi/o*   *opt/o*

Match the following terms and abbreviations with their synonyms or meanings.

59. _____ venipuncture   a. calculations done to classify anemia

60. _____ HCT   b. thrombocytes

61. _____ WBC   c. protein

62. _____ SpGr   d. count of erythrocytes

63. _____ occult blood   e. count of leukocytes

64. _____ nitrite   f. glucose

65. _____ metabolic panel   g. measure of packed RBCs

66. _____ platelets   h. hidden red blood cells

67. _____ RBC   i. measure of urine concentration

68. _____ blood indices   j. phlebotomy

69. _____ BS   k. presence indicates bacteria

70. _____ albumin   l. blood tests used to screen for disease

MEDICAL RECORD EXERCISES

Medical Record 5-1

X-Ray Report

Jay Dorn, a retired construction worker, has had intermittent back pain for the past 2 months. When he began also having shooting pains in his legs, he went to see Dr. Spaulding, his doctor at Central Medical Center. After a physical examination, Mr. Dorn underwent a series of back x-rays. Medical Record 5-1 (page 260) is the radiographic report dictated by Dr. Mary Volz, the radiologist, after studying Mr. Dorn's x-rays. Read the report and answer the following questions.

Questions about Medical Record 5-1

1. Below are medical terms used in this record that you have not yet encountered in the text. Underline each term where it appears in the record and, using a medical dictionary, define the terms below.

   lumbosacral _____

   lipping _____

   S1 joint _____

   spondylolisthesis _____

   spondylolysis _____

   dextroscoliosis _____

   eburnation _____

   articulating facets _____

   discogenic _____

2. What phrase in the report indicates that more than one x-ray was taken?

   _____

   Does the report state how many x-rays were taken? _____ yes   _____ no
   If yes, how many? _____

3. In your own words, not using medical terminology, describe the three diagnoses that Dr. Volz makes.

   a. _____

   b. _____

   c. _____

4. Without using abbreviations, explain what test Dr. Volz says may be useful for Mr. Dorn to have next.

_____

5. Which of the following is not mentioned in the report as a finding?

   a. lateral curvature of the spine
   b. forward slipping of a vertebra
   c. immobile condition of the spine
   d. inflammation of the bone marrow
   e. inflammation of joints in both hips

CENTRAL MEDICAL CENTER

211 Medical Center Drive · Central City, US 90000-1234 · PHONE: (012) 125-6784 · FAX: (012) 125-9999

X-RAY REPORT

LUMBOSACRAL SPINE:
Multiple views reveal no evidence of fracture. There is slight lumbar spondylosis with slight lipping and minimal bridging. The disc spaces appear maintained except for slight narrowing at L4-L5 and L5-S1. There is also a Grade I spondylolisthesis of L5 on S1 and evidence of spondylolysis at L5 on the left. There is also slight dextroscoliosis in the lumbar region and slight increased lordosis in the lumbosacral region. The bony architecture is unremarkable except for eburnation between the articulating facets at L5-S1. The SI joints appear unremarkable. Incidentally noted are slight osteoarthritic changes involving both hips.

CONCLUSION:

1. Slight lumbar spondylosis with hypertrophic lipping and slight narrowing of the L4-L5 and L5-S1 disc spaces, rule out discogenic disease. If clinically indicated, CT of the lumbosacral spine may prove helpful in further evaluation.

2. Grade I spondylolisthesis of L5 on S1 with evidence of spondylolysis at L5 on the left.

3. Slight dextroscoliosis in the lumbar region and slight increased lordosis in the lumbosacral region.

M. Volz MD

M. Volz, M.D.

MV:ti

D: 10/19/20xx
T: 10/20/20xx

X-RAY REPORT		
	PT. NAME:	DORN, JAY F.
	ID NO:	RL-483091
	ATT. PHYS:	T. LIGHT, M.D.

MEDICAL RECORD 5-1 X-ray Report

Medical Record 5-2

Endoscopy Laboratory Report

In the Meet the Patient vignette earlier in this chapter, you learned that Mr. Antonio Villata undergoes a comprehensive physical examination each year as part of a wellness program promoted by his employer. This year, after a routine sigmoidoscopic exam revealed a polyp in his intestine, Dr. Spaulding referred him to Dr. Blain, a gastroenterologist at Central Medical Center, for evaluation. Medical Record 5-2 (page 263) is a documentation of the procedure dictated by Dr. Blain after his evaluation and treatment of Mr. Villata in the endoscopy suite. Read the report and answer the following questions.

Questions about Medical Record 5-2

1. 📖 Below are medical terms used in this record that you have not yet encountered in this text. Underline each term where it appears in the record and, using a medical dictionary, define the terms below.

polyp _____

lesions _____

sedative _____

masses (mass) _____

cecum _____

ileum _____

cannulated (cannula) _____

diverticula _____

pediculated _____

verge _____

snare _____

aspirated _____

hemorrhoids _____

adenomatous _____

hyperplastic _____

2. Describe the screening procedure performed by Dr. Spaulding prior to Mr. Villata's referral to Dr. Blain.

_____

_____

_____

3. In your own words, without using medical terminology, briefly describe the procedure performed by Dr. Blain and the indications for which the patient was referred.

_____

_____

_____

4. What position was Mr. Villata in when the procedure was performed?
   a. lying flat, face-down
   b. lying flat, face-up
   c. lying on his side
   d. sitting

5. Copy the sentence from the medical record that indicates how the polypectomy was performed.

_____

_____

_____

6. Name and describe the condition for which a high-fiber diet was indicated in the plan.

_____

_____

_____

7. In your own words, describe the recommendations outlined in the plan that will be made depending on the results of the biopsy.

_____

_____

_____

CENTRAL MEDICAL CENTER

211 Medical Center Drive   •   Central City, US 90000-1234   •   PHONE: (012) 125-6784   •   FAX: (012) 125-9999

ENDOSCOPY LABORATORY REPORT

PATIENT: Villata, Antonio   DATE: 4/29/20xx

PROCEDURE PERFORMED: COLONOSCOPY WITH BIOPSY

INDICATIONS: This is a 54-year-old white male referred to me for evaluation of a polyp found during a screening sigmoidoscopy by Dr. Spaulding. A complete colonoscopy is being done to remove the polyp and rule out other concurrent lesions.

CONSENT: The procedure and its risks including bleeding, infection, perforation, and sedative reaction have been explained to the patient, and informed consent was obtained.

INSTRUMENT USED: Olympus video colonoscope.

MEDICATIONS GIVEN: Demerol 50 mg and Versed 3 mg in divided doses. The patient had stable vital signs. A Fleets Phospho-Soda prep provided good visualization.

PROCEDURE: The patient was placed in the left lateral decubitus position. After adequate sedation, a rectal examination was performed. No masses were felt. The video colonoscope was inserted in the rectum and advanced carefully to the cecum. The location of the cecum was confirmed by internal and external landmarks and photographic documentation was obtained. The terminal ileum was then cannulated. This was normal to about 2 cm. The scope was brought back to the cecum and then gradually withdrawn. The lining of the colon was thoroughly inspected. There were scattered diverticula noted in the sigmoid colon. A pediculated 4 mm polyp was seen in the sigmoid colon at 30 cm from the anal verge. This was removed using a snare and submitted to pathology lab for biopsy. The scope was brought back to the rectum and retroflexed. Minimal hemorrhoids were noted. The scope was straightened, air was aspirated, and withdrawn. The patient tolerated the procedure well.

IMPRESSION:
1. POLYP ON SIGMOID COLON AT 30 CM.
2. SIGMOID DIVERTICULAR DISEASE.
3. HEMORRHOIDS.

PLAN:
1. A high-fiber diet is indicated.
2. Await pathology results. If adenomatous, a full colonoscopy is indicated in 3 years. If hyperplastic or normal, a colonoscopy is indicated in 10 years.

T. Blain, M.D.
Roger Blain, M.D.

RB:mw
D: 4/29/xx
T: 5/1/xx

cc: J. Spaulding, M.D.

MEDICAL RECORD 5-2   Endoscopy Laboratory Report

Medical Record 5-3

Hematology Laboratory Report

You read about Mr. Lin in the Meet the Patient vignette at the beginning of the chapter. Medical Record 5-3 (page 265) is a hematology laboratory report performed to monitor his treatment for leukemia. Read the report and answer the following question.

Questions about Medical Record 5-3

1. Study the April 15 laboratory report carefully and complete the following table of selected test results. Write out the full name of the abbreviated measurement, and circle N (normal) if the result for Mr. Lin is within normal range or A (abnormal) if the result is outside of the normal range.

	Measurement	Test Name	Result Range	
a.	WBC		N	A
b.	RBC		N	A
c.	HGB		N	A
d.	HCT		N	A
e.	MCV		N	A
f.	MCH		N	A
g.	MCHC		N	A
h.	PLT		N	A
i.	lymph		N	A
j.	mono		N	A
k.	neutro		N	A
l.	eos		N	A
m.	baso		N	A

CENTRAL MEDICAL CENTER
211 Medical Center Drive • Central City, US 90000-1234 • PHONE: (012) 125-6784 • FAX: (012) 125-9999

04/15/20xx
14:27

NAME   : Lin, Henry   LOC: TEST   DOB: 2/2/xx   AGE: 69Y
MR#   : TEST-226   SEX: M
ACCT#   : 168946701

M63558 COLL: 04/15/20xx 13:23   REC: 04/15/20xx 13:25

HEMOGRAM

CBC
WBC	4.1	[4.5 - 10.5]	K/UL
RBC	2.93	[4.6 - 6.2]	M/UL
HGB	9.1	[14.0 - 18.0]	G/DL
HCT	25.3	[42.0 - 52.0]	%
MCV	86.2	[82 - 92]	FL
MCH	31.1	[27 - 31]	PG
MCHC	36.0	[32 - 36]	G/DL
PLT	90	[150 - 450]	K/UL
Auto Lymph %	8.3	[20 - 40]	%
Auto Mono %	32.6	[1 - 11]	%
Auto Neutro %	57.8	[50 - 75]	%
Auto Eos %	1.0	[0 - 6]	%
Auto Baso %	0.3	[0 - 2]	%
Auto Lymph #	0.3	[1.5 - 4.0]	K/UL
Auto Mono #	1.3	[0.2 - 0.9]	K/UL
Auto Neutro #	2.4	[1.0 - 7.0]	K/UL
Auto Eos #	0.0	[0 - 0.7]	K/UL
Auto Baso #	0.0	[0 - 0.2]	K/UL

TEST, PATIENT   TEST-221   END OF REPORT   PAGE 1
04/15/20xx 14:27   INTERIM REPORT

INTERIM REPORT COMPLETE

MEDICAL RECORD 5-3   Hematology Laboratory Report

Answers to Examine Your Understanding

1. sono/graph
   <u>sound</u> / <u>instrument for recording</u>
     CF   S

2. cysto/scopy
   <u>bladder or sac</u> / <u>process of examination</u>
       CF   S

3. mammo/graphy
   <u>breast</u> / <u>process of recording</u>
     CF   S

4. spiro/metry
   <u>breathing</u> / <u>process of measuring</u>
      CF   S

5. patho/logy
   <u>disease</u> / <u>study of</u>
     CF   S

6. stetho/scope
   <u>chest</u> / <u>instrument for examination</u>
     CF   S

7. poly/somno/graphy
   <u>many</u> / <u>sleep</u> / <u>process of recording</u>
     P   CF   S

8. audio/metry
   <u>hearing</u> / <u>process of measuring</u>
     CF   S

9. electro/encephalo/gram
   <u>electricity</u> / <u>entire brain</u> / <u>record</u>
      CF   CF   S

10. trans/esophag/eal
    <u>across or through</u> / <u>esophagus</u> / <u>pertaining to</u>
          P   R   S

11. d
12. b
13. a
14. b
15. b
16. d
17. angi/o means vessel; arteri/o means artery, a type of blood vessel
18. spri/o is a combining form meaning breathing; -pnea is a suffix meaning breathing

19. endo- is a prefix meaning within; trans- is a prefix meaning across or through
20. ot/o is a combining form meaning ear; opt/o is a combining form meaning eye
21. f
22. h
23. d
24. e
25. g

26. b
27. a
28. c
29. electroencephalogram
30. magnetic resonance imaging
31. echocardiogram
32. biopsy
33. computed tomography
34. electromyogram
35. ultrasound
36. culture and sensitivity
37. complete blood count

38. electrocardiogram
39. urinalysis
40. e
41. d
42. a
43. b
44. c
45. bronchoscope
46. colonoscope
47. ophthalmoscope
48. laparoscope
49. otoscope
50. cystoscope
51. ren/o
52. rect/o
53. bi/o
54. ophthalm/o
55. audi/o
56. pharyng/o
57. ven/o
58. ot/o
59. j
60. g
61. e
62. i
63. h
64. k
65. l
66. b
67. d
68. a
69. f
70. c

ANSWERS TO MEDICAL RECORD EXERCISE 5-1

1. See medical dictionary.
2. "Multiple views reveal no evidence of fracture." No, the report does not state how many x-rays were taken.
3. Dr. Volz makes the following diagnoses:
   a. slight degeneration (deterioration) of the vertebrae in the lower back, including the formation of enlarged, lip-like structures between the joint spaces with narrowing of the spaces between the fourth and fifth lumbar vertebrae in the lower back and narrowing between the fifth lumbar vertebra and the sacrum
   b. forward slipping of the fifth vertebra of the lumbar spine, slipping onto the sacrum, with signs of a breaking down of the fifth lumbar vertebra on the left
   c. slight right lateral curve of the spine in the lumbar region and increased forward bend of the vertebrae in the lower back at the base of the spine
4. computed tomography (procedure using computers to compile cross-sectional x-ray pictures into a three-dimensional image)
5. d

ANSWERS TO MEDICAL RECORD EXERCISE 5-2

1. See medical dictionary.
2. Inspection through an endoscope of the interior of the sigmoid colon.
3. Visual examination of the inner surface of the colon by means of a colonoscope for removal and pathological examination of a polyp known to be located in the sigmoid colon, and further examination to check for any other possible lesions anywhere else in the colon.
4. c
5. "This was removed using a snare and submitted to pathology lab for biopsy."
6. Diverticulosis—a condition of abnormal side pockets in the sigmoid colon.
7. If the polyp is composed of noncancerous glandular tissue, a follow-up colonoscopy will be necessary in 3 years. If the polyp is found to be normal or there is an

overgrowth tissue that is not related to tumor formation, a follow-up colonoscopy is not necessary for 10 more years.

ANSWERS TO MEDICAL RECORD EXERCISE 5-3

a. white blood cell count-A
b. red blood cell count-A
c. hemoglobin-A
d. hematocrit-A
e. mean cell volume-N
f. mean cell hemoglobin-A
g. mean cell hemoglobin concentration-N
h. platelet count-A
i. lymphocytes-A
j. monocytes-A
k. neutrophils-N
l. eosinophils-N
m. basophils-N

CHAPTER 6

OPERATIVE AND THERAPEUTIC TERMS

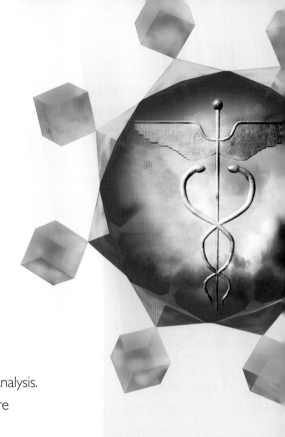

OBJECTIVES

1. Identify common operative, or surgical, suffixes.
2. Define common operative terms using term structure analysis.
3. Define common therapeutic terms using term structure analysis.
4. Identify common drug classifications.

CHECKLIST

CHECKLIST	LOCATION
☐ Complete Chapter 6 Self-Instruction and Programmed Review sections	pages 270–314 📖
☐ Review the Flash Cards related to Chapter 6	FC
☐ Complete the Chapter 6 Examine Your Understanding exercises	pages 318–323 📖
☐ Complete Medical Record Exercises 6-1 and 6-2	pages 324–330 📖
☐ Practice saying the Chapter 6 terms out loud with the Audio Pronunciation Glossary on the Student Resource CD-ROM	CD-ROM
☐ Complete the Chapter 6 Interactive Exercises on the Student Resource CD-ROM	CD-ROM
☐ Take the Chapter 6 Quiz on the Student Resource CD-ROM	CD-ROM
☐ When you receive 70% or higher on the Quiz, move on to the Final Assessment on the Student Resource CD-ROM	CD-ROM

MEET THE PATIENT   Larry Phelps, age 31, has been happily married to his wife, Nancy, for almost 5 years, and they have two children. The second pregnancy caused some health problems for Nancy, and her obstetrician recommended that they have no more children because of the risk to her health. After trying different forms of birth control, Nancy and Larry decided that he should have a vasectomy. Dr. Spaulding referred him to Dr. Jerard Derrick in the urology department at Central Medical Group. He eventually underwent a vasectomy, which you'll read about in **Medical Record 6-1.**

In Chapter 3, you learned that a provider's plan outlines the strategies designed to prevent and/or treat a patient's condition. This chapter focuses on common treatments, including procedures, such as operations, and various therapies, including medications.

Operative Terms

An operation (also called a surgery) is the treatment of a disease, injury, or deformity by performing a procedure using either major (invasive) or minor (minimally invasive) techniques under sterile conditions. Note that the terms "operative" and "surgical" are synonymous. Operative suffixes are word endings used in terms that describe specific surgical techniques, whether they are major or minor. A summary list of common operative suffixes is presented below, followed by learning segments that show how each is used in surgical terms.

SUFFIX	MEANING	FLASH CARD ID
-centesis	puncture for aspiration	S-4
-desis	binding	S-5
-ectomy	excision or removal	S-6
-graft	transfer	S-10
-pexy	suspension or fixation	S-32
-plasty	surgical repair or reconstruction	S-35
-rrhaphy	suture	S-41
-scope	instrument for examination	S-43
-scopy	process of examination	S-44
-stomy	creation of an opening	S-47
-tomy	incision	S-48
-tripsy	crushing	S-49

SELF-INSTRUCTION: -tomy (incision)

Add the following combining forms to your study of -tomy before starting the Programmed Review below.

COMBINING FORM	MEANING	FLASH CARD ID
lapar/o	abdomen	CF-1
myring/o	eardrum or tympanic membrane	CF-66
thorac/o	chest	CF-63
tom/o	to cut	
trache/o	trachea (windpipe)	

PROGRAMMED REVIEW: -tomy (incision)

ANSWERS	REVIEW
ending surgical cut process of -tomy	**6.1** An operative suffix is a term _____ used to describe a major or minor operative, or _____, procedure. Traditional surgical procedures require an incision. Formed by the link of *tom/o,* a combining form meaning to _____, and *-y,* the simple suffix meaning condition or_____ ____, the compound operative suffix meaning incision is _____.
abdomen laparotomy examination	**6.2** An incision is the first step in most surgical procedures. For example, *lapar/o,* the combining form meaning _____, is linked to *-tomy* in the term referring to an incision into the abdomen: _____. Laparotomy is performed for the purpose of exploring the abdominal cavity for both diagnostic and therapeutic reasons. It often includes the insertion of a laparoscope, an instrument for _____ of the abdomen.

trachea

6.3 You'll recall that *trache/o* is the combining form meaning _____, which can also be referred to as the "windpipe." Blockage of the trachea may necessitate a surgical incision in it to allow air into the lungs. Using the surgical suffix meaning incision, the term used to describe the process of making an incision in the trachea is

tracheotomy

_____ (Fig. 6-1A).

A **Tracheotomy**
Incision of the trachea for exploration, for removal of a foreign body, or for obtaining a biopsy specimen

Incision

B **Tracheostomy**
Incision of the trachea and insertion of a tube to facilitate passage of air or removal of secretions

Placement of tracheostomy tube

Sagittal view, with tracheostomy tube in place

Tracheostomy tube

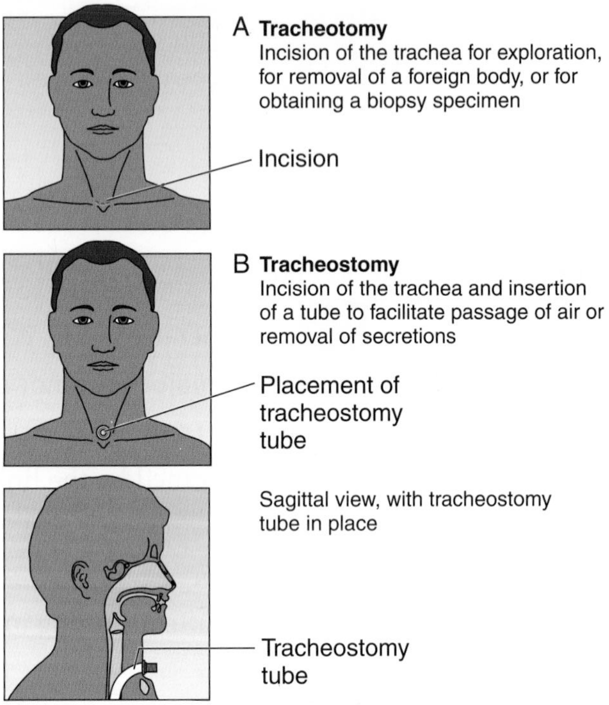

FIGURE 6-1   Operative procedures related to the trachea. **A.** Tracheotomy. **B.** Tracheostomy.

chest

thoracotomy

6.4 When *-tomy* is linked to *thorac/o,* a combining form meaning _____, it forms the term for an incision in the chest, called a _____.

eardrum

incision

6.5 When *myring/o,* a combining form referring to the tympanic membrane, or _____, is linked to *-tomy,* the suffix meaning _____, it forms the term

myringotomy	describing a surgical incision into the eardrum: _____. A myringotomy is performed to relieve pressure caused by the buildup of fluid in the ear canal. This accumulation of fluid is typically the result of
inflammation	otitis media, a condition of _____ of the middle ear.

SELF-INSTRUCTION: -stomy (creation of an opening)

Add the following combining forms to your study of -stomy before starting the Programmed Review below.

COMBINING FORM	MEANING	FLASH CARD ID
col/o, colon/o	colon (large intestine)	
ile/o	ileum (third portion of small intestine)	
salping/o	uterine or fallopian tube	CF-56
ur/o	urine	CF-67

PROGRAMMED REVIEW: -stomy (creation of an opening)

ANSWERS	REVIEW
	6.6 Recall that -tomy, the surgical suffix meaning
incision	_____, is formed by a link of tom/o, meaning
cut, -y	to _____, with ____, the simple suffix meaning
	condition or process of. -stomy, the suffix meaning
creation, opening	_____ of a/an _____, is formed by
	a link of stoma, the Greek word for mouth or opening, with
	-y, the suffix referring to a condition or _____
process	
of	_____. -stomy is used to modify the meaning of a surgical
	term when it is necessary to keep an incision open, such as
	is required to insert a tube.

incision, trachea	**6.7** You'll recall that a tracheotomy refers to a/an _____ in the _____. If it is necessary to keep the trachea (windpipe) open for any length of time, a tube is inserted, and the incision is left open. The term for this procedure is formed by the link of *trache/o* with *-stomy*: _____ (Fig. 6-1B).
tracheostomy	
thoracotomy	**6.8** As you've learned, an incision in the chest is termed _____; however, when an incision is made in the chest for the purpose of creating an opening, such as may be necessary to insert a tube, the term to describe this surgical opening is _____.
thoracostomy	
uterine	**6.9** *salping/o*, a combining form referring to the fallopian or _____ tube, is used in salpingotomy to refer to a/an _____ in the uterine tube. Salpingostomy refers to the _____ of a/an _____ in the uterine tube. This is most commonly done to remove products of conception in cases of tubal pregnancy, which is a type of ectopic pregnancy.
incision	
creation	
opening	
cut	**6.10** Sometimes it is necessary to create an artificial stoma, or opening, in a structure to provide for temporary or permanent functional diversion, such as to reroute the passage of stool from the colon or small intestine or urine from the bladder. The opening is referred to as an ostomy (a term coined by a link of os, a Latin word for opening, with *tom/o*, the combining form meaning to _____, and *-y*, the suffix meaning condition or _____ ____). The most common ostomies include colostomy, the creation of an opening in the _____; ileostomy, the
process	
of	
colon	

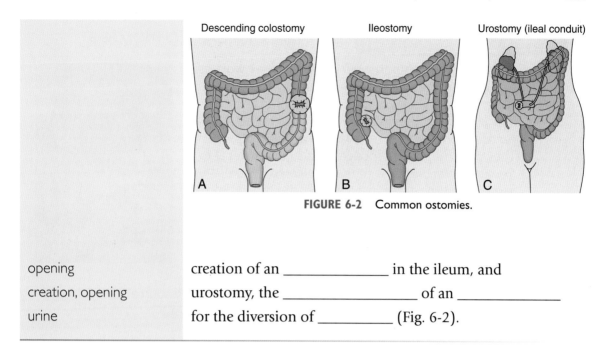

FIGURE 6-2   Common ostomies.

opening	creation of an _____ in the ileum, and
creation, opening	urostomy, the _____ of an _____
urine	for the diversion of _____ (Fig. 6-2).

SELF-INSTRUCTION: *-ectomy* (excision or removal)

Add the following term components to your study of *-ectomy* before starting the Programmed Review.

PREFIX	MEANING	FLASH CARD ID
ec-	out or away	P-13
hemi-	half	P-18
trans-	across or through	P-11

COMBINING FORM	MEANING	FLASH CARD ID
append/o	appendix	
chol/e	bile	CF-14
gastr/o	stomach	CF-26
mast/o	breast	CF-38
oophor/o, ovari/o	ovary	
prostat/o	prostate gland	
uter/o, metr/o, hyster/o	uterus	
vas/o	vessel	CF-5

Health Care Professionals   MEET THE SURGICAL TECHNOLOGIST

Surgical technologists are well known for their work as part of the surgical team in the operating room. During surgery, the surgical technologist is responsible for ensuring that the instruments and equipment needed for that particular procedure are available and working properly. They pass instruments, sponges, and suture material to the surgeon and assist with the surgical procedure—always maintaining sterility to protect the patient from infection. Surgical technologists are employed in settings such as hospital surgical suites, outpatient surgical centers, trauma centers, surgeon's offices, and surgical equipment companies.

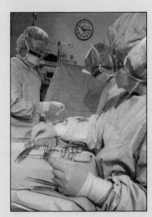

A more detailed description of surgical technologist as a health care career can be found on the Student Resource CD-ROM and at the companion website at www.thePoint.lww.com/WillisQC.

PROGRAMMED REVIEW: *-ectomy* (excision or removal)

ANSWERS	REVIEW
	6.11 When *-ectomy* appears at the end of a term, it indicates
excision, removal	a/an _____ or _____. This
	compound suffix is formed by linking *ec-*, the prefix
out, away	meaning _____ or _____, to *tom/o*, the combining
cut	form meaning to _____, and *-y*, the simple suffix meaning
process of	condition or _____ ____. Excision is the act of
	cutting out and removing all or part of a structure or organ.
	Most terms related to excision are formed by a link of the
	combining form for the structure or organ to be removed
-ectomy	with _____, the suffix meaning excision or
	removal.
	6.12 Simply termed, a lumpectomy is the
excision, removal	_____ or _____ of a lump,

breast mastectomy	specifically a cancerous or benign lump from the breast. Using *mast/o*, a combining form meaning _____, the excision of a breast is called _____.
inflammation appendix appendectomy	**6.13** *append/o* is a combining form for appendix. A patient diagnosed with appendicitis suffers from a/an _____ of his or her _____ and must receive immediate surgery to have it removed. This procedure is called a/an _____.
colon colectomy excision, removal, half	**6.14** *colon/o* and *col/o* are combining forms meaning _____. The latter combining form is used in the term for a partial or complete removal of the colon: _____. Hemicolectomy is defined as an _____ or _____ of _____ of the colon.
bile presence of, stones itis cholecystectomy	**6.15** You'll recall that *chol/e* is a combining from meaning _____. Bile is produced in the liver and stored in the cholecyst, or gallbladder. In Chapter 4, you learned that cholelithiasis refers to the formation of or _____ ____ bile or gall _____. Inflammation of the gallbladder, or cholecyst, is called cholecyst_____. A surgical removal of the gallbladder is often a remedy for cholelithiasis or cholecystitis; the term for this operation is _____.
	6.16 You'll recall that there are three combining forms meaning uterus: *uter/o, metr/o,* and *hyster/o.* Using the latter,

hysterectomy	the term for excision or removal of the uterus is _____. You'll recall that the combining form for the fallopian or uterine tube is
salping/o	_____. Salpingectomy refers to the
excision, removal	_____ or _____ of a uterine tube. There are two combining forms for ovary: *ovari/o* and
oophor/o	_____. Using the latter, the term for excision or
oophorectomy	removal of an ovary is _____. A salpingo-oophorectomy refers to the removal of a uterine
tube, ovary	_____ and _____. A bilateral salpingo-oophorectomy describes the excision or removal of uterine
both	tube and ovary on two or _____ sides.

6.17 Cancer of the stomach often requires partial or complete removal of that organ. Using the combining form for stomach, the term for its surgical removal is

gastrectomy

_____. Gastric resection is a similar term used to indicate a removal of only the diseased sections

stomach

of the _____.

vessel

6.18 *vas/o* is a combining form meaning _____. The vas deferens is the vessel that carries sperm to the urethra during ejaculation. The surgery to produce male sterility by excision of part of the vas deferens is formed by linking *vas/o* with *-ectomy*, the suffix meaning

excision, vasectomy

_____ or removal: _____ (Fig. 6-3).

6.19 Using *prostat/o,* the combining form meaning

prostate

_____ gland, the term for the excision of the prostate gland, such as commonly done to treat prostate

prostatectomy

cancer, is _____. In a condition

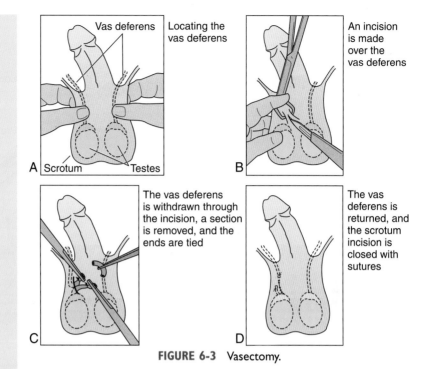

FIGURE 6-3   Vasectomy.

known as benign prostatic hyperplasia (BPH), a non-cancerous condition of excessive formation of prostate tissue, the surgical remedy is often a resection of the prostate. In a surgical resection, only the overgrown sections of the _____ gland are removed. This procedure is called transurethral resection of the prostate (TURP) (Fig. 6-4). You'll recall that *trans-* is a prefix meaning across or _____, and *urethr/o* is a combining form referring to the _____ (the structure that carries urine from the bladder to the outside of the body). In a TURP, an endoscope equipped with cutting instruments is passed through the urethra to the prostate, encircling the bladder, in order to cut away the overgrown tissue.

prostate

through

urethra

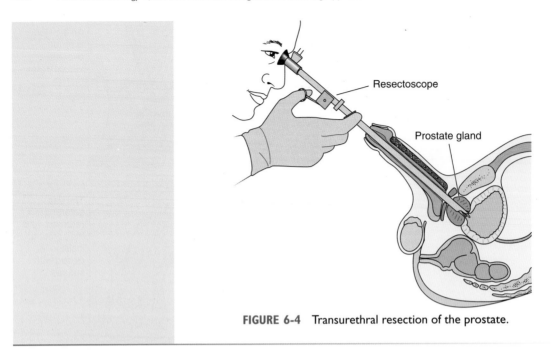

FIGURE 6-4 Transurethral resection of the prostate.

Rx for Success

It is important to understand the difference between a diagnosis and a surgical treatment. A good way to do this is to put special emphasis on memorizing surgical suffixes; when you see one in a term, you'll know it relates to an operation. Then, by process of elimination, you'll recognize terms such as appendectomy and tonsillectomy as surgical terms and terms such as appendicitis and tonsillitis as diagnostic terms.

SELF-INSTRUCTION: *-centesis* (puncture for aspiration)

Add the following term components to your study of *-centesis* before starting the Programmed Review.

PREFIX	MEANING	FLASH CARD ID
para-	alongside of or abnormal	P-31

COMBINING FORM	MEANING	FLASH CARD ID
abdomin/o	abdomen	CF-1
arthr/o	joint	CF-6

PROGRAMMED REVIEW: -*centesis* (puncture for aspiration)

ANSWERS	REVIEW
puncture aspiration	**6.20** -*centesis*, meaning _____ for _____, is a surgical suffix used in terms related to treatment and testing. A needle with a suction device is inserted into a body cavity so that the gas or fluid within can be drawn out, or aspirated.
abdomen abdominocentesis alongside of	**6.21** Combined with *abdomin/o,* the combining form meaning _____, the procedure involving puncture for aspiration of the abdominal cavity is _____; this is also known as paracentesis or abdominal paracentesis (*para-* is the prefix meaning abnormal or _____ ____). Abdominal paracentesis is most commonly done to remove fluid that has accumulated in the abdominal cavity, a condition known as ascites.
chest thoracocentesis	**6.22** You'll recall that *thorac/o* is a combining form meaning _____. Combined with -*centesis,* it forms the term for a puncture of the chest to remove fluid or air from the pleural space, which is the lining of the lungs. This procedure called is called _____ and is also known as thoracentesis.
puncture aspiration	**6.23** In amniocentesis, the _____ for _____ is of fluid from the amniotic sac. (The amniotic sac is the membrane in the pregnant uterus that surrounds the embryo and later the fetus; it is filled with amniotic fluid.) This procedure is done to test for fetal abnormalities and requires the transabdominal insertion of

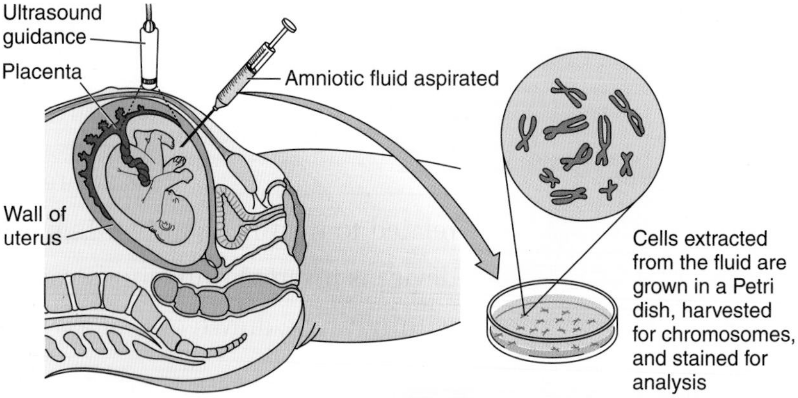

FIGURE 6-5   Amniocentesis.

	a needle into the sac (Fig. 6-5). Remember, *trans-*
across, through	is a prefix meaning _____ or _____.
joint	**6.24** *arthr/o* is the combining form meaning _____.
	A puncture for aspiration of fluid from a joint is called
arthrocentesis	_____.

SELF-INSTRUCTION: -desis (binding)

Add the following term components to your study of *-desis* before starting the Programmed Review.

PREFIX	MEANING	FLASH CARD ID
syn-	together or with	P-37

COMBINING FORM	MEANING	FLASH CARD ID
spondyl/o, vertebr/o	vertebra	CF-69

PROGRAMMED REVIEW: -desis (binding)

ANSWERS	REVIEW
binding	**6.25** -desis, meaning _____, is a surgical
suffix	_____ that is often used to name orthopedic procedures. arthr/o, the combining form meaning
joint	_____, is used in the term for binding or fusing joint
arthrodesis	surfaces: _____. Tenodesis describes
binding	the _____ of tendons. You'll recall that
spondyl/o	vertebr/o and _____ are combining forms
vertebra, prefix	meaning _____, and syn- is a _____
together	meaning _____ or with. These components are combined with -desis in spondylosyndesis, the term
binding	referring to a _____ together of vertebrae (also known as a spinal fusion) (Fig. 6-6).

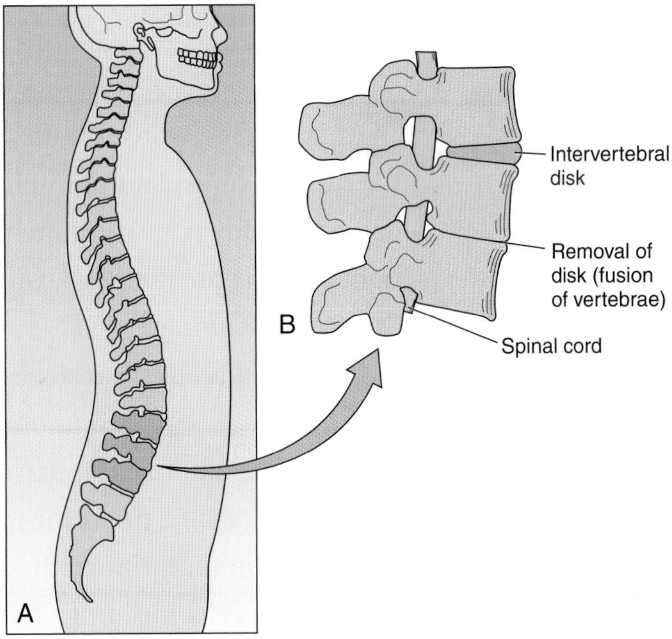

FIGURE 6-6   Spondylosyndesis. **A.** Spinal column. **B.** Spinal fusion.

SELF-INSTRUCTION: *-graft* (transfer)

Add the following term components to your study of *-graft* before starting the
Programmed Review below.

PREFIX	MEANING	FLASH CARD ID
allo-	other	P-4
auto-	self	P-8
hetero-	different	P-19
homo-	same	P-20
xeno-	strange or foreign	P-40

COMBINING FORM	MEANING	FLASH CARD ID
coron/o	circle or crown	

PROGRAMMED REVIEW: *-graft* (transfer)

ANSWERS	REVIEW
	6.26 Graft is a word or suffix used in terms to indicate the surgical transplant or implant of tissue to replace a damaged body part or compensate for a defect. Skin and bone grafting are the most common types of grafts. *auto-*,
self	the prefix meaning _____, is used to name the type of graft that involves transfer of the patient's own tissue:
autograft	_____. A homograft is a transfer of tissue from one human to another (*homo-* is a prefix meaning
same, other	_____). *allo-*, a prefix meaning _____, is used
allograft	in a synonym for homograft: _____.
different	*hetero-*, the prefix meaning _____, is

used to name the graft of tissue from one species to another, such as animal to human. *xeno-*, a prefix meaning strange or _____, is used in the synonym for heterograft: _____.

foreign

xenograft

6.27 To bypass something is to go around it. *coron/o*, the combining form meaning _____ or _____ was used to name the coronary arteries because they circle the heart to provide oxygen and nutrition to heart muscle. The surgical procedure involving the graft of vessels harvested elsewhere in the body to bypass a coronary artery that is occluded by atherosclerotic buildup is called a _____ _____ _____ _____ (CABG) (Fig. 6-7).

circle

crown

coronary

artery bypass graft

MEET THE PATIENT Alice Toohey is a 56-year-old woman who enjoys spending time with her 3-year-old granddaughter Katey. One afternoon, while playing with Katey, Alice stepped on a toy and fell down the porch steps, violently wrenching her ankle. Worried that her mother may have sustained a neck or back injury in the fall, Alice's daughter called 9-1-1. An **Emergency Medical Technician (EMT)** responded in a matter of minutes and cared for Mrs. Toohey at the scene. Because of the sharp pain and immediate swelling, she was transported to the hospital. After being seen by the emergency department physician, Alice learned that her most serious injury was a fracture dislocation of her right ankle. She was admitted that day and scheduled for surgery. **Medical Record 6-2** is the operative report dictated by the surgeon, Dr. Ricardo Rodriguez, immediately after the operation.

A. Common sites for bypass grafts

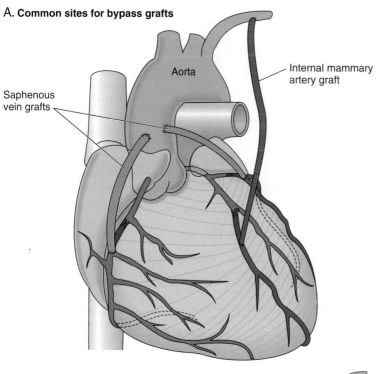

Aorta

Internal mammary
artery graft

Saphenous
vein grafts

B. Bypass process

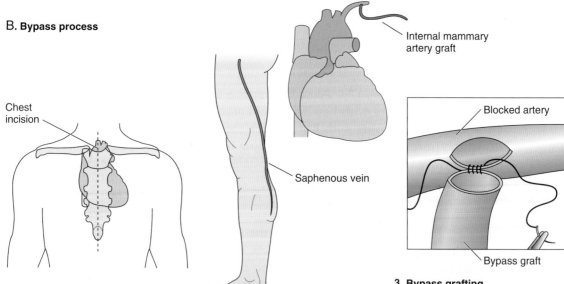

Internal mammary
artery graft

Chest
incision

Saphenous vein

Blocked artery

Bypass graft

1. Bypass incisions
An incision is made in the chest, dividing the sternum to allow access to the heart.

2. Bypass vessels
The long saphenous vein in the leg can be used to make several bypasses, if needed. The internal mammary artery may also be used as a graft. Both are "excess" blood vessels the body does not need.

3. Bypass grafting
Grafting is performed under magnification using extremely fine sutures. Each graft is sewn to the aorta, except for the internal mammary artery, which already originates from a branch of the aorta. The other end is sewn to the artery below the blockage.

FIGURE 6-7 Traditional method of coronary artery bypass graft (CABG).

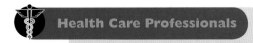 **Health Care Professionals**

MEET THE EMERGENCY MEDICAL TECHNICIAN (EMT)

When an individual is extremely ill or injured and a loved one or bystander calls 9-1-1, a dispatcher sends emergency medical services (EMS) providers to the scene. An emergency medical technician (EMT) is a health care professional who is specially trained to manage medical emergencies. EMTs employ skills such as opening a patient's airway, defibrillating a patient's heart, controlling bleeding, and splinting extremities. They often then transport 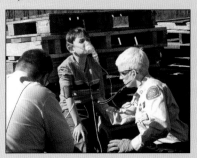 the patient to a hospital for further care. EMTs can pursue additional education and training to become more advanced providers, such as EMT-intermediates and paramedics. All of these emergency care providers work under protocols approved by local physicians who oversee the care of patients in EMS systems.

🔬 A more detailed description of emergency medical technician as a health care career can be found on the Student Resource CD-ROM and at the companion website at www.thePoint.lww.com/WillisQC.

SELF-INSTRUCTION: -pexy (suspension or fixation)

Add the following combining form to your study of *-pexy* before starting the Programmed Review below.

COMBINING FORM	MEANING	FLASH CARD ID
orchi/o	testis or testicle	CF-61

PROGRAMMED REVIEW: -pexy (suspension or fixation)

ANSWERS	REVIEW
-pexy	**6.28** Suspension or fixation is a condition of being firmly attached or set. The surgical suffix indicating the process of suspension or fixation is _____.

breast	**6.29** *mast/o*, a combining form meaning _____, is used in the term for surgical fixation of pendulous
mastopexy	(loosely hanging) breast(s): _____.

6.30 You'll recall that *orchi/o* is a Greek combining

testicle or testis   form meaning _____, and *-ism* is a suffix

condition of   referring to a _____ ____. The

combination of these components with *crypt/o*, meaning to hide, forms cryptorchism, the medical term describing the failure of one or more testes to descend into the scrotal sac during fetal development (Fig. 6-8). This condition can necessitate surgery soon after birth to move the testicle down to its proper location in the scrotum. The surgical term for this procedure is

orchiopexy   _____ (formed by linking the

combining form for testicle with *-pexy*, to indicate its

fixation   suspension or _____).

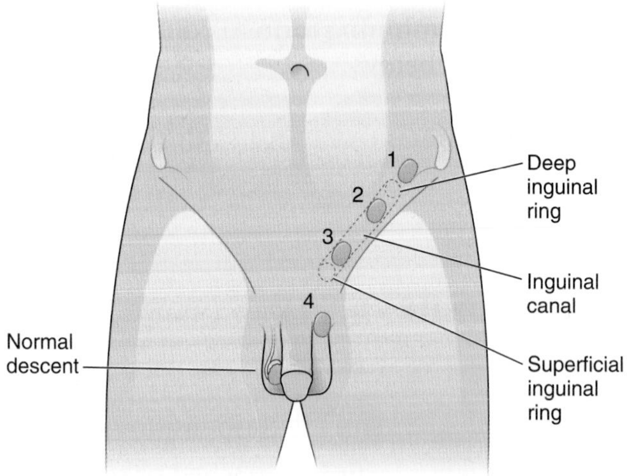

FIGURE 6-8 Cryptorchism, a condition requiring orchiopexy, the surgical procedure to position the undescended testicle to its proper place in the scrotum.

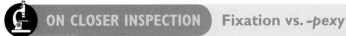

ON CLOSER INSPECTION Fixation vs. -pexy

The word fixation is used instead of -pexy in the term describing the surgical repair of a complex fracture: open reduction, internal fixation (ORIF). In this surgery, an open incision is made, and the broken bone(s) are brought into alignment and fixed in place using devices such as plates, screws, and pins.

This x-ray was taken of Mrs. Alice Toohey's right ankle after an ORIF (see **Medical Record Exercise 6-2**).

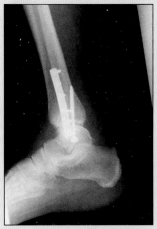

Postoperative x-ray of Alice Toohey's open reduction, internal fixation (ORIF).

SELF-INSTRUCTION: -plasty (surgical repair or reconstruction)

Add the following term components to your study of -plasty before starting the Programmed Review.

PREFIX	MEANING	FLASH CARD ID
hyper-	above or excessive	P-21
hypo-	below or deficient	P-22
macro-	large	P-24
micro-	small	P-26
per-	by	P-32
trans-	across or through	P-11

COMBINING FORM	MEANING	FLASH CARD ID
angi/o	vessel	CF-5
cutane/o	skin	CF-21
my/o	muscle	CF-40
nas/o, rhin/o	nose	CF-43

PROGRAMMED REVIEW: *-plasty* (surgical repair or reconstruction)

ANSWERS	REVIEW
-plasty	**6.31** The operative suffix that indicates a surgical repair or reconstruction is _____. It is used to name a variety of surgical procedures.
reconstruction joint repair muscle	**6.32** Related to orthopedics, arthroplasty is the surgical repair or _____ of a _____ (Fig. 6-9). Myoplasty describes the surgical _____ or reconstruction of _____.

FIGURE 6-9 Total knee arthroplasty. Postoperative anteroposterior radiograph of total knee replacement.

ANSWERS	REVIEW
nose rhino	**6.33** *nas/o* (Latin) and *rhin/o* (Greek) are combining forms meaning _____. Using the Greek combining form for nose, the term describing the cosmetic surgery to reconstruct the nose is _____plasty.

6.34 Surgical repair of breast tissue is common. You'll recall that there are two combining forms meaning breast:

mamm/o and _____. The latter is used more frequently in diagnostic terms. For example, *mast/o,*

combined with *micro-,* the prefix meaning _____,

and *-ia,* the suffix meaning _____ _____,

names the condition of small breast:

_____. This condition is also called

hypomastia (*hypo-* means below or

_____). In contrast, macromastia is a

condition of a _____ breast, also called hypermastia

(*hyper-* means above or _____).

mast/o	
small	
condition of	
micromastia	
deficient	
large or long	
excessive	

6.35 Mammoplasty, or surgical repair or

_____ of the _____

is a remedy for both conditions. Patients with micromastia (hypomastia) may elect to have tissue added to the breast in the surgery known as augmentation

_____. Reconstruction that takes

away excessive breast tissue in cases of macromastia (also

known as _____) is called reduction

_____.

reconstruction, breast

mammoplasty

hypermastia
mammoplasty

6.36 Angioplasty, a surgical repair or

_____ of a _____, is

performed to restore blood through narrowed arteries. Percutaneous transluminal angioplasty (PTA) is the most common technique, using instruments passed through the skin into a vessel. Percutaneous is an adjective formed by linking *per-,* the prefix meaning _____, with *cutane/o,* a

combining form meaning _____, and *-ous,* the simple

suffix meaning _____ _____.

reconstruction, vessel

by
skin
pertaining to

through	**6.37** Transluminal is an adjective formed by *trans-*, a prefix meaning across or _____, with luminal, an adjective that pertains to a lumen (the inner space of a tubular structure). Coronary is a term formed by a link of *coron/o*, a combining form meaning crown or
circle	_____, and *-ary*, a suffix meaning
pertaining to	_____ _____. The coronary arteries are
circle	those that _____ the heart. Percutaneous transluminal coronary angioplasty (PTCA) is a procedure
coronary	to repair an occluded _____ artery (Fig. 6-10).

SELF-INSTRUCTION: -rrhaphy (suture)

Add the following combining forms to your study of *-rrhaphy* before starting the Programmed Review below.

COMBINING FORM	MEANING	FLASH CARD ID
gloss/o	tongue	CF-36
herni/o	hernia	
splen/o	spleen	

PROGRAMMED REVIEW: -rrhaphy (suture)

ANSWERS	REVIEW
	6.38 Suture refers to the thread-like material used to sew or stitch surfaces together during a surgical procedure. The operative suffix used to indicate the process of suturing is
-rrhaphy	_____. Suturing is used to close a wound or to stitch together a torn or injured part (Fig. 6-11).

ANTERIOR VIEW OF CORONARY ARTERIES

Superior vena cava

Arch of aorta

Pulmonary trunk

Left coronary artery

Circumflex branch

Right coronary artery

Left anterior descending artery

Left marginal artery

Diagonal artery

Right marginal artery

PLACEMENT OF STENT TO KEEP ARTERY OPEN AFTER ANGIOPLASTY

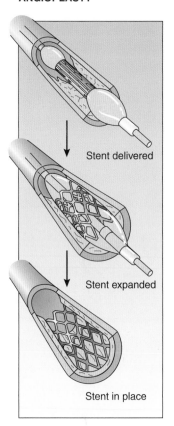

Stent delivered

Stent expanded

Stent in place

PERCUTANEOUS TRANSLUMINAL CORONARY ANGIOPLASTY (PTCA)

Predilation angiogram revealing 99% stenosis of the right coronary artery (RCA)

PTCA procedure showing catheter placement and straddling of the balloon at the occluded site.

Post-PTCA angiogram showing successful dilation

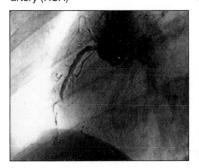

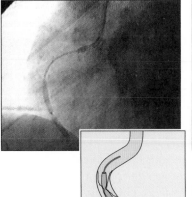

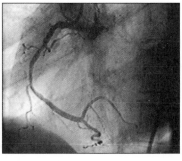

Catheter and wire placement with balloon inflation.

FIGURE 6-10 Percutaneous transluminal coronary angioplasty (PTCA). **A.** Coronary arteries and angiograms illustrating angioplasty. **B.** Placement of stent after angioplasty to keep artery open.

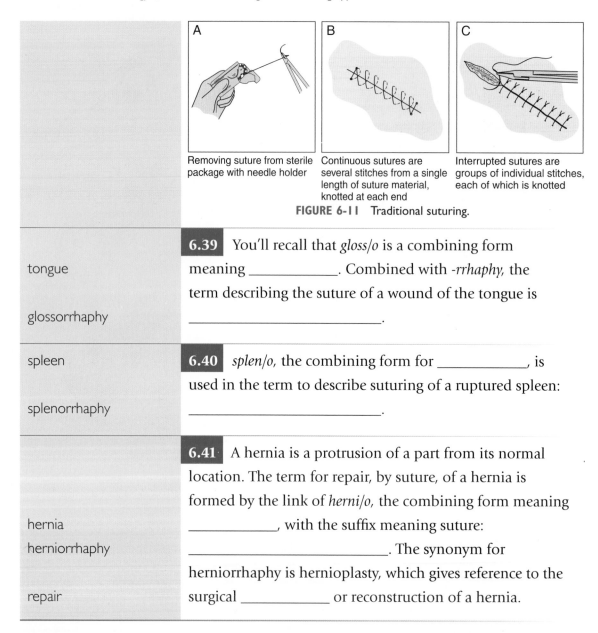

A — Removing suture from sterile package with needle holder

B — Continuous sutures are several stitches from a single length of suture material, knotted at each end

C — Interrupted sutures are groups of individual stitches, each of which is knotted

FIGURE 6-11 Traditional suturing.

---

tongue

glossorrhaphy

6.39 You'll recall that *gloss/o* is a combining form meaning _____. Combined with *-rrhaphy,* the term describing the suture of a wound of the tongue is _____.

---

spleen

splenorrhaphy

6.40 *splen/o,* the combining form for _____, is used in the term to describe suturing of a ruptured spleen: _____.

---

hernia

herniorrhaphy

repair

6.41 A hernia is a protrusion of a part from its normal location. The term for repair, by suture, of a hernia is formed by the link of *herni/o,* the combining form meaning _____, with the suffix meaning suture: _____. The synonym for herniorrhaphy is hernioplasty, which gives reference to the surgical _____ or reconstruction of a hernia.

 ON CLOSER INSPECTION   **Greek Origins of Operative Suffixes**

Most operative suffixes are Greek in origin, and they are typically linked to Greek combining forms in surgical terms. For example, *uter/o* is the Latin combining form for uterus, but *hyster/o,* from Greek, is used in hysterectomy, which is the surgical term for excision of the uterus. Other examples include the use of *orchi/o* in orchiopexy, the term for fixation of the testicle, and *spondyl/o* in spondylosyndesis, the term for the fusion of vertebrae.

SELF-INSTRUCTION: -tripsy (crushing)

Add the following term components to your study of -tripsy before starting the
Programmed Review below.

PREFIX	MEANING	FLASH CARD ID
extra-	outside	P-17
intra-	within	P-14

COMBINING FORM	MEANING	FLASH CARD ID
lith/o	stone	CF-37
nephr/o, ren/o	kidney	CF-45

PROGRAMMED REVIEW: -tripsy (crushing)

ANSWERS	REVIEW
crushing stone presence of	**6.42** -tripsy, the suffix meaning _____, is most commonly used to describe methods of crushing stones. lith/o is the combining form for _____. Linked with -iasis, the suffix referring to a formation of or _____ _____, lithiasis refers to the presence of stones, such as those formed in the gallbladder and kidney.
bile	**6.43** You'll recall that cholelithiasis is the name for the presence of _____ stones.
kidney nephrolithiasis	**6.44** nephr/o, from Greek, and ren/o, from Latin, are combining forms for _____. Using the Greek combining form, the term for the presence of kidney stones is _____. A common treatment for nephrolithiasis is extracorporeal shock wave

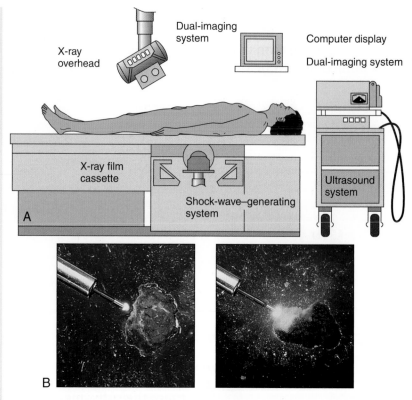

FIGURE 6-12   Lithotripsy. **A.** System for extracorporeal shock wave lithotripsy (ESWL) of kidney stones. High-energy sound waves penetrate the body from outside to bombard and disintegrate a stone from within; most commonly used to treat kidney stones above the bladder. **B.** Intracorporeal lithotripsy. Simulation shows method of destroying stones within the urinary tract using electrical discharges transmitted to a probe within a flexible endoscope; most commonly used to pulverize bladder stones.

lithotripsy (ESWL), a method termed by linking *extra-*, a

outside

prefix meaning _____, with corporeal, a term

that means pertaining to the body. Ultrasonic shock waves

penetrate from outside the body to crush kidney stones that

have formed above the bladder. A similar term uses *intra-*,

within

a prefix meaning _____; intracorporeal lithotripsy

describes the technique using a lithotripter within an

endoscope to directly pulverize a stone, such as those

found in the lower urinary tract (e.g., in the bladder or

ureter) (Fig. 6-12).

SELF-INSTRUCTION: Terms Related to Operation

Add the following term components and list of terms related to operation, or surgery, to your study before starting the Programmed Review below.

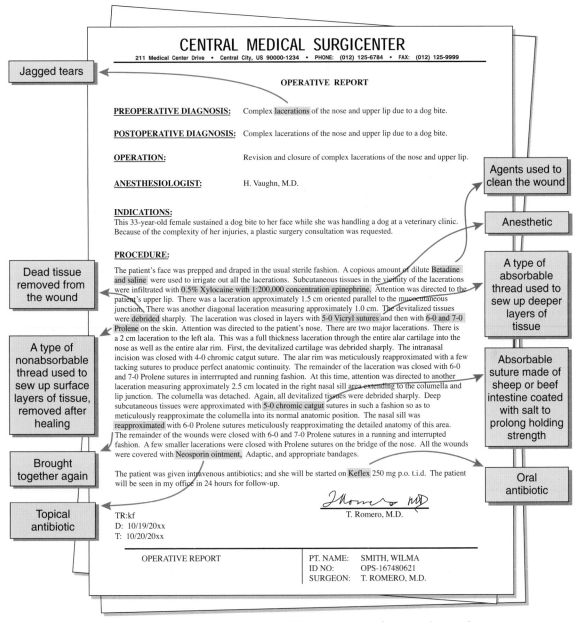

Jagged tears

Agents used to clean the wound

Anesthetic

Dead tissue removed from the wound

A type of absorbable thread used to sew up deeper layers of tissue

A type of nonabsorbable thread used to sew up surface layers of tissue, removed after healing

Absorbable suture made of sheep or beef intestine coated with salt to prolong holding strength

Brought together again

Topical antibiotic

Oral antibiotic

CENTRAL MEDICAL SURGICENTER
211 Medical Center Drive • Central City, US 90000-1234 • PHONE: (012) 125-6784 • FAX: (012) 125-9999

OPERATIVE REPORT

PREOPERATIVE DIAGNOSIS: Complex lacerations of the nose and upper lip due to a dog bite.

POSTOPERATIVE DIAGNOSIS: Complex lacerations of the nose and upper lip due to a dog bite.

OPERATION: Revision and closure of complex lacerations of the nose and upper lip.

ANESTHESIOLOGIST: H. Vaughn, M.D.

INDICATIONS:
This 33-year-old female sustained a dog bite to her face while she was handling a dog at a veterinary clinic. Because of the complexity of her injuries, a plastic surgery consultation was requested.

PROCEDURE:
The patient's face was prepped and draped in the usual sterile fashion. A copious amount of dilute Betadine and saline were used to irrigate out all the lacerations. Subcutaneous tissues in the vicinity of the lacerations were infiltrated with 0.5% Xylocaine with 1:200,000 concentration epinephrine. Attention was directed to the patient's upper lip. There was a laceration approximately 1.5 cm oriented parallel to the mucocutaneous junction. There was another diagonal laceration measuring approximately 1.0 cm. The devitalized tissues were debrided sharply. The laceration was closed in layers with 5-0 Vicryl sutures and then with 6-0 and 7-0 Prolene on the skin. Attention was directed to the patient's nose. There are two major lacerations. There is a 2 cm laceration to the left ala. This was a full thickness laceration through the entire alar cartilage into the nose as well as the entire alar rim. First, the devitalized cartilage was debrided sharply. The intranasal incision was closed with 4-0 chromic catgut suture. The alar rim was meticulously reapproximated with a few tacking sutures to produce perfect anatomic continuity. The remainder of the laceration was closed with 6-0 and 7-0 Prolene sutures in interrrupted and running fashion. At this time, attention was directed to another laceration measuring approximately 2.5 cm located in the right nasal sill area extending to the columella and lip junction. The columella was detached. Again, all devitalized tissues were debrided sharply. Deep subcutaneous tissues were approximated with 5-0 chromic catgut sutures in such a fashion so as to meticulously reapproximate the columella into its normal anatomic position. The nasal sill was reapproximated with 6-0 Prolene sutures meticulously reapproximating the detailed anatomy of this area. The remainder of the wounds were closed with 6-0 and 7-0 Prolene sutures in a running and interrupted fashion. A few smaller lacerations were closed with Prolene sutures on the bridge of the nose. All the wounds were covered with Neosporin ointment, Adaptic, and appropriate bandages.

The patient was given intravenous antibiotics; and she will be started on Keflex 250 mg p.o. t.i.d. The patient will be seen in my office in 24 hours for follow-up.

T. Romero, M.D.

TR:kf
D: 10/19/20xx
T: 10/20/20xx

OPERATIVE REPORT

PT. NAME: SMITH, WILMA
ID NO: OPS-167480621
SURGEON: T. ROMERO, M.D.

Anatomy of an operative report; typical documentation of a surgical procedure.

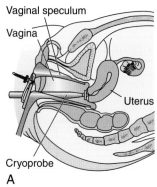

Vaginal speculum
Vagina
Uterus
Cryoprobe

A
Cryosurgical probe is passed through speculum into vagina

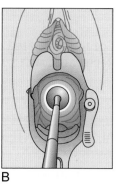

B
Placement of probe at treatment site on cervix

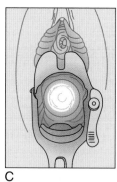

C
Ice crystals seen immediately after freezing treatment

FIGURE 6-13 Cryosurgical procedure to treat cervical dysplasia.

PREFIX	MEANING	FLASH CARD ID
endo-	within	P-14

COMBINING FORM	MEANING	FLASH CARD ID
cry/o	cold	
electr/o	electricity	

TERM	MEANING
cryosurgery	destruction of tissue by freezing with application of an extremely cold chemical, such as liquid nitrogen (Fig. 6-13)
electrosurgery	use of electric currents to destroy tissue; strength of the current and method of application vary
electrocautery	use of an instrument heated by electric current (cautery) to coagulate bleeding areas by burning the tissue (e.g., to sear a blood vessel) (Fig. 6-14)

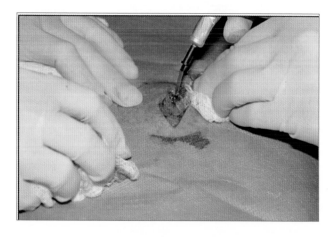

FIGURE 6-14 Electrocautery. A cautery device is used to perform hemostasis (stop bleeding) during a surgical procedure.

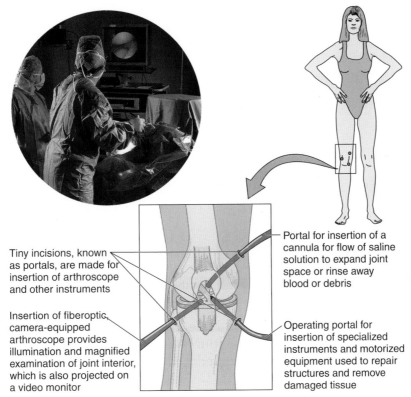

FIGURE 6-15   Arthroscopic knee surgery showing projection of surgeon's view on video monitor.

Tiny incisions, known as portals, are made for insertion of arthroscope and other instruments

Insertion of fiberoptic, camera-equipped arthroscope provides illumination and magnified examination of joint interior, which is also projected on a video monitor

Portal for insertion of a cannula for flow of saline solution to expand joint space or rinse away blood or debris

Operating portal for insertion of specialized instruments and motorized equipment used to repair structures and remove damaged tissue

endoscopic surgery	procedure using an endoscope that includes examination and operative treatment; used in a variety of procedures
arthroscopic surgery	procedure using an arthroscope to examine, diagnose, and repair a joint from within (Fig. 6-15)
laparoscopic surgery	operative procedures within the abdominal and pelvic regions after insertion of a laparoscope (commonly referred to as "key hole" surgery because of the small incision that is made as opposed to traditional laparotomy); common laparoscopic procedures include appendectomy, cholecystectomy, and tubal ligation (female sterilization by cutting and tying uterine tubes)
endovascular surgery	minimally invasive interventional techniques performed within a vessel (e.g., an artery) most commonly done at the same time as a diagnostic procedure such as cardiac catheterization or diagnostic neuroradiological exam; percutaneous transluminal coronary angioplasty (PTCA) is an example (see Fig. 6-10)

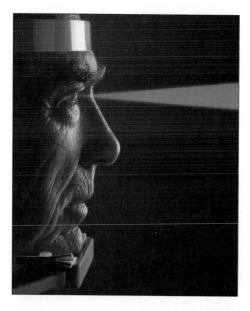

FIGURE 6-16 Simulation of laser application in the eye.

laser surgery	surgical use of a laser to make incisions or destroy tissues (e.g., to create fluid passages and obliterate tumors); commonly applied to delicate tissues such as in the eye (Fig. 6-16)
LASER	acronym for light amplification by stimulated emission of radiation; the instrument produces a small, extremely intense beam that is precise in depth and diameter; it is applied to body tissues to destroy lesions or for dissection (cutting of parts for study)

PROGRAMMED REVIEW: Terms Related to Operation

ANSWERS	REVIEW
cold freezing	**6.45** *cry/o* is a combining form meaning _____. Cryosurgery destroys tissue by _____ it, usually with an extremely cold chemical, such as liquid nitrogen.
electrosurgery	**6.46** Electricity is used in many procedures to destroy unwanted tissue. The general term for such procedures is _____. The use of an

electrically heated instrument to coagulate a bleeding area by burning tissue is called

electrocautery _____.

6.47   You'll recall from Chapter 5 that *-scopy,* the suffix

process, examination   meaning _____ of _____,

is used in the general term that describes the process of

endoscopy   examination within the body: _____

(particularly the interior of a tubular or hollow organ).

Surgical repair of a body part done at the same time as

endoscopic   endoscopic examination is called _____

joint   surgery. *arthr/o,* a combining form meaning _____,

is used in the procedure that includes both examination and

arthroscopy   surgical repair of a joint: _____.

6.48   *lapar/o,* a combining form meaning

abdomen   _____, is used to name the surgical procedures

performed within the abdominal and pelvic cavities using a

laparoscopic   laparoscope: _____ surgery

hole   (commonly referred to as "key _____" surgery

because of the small incision that is made). Common

laparoscopic procedures include appendectomy

excision, removal   (_____ or _____ of the appendix),

cholecystectomy (removal of the

gallbladder   _____), and tubal ligation (female

cutting, tying   sterilization by _____ and _____ the

uterine tubes).

6.49   The combination of *endo-,* a prefix meaning

within   _____, with *vascul/o,* a combining form meaning

vessel   _____, and *-ar,* a suffix meaning

pertaining to   _____ _____, forms the general term for

endovascular reconstruction vessel	minimally invasive interventional techniques performed within a vessel: _____ surgery. A common endovascular surgery is angioplasty, which involves the repair or _____ within a _____ (commonly an artery).
LASER laser	**6.50** The acronym for light amplification by stimulated emission of radiation is _____. This technology is used in an instrument that produces a small, extremely intense beam that is precise in depth and diameter; it is applied to body tissues to destroy lesions or for dissection in the operative technique known as _____ surgery.

Therapeutic Terms

Therapy is a Greek word referring to the nonsurgical treatment of a disease or disorder. Common therapies are presented in the Self-Instruction and Programmed Review sections that follow.

SELF-INSTRUCTION: Common Therapies

Add the following terms related to therapy to your study before starting the Programmed Review below.

TERM	MEANING
chemotherapy	treatment of malignancies, infections, and other diseases with chemical agents that destroy selected cells or impair their ability to reproduce
psychotherapy	treatment of psychiatric disorders using verbal and nonverbal interaction with patients, individually or in a group, employing specific actions and techniques
radiation therapy	treatment of disease, especially cancer, using ionizing radiation to impede the proliferation of abnormal cells
physical medicine and rehabilitation therapy	therapy to restore function and prevent disability resulting from illness or injury; provided by physicians, known as physiatrists, and therapists in specialized areas including physical therapy, occupational therapy, speech therapy, and massage therapy

physical therapy (PT), *syn.* physiotherapy	treatment to rehabilitate patients who are disabled by illness or injury; involves many different modalities (methods), such as exercise, hydrotherapy, and therapeutic ultrasound
occupational therapy (OT)	rehabilitation of individuals suffering from physical, developmental, mental, or emotional disabilities to regain or improve functions in areas of self-care and tasks needed to perform everyday activities independently
speech-language therapy	therapy to assess, diagnosis, treat, and prevent communication disorders related to speech (voice or sound) or language (words)
massage therapy	manipulation of the soft muscle tissues of the body to improve circulation and remove waste products; used to treat overworked muscles as a result of sports injuries, reduce stress, and promote general health; considered a practice of complementary and alternative medicine (CAM)

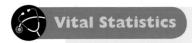

Vital Statistics   COMPLEMENTARY AND ALTERNATIVE MEDICINE

Complementary and alternative medicine (CAM) refers to various medical and health care systems, practices, and products that are not currently considered to be part of "conventional medicine" (that is, medicine as practiced by medical doctors, doctors of osteopathy, and other health care professionals, such as physical therapists, psychologists, and nurses).

The main difference between complementary and alternative medicine is based on how a treatment is used. A nontraditional therapy is called **complementary** when it is used *together with* conventional medicine. An example of this is using aromatherapy (in which a patient inhales the scent of essential oils from flowers, herbs, and trees to promote health and well-being and to alleviate discomfort) in conjunction with traditional pain medications following surgery. A nontraditional therapy is considered **alternative** when it is used *in place of* conventional medicine. Using a special diet to treat cancer instead of undergoing surgery, radiation, or chemotherapy is an example of an alternative therapy.

As CAM therapies prove to be effective, they are being incorporated more often with conventional care. **Integrative medicine** is an approach to healing in which two or more modalities or systems are combined, designed to treat the person as a whole. For example, an integrative medicine approach to reduce a patient's cholesterol levels may include adhering to an Ayurvedic diet and receiving acupuncture therapy, as well as taking medications prescribed by his or her conventional doctor.

The list of what is considered to be CAM is constantly changing, but the major types of CAM include:

- **Whole medical systems**—Complete systems of theory and practice, such as homeopathic medicine, naturopathic medicine, traditional Chinese medicine, and Ayurveda.
- **Mind-body medicine**—A variety of techniques designed to enhance the mind's ability to affect bodily functions and symptoms, such as yoga, meditation, prayer, mental healing, and therapies that use creative outlets such as art, music, or dance.
- **Biologically based practices**—Use of substances found in nature, such as herbs, foods, and vitamins, to treat illness.
- **Manipulative and body-based practices**—Practices based on manipulation, such as chiropractic medicine and massage.
- **Energy medicine**—Treatment that involves the use of energy fields, including biofield therapy (e.g., Reiki and therapeutic touch) and bio-electromagnetic-based therapy (e.g., pulsed fields, magnetic fields, or AC/DC fields).

Although some CAM therapies are supported with scientific evidence, most therapies have not been tested through well-designed scientific studies. Such studies would address whether these therapies are safe and whether they work for the diseases or medical conditions for which they are used.

 Health Care Professionals   MEET THE MASSAGE THERAPIST

Massage therapy is a highly versatile field with a wide range of applications and settings. Massage therapists perform various types of touch-based modalities to benefit the health of their clients, such as Swedish massage, deep tissue work, myofascial release, craniosacral therapy, trigger point work, lymphatic drainage techniques, polarity, reflexology, and many others. One of the attractive things about massage therapy and other types of bodywork is that these professions can be practiced in a wide variety of settings.

A more detailed description of massage therapy as a health care career can be found on the Student Resource CD-ROM and at the companion website at www.thePoint.lww.com/WillisQC.

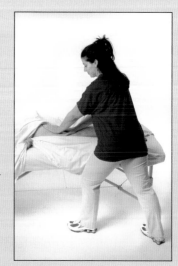

PROGRAMMED REVIEW: Common Therapies

ANSWERS	REVIEW
chemotherapy	**6.51** The combining form referring to chemical agents is *chem/o*. The treatment of malignancies, infections, and other diseases with chemical agents that destroy targeted cells is called _____.
mind psychotherapy	**6.52** *psych/o*, the combining form meaning _____, is used to name the therapy to treat psychiatric disorders that emphasizes verbal and nonverbal communication and interaction with patients: _____.
radiation therapy	**6.53** Some kinds of cancer are treated with radiation, which deters the proliferation of abnormal cells. This is called _____ _____.
function, prevent	**6.54** Physiatrists, physical therapists, occupational therapists, speech therapists, and massage therapists are rehabilitation specialists who provide therapy designed to restore _____ and _____ disability in injured or ill patients.

Pharmacotherapy

A drug is a therapeutic agent used to prevent or treat an abnormal condition. Pharmakon, a Greek word meaning medicine, is used in terms referring to a medication or drug. Pharmacology is the study of medications or drugs, and pharmacotherapy describes the treatment of disease using drugs. Because drugs are so often prescribed for the treatment of illness and injury, it is important to know about common drug classifications and pharmacotherapies.

SELF-INSTRUCTION: Common Therapeutic Drug Classifications

Add the following suffixes, prefixes, and combining forms to your study before learning terms related to the common therapeutic drug classifications that follow.

SUFFIX	MEANING	FLASH CARD ID
-lytic (adjective form of -lysis)	pertaining to breakdown or dissolution	
-emetic (adjective form of -emesis)	pertaining to vomiting	

PREFIX	MEANING	FLASH CARD ID
a-, an-	without	P-1
anti-, contra-	against, or opposed to	P-7

COMBINING FORM	MEANING	FLASH CARD ID
anxi/o	anxiety	
bi/o	life	
bronch/o	bronchus (airway)	
cardi/o	heart	CF-11
coagul/o	clotting	
esthesi/o	sensation	CF-25
hypn/o	sleep	CF-32
narc/o	stupor or sleep	CF-42
pyret/o	fever	CF-55
thromb/o	clot	CF-64
ton/o	tone or tension	

A drug's classification is key to understanding what symptom or diagnosis a specific drug treats. Add the following common therapeutic drug classifications to your study before starting the Programmed Review.

CLASSIFICATION	DESCRIPTION
analgesic	a drug that relieves pain
narcotic	a potent analgesic with addictive properties
anesthetic	a drug that temporarily blocks transmission of nerve conduction to produce a loss of sensation, such as pain
antacid	a drug that neutralizes stomach acid
antianginal	a drug that dilates coronary arteries, restoring oxygen to the tissues to relieve the pain of angina pectoris, or chest pain
antianxiety agent, *syn.* anxiolytic agent	a drug used to reduce anxiety

antiarrhythmic	a drug that counteracts cardiac arrhythmia
antibiotic	a drug that kills or inhibits the growth of microorganisms
anticoagulant	a drug that prevents clotting of the blood
anticonvulsant	an agent that prevents or lessens convulsions, or seizures; commonly used to treat epilepsy
antidiabetic	any of several agents used to control blood sugar levels in the treatment of diabetes mellitus
antidepressant	an agent that counteracts depression
antiemetic	a drug that prevents or stops vomiting
antifungal	a drug that kills or prevents the growth of fungi
antihistamine histamine	a drug that blocks the effects of histamine in the body a regulating body substance released in excess during allergic reactions, causing swelling and inflammation of tissues; seen in hay fever and urticaria, or hives
antihyperlipidemic	a drug that reduces serum fat and cholesterol
antihypertensive	a drug that lowers blood pressure
antiinflammatory	a drug that reduces inflammation
antipruritic	a drug that relieves itching
antipyretic	a drug that relieves fever
antiseptic	an agent that inhibits the growth of infectious micro-organisms
antispasmodic	a drug that prevents or relieves muscle spasm
antithyroid drug	an agent that blocks the production of thyroid hormones; used to treat hyperthyroidism
antiviral	an agent that destroys a virus or weakens its action
bronchodilator	a drug that dilates the muscular walls of the bronchi
cardiotonic	a drug that increases the force of myocardial contractions in the heart; commonly used to treat congestive heart failure (CHF)
cathartic	a drug that causes movement of the bowels; also called a laxative
decongestant	a drug that reduces congestion and swelling of membranes, such as those of the nose and eustachian tube during an infection
diuretic	a drug that increases the secretion of urine; commonly prescribed in treating hypertension

expectorant	a drug that breaks up mucus and promotes coughing
hypnotic	an agent that induces sleep
hypoglycemic, *syn.* antihyperglycemic	a drug that lowers blood glucose level (e.g., insulin)
nonsteroidal antiinflammatory drug (NSAID)	a group of drugs with analgesic, antiinflammatory, and antipyretic properties (e.g., ibuprofen and aspirin) commonly used to treat arthritis
psychotropic drug	a medication capable of affecting the mind, emotions, and behavior; used to treat mental illness (*trop/o* = a turning)
antipsychotic agents	a class of psychotropic drugs used to treat psychosis, especially schizophrenia
sedative	an agent that has a calming effect and quiets nervousness
thrombolytic agents	a drug used to dissolve thrombi (blood clots), such as streptokinase and tissue plasminogen activator (TPA or tPA); used in acute management of myocardial infarction (MI) and ischemic stroke; commonly called "clot busters"
vasoconstrictor	a drug that causes a narrowing of the blood vessels, thereby decreasing blood flow
vasodilator	a drug that causes dilation of the blood vessels, thereby increasing blood flow

PROGRAMMED REVIEW: Common Therapeutic Drug Classifications

ANSWERS	REVIEW
	6.55 Anesthetic, the term for the class of drugs that temporarily block transmission of nerve conduction to produce a loss of sensations, is derived from the combination of *esthesi/o*, a combining form meaning
sensation	_____, the suffix -*tic*, meaning
pertaining to	_____ ____, and the prefix *an-*,
without	meaning _____.
	6.56 The Greek word algesis means pain. A drug that
analgesic	relieves pain is called a/an _____

pertaining to	(using *-ic*, the suffix meaning _____ ____, and the prefix *an-*). *narc/o*, a combining form meaning
stupor	_____ or sleep, was used to name a type of potent,
narcotic	addictive analgesic drug known as a _____ (also using the suffix *-ic*).

	6.57 Many drug classifications are named according to their action against a condition or symptom. The prefix
against, opposed to	*anti-*, meaning _____ or _____ ____, is key to understanding the action. For instance, a drug that works against excess stomach acid by
antacid	neutralizing it is a/an _____. (This term applies the rule for forming medical terms that occasionally, when a prefix [such as *anti-*] ends in a vowel and the root begins with a vowel, the final vowel
dropped	is _____ from the prefix.) In the term antacid, the suffix *-ic* is not used.

chest	**6.58** Angina pectoris, you recall, is _____
pain	_____. Drugs that treat anginal pain are classified as
antianginal	_____ drugs. Nitroglycerin is a common
dilator	antianginal medication. It acts as a vaso_____, causing the coronary arteries to expand and increasing the flow of blood to the heart muscle tissue, or
myocardium	_____.

	6.59 A drug that acts against or opposed to anxiety in order to reduce it is classified as an
antianxiety	_____ or anxiolytic agent. *-lytic* is the adjective form of *-lysis*, a suffix meaning
breakdown, dissolution	_____ or _____.

arrhythmic	**6.60** A drug that counteracts a cardiac arrhythmia is called an anti_____.
life antibiotic	**6.61** *bi/o*, the combining form meaning _____, is modified by *-tic* and *anti-* to denote a drug class that acts to kill or inhibit microbial life. This drug is a/an _____.
against opposed to clotting	**6.62** Formed by a link of *anti-*, meaning _____ or _____ ____, with *coagul/o*, a combining form meaning _____, anticoagulants work to prevent clot formation.
anticonvulsant	**6.63** The prefix *anti-* is also linked to convulsion to name a type of drug used to prevent or lessen seizures: _____.
diabetes mellitus	**6.64** An antidiabetic drug is used to treat _____ _____ (DM).
antidepressant	**6.65** A drug that counteracts depression is classified as a/an _____.
vomiting	**6.66** An antiemetic is used to stop or prevent _____.
antifungal against, opposed to	**6.67** Fungus infections are common and affect many parts of the body, including the skin and nails. A drug that kills or prevents the growth of such infections is called a/an _____, using the prefix *anti-*, which means _____ or _____ ____.

6.68 Histamine is a body substance released in excess during an allergic reaction. A drug that blocks the effects of this substance is called a/an _____.
Such drugs are used to combat allergic reactions such as hives and hay fever.

antihistamine

6.69 A drug that lowers high blood pressure is called an anti_____. One type of antihypertensive drug, called a diuretic, works by increasing the secretion of _____ from the body.

hypertensive

urine

6.70 A drug that reduces inflammation is called a/an _____.

antiinflammatory

6.71 The term for itching is pruritus, and a drug that relieves itching is called a/an _____.

antipruritic

6.72 *pyret/o*, a combining form meaning fire or _____, is modified by the prefix *anti-*, meaning against or _____ ____, in the name for the class of drugs that relieve fever: _____.

fever

opposed to

antipyretic

6.73 Sepsis is an infection by microorganisms; a drug that inhibits the growth of such microorganisms is a/an _____.

antiseptic

6.74 Simply put, a drug that relieves spasm is called a/an _____.

antispasmodic

6.75 An agent that blocks the production of thyroid hormones is called a/an _____ drug.

antithyroid

antiviral	**6.76** The drug that works against the ill effects of a virus by destroying it or weakening its actions is referred to as a/an _____ agent.
bronchodilator	**6.77** A person with asthma can experience constriction of the bronchi during an attack. A therapeutic drug that counteracts this constriction by dilating the muscular walls of the bronchi is a/an _____.
tonic	**6.78** Congestive heart failure is often treated with drugs that increase the force of ventricular contractions. These drugs are called cardio_____ agents.
cathartic	**6.79** The Greek word katharsis means purification by purging. A drug that purges the large intestine by stimulating a bowel movement is called a/an _____; such a drug is also called a laxative.
not decongestant	**6.80** The prefix *de-* means from, down, or _____. A drug that is given to reduce congestion, such as may occur in the eustachian, or auditory, tube during an infection, is a/an _____.
expectorant	**6.81** Expectoration means coughing up and spitting out material from the lungs. A type of drug that breaks up mucus to promote coughing is a/an _____.
hypn/o hypnotic	**6.82** The combining forms for sleep are *somn/i, somn/o,* and _____. Formed from the last of these, the term for an agent that induces sleep is a/an _____.

hyperglycemia	**6.83** Recall that the condition of high blood sugar is called _____. A drug that works against this condition by lowering the blood glucose level
antihyperglycemic	is a/an _____ drug.
hypoglycemic	Another term for this is a/an _____ drug.

6.84 Lipids, you'll recall, are fats. Hyperlipidemia refers
excessive to condition of _____ level of fat in
blood the _____. Using the prefix *anti-*, drugs that work
against this condition by lowering the amount of fat in
antihyperlipid the blood are called _____emic
agents.

6.85 The suffix *-tropic*, meaning pertaining to turning,
is used in a link to *psych/o*, the combining form meaning
mind _____, to name the general classification of
medications used to treat mental illness:
psychotropic _____ drugs. You'll recall from
mind Chapter 4 that psychosis is a condition of the _____
in which the patient has lost touch with reality; the
patient is said to be psychotic. When *anti-*, the prefix
against meaning opposed to or _____, is combined
with psychotic, it forms the name for the class of
psychotropic drugs used to act against psychoses, especially
antipsychotic schizophrenia: _____.

6.86 There are several types of analgesic and
antiinflammatory drugs. The group that includes aspirin
nonsteroidal and ibuprofen is called _____
antiinflammatory _____ drugs (NSAIDs).

sedative	**6.87** Sedatio, a Latin word meaning to calm, is used to name the agent that has a calming effect and quiets nervousness: _____.
breaking down, dissolution	**6.88** -*lysis* is a suffix meaning _____
clots	_____ or _____. Drugs that work to dissolve thrombi or _____ in the blood are called
thrombo	_____lytic agents.
vessel	**6.89** *vas/o* is a combining form referring to _____. A drug that causes a narrowing of the blood vessels and decreases blood flow is classified as
vaso	a/an _____constrictor.
vaso	**6.90** An antianginal agent works to counteract chest pain by causing dilation of the coronary arteries. Any drug that causes dilation of the blood vessels and increases blood flow is classified as a/an _____dilator.

Pronunciation Summary

Below you'll find a list of medical terms that you have learned to build and spell in this chapter, followed by the page number on which each term can be found and its written pronunciation. 🎧 Take a minute to listen to the audio pronunciations of these terms on the Student Resource CD-ROM, and then practice pronouncing them out loud. For additional practice and reinforcement, write the definition of each term on a separate piece of paper.

abdominocentesis/281
ab-dom′i-nō-sen-tē′sis

allograft/284
al′ō-graft

amniocentesis/281
am′nē-ō-sen-tē′sis

analgesic/306
an′ăl-jē′zik

anesthetic/306
an′es-thet′ik

angioplasty/291
an′jē-ō-plas-tē

antacid/306
ant-as'id

antianginal/306
an'tē-an'ji-năl

antianxiety agent/306
an'tē-ang-zī'ĕ-tē ā'jĕnt

antiarrhythmic/307
an'tē-ă-rith'mik

antibiotic/307
an'tē-bī-ot'ik

anticoagulant/307
an'tē-kō-ag'yū-lănt

anticonvulsant/307
an'tē-kŏn-vŭl'sănt

antidiabetic/307
an'tē-dī-ă-bet'ik

antidepressant/307
an'tē-dĕ-pres'ănt

antiemetic/307
an'tē-ĕ-met'ik

antifungal/307
an'tē-fŭng'găl

antihistamine/307
an-tē-his'tă-mēn

antihyperglycemic/308
an'tē-hī'per-glī-sē'mik

antihyperlipidemic/307
an'tē-hī-per-lip'i-dē'mik

antihypertensive/307
an'tē-hī-per-ten'siv

antiinflammatory/307
an'tē-in-flam'ă-tor-ē

antipruritic/307
an'tē-prū-rit'ik

antipyretic/307
an'tē-pī-ret'ik

antiseptic/307
an'ti-sep'tik

antispasmodic/307
an'ti-spaz-mod'ik

antithyroid/307
an'tē-thī'royd

antiviral/307
an'tē-vī'răl

anxiolytic agent/306
ang'zē-ō-lit'ik ā'jĕnt

appendectomy/277
ap'pĕn-dek'tŏ-mē

arthrocentesis/282
ahr'thrō-sen-tē'sis

arthrodesis/283
ahr-throd'ĕ-sis

arthroplasty/290
ahr'thrō-plas-tē

arthroscopic surgery/299
ahr'thrō-skop-ik sŭr'jĕr-ē

augmentation mammoplasty/291
awg'men-tā'shŭn mam'ō-plas-tē

autograft/284
aw'tō-graft

bronchodilator/307
brong'kō-dī'lā-tŏr

bypass graft/285
bī'pas graft

cardiotonic/307
kar'dē-ō-ton'ik

cathartic/307
kă-thar'tik

chemotherapy/302
kē'mō-thār'ă-pē

cholecystectomy/277
kō'lĕ-sis-tek'tŏ-mē

colectomy/277
kŏ-lek'tŏ-mē

colostomy/274
kō-los'tŏ-mē

coronary artery/285
kōr'ŏ-nār-ē ahr'tĕr-ē

cryosurgery/298
krī-ō-ser'jer-ē

decongestant/307
dē-kon-jes'tant

diuretic/307
dī-yū-ret'ik

electrocautery/298
ē-lek'trō-caw'ter-ē

endoscopic surgery/299
en'dō-skop'ik sŭr'jĕr-ē

endovascular surgery/299
en'dō-vas'kyū-lăr sŭr'jĕr-ē

expectorant/308
ek-spek'tō-rănt

extracorporeal shock wave lithotripsy (ESWL)/295
eks'tră-kōr-pōr'ē-ăl shok wāv lith'ō-trip'sē

gastrectomy/278
gas-trek'tŏ-mē

glossorrhaphy/294
glos-ōr'ă-fē

herniorrhaphy/294
hĕr'nē-ōr'ă-fē

heterograft/284
het'ĕr-ō-graft

histamine/307
his'tă-mēn

homograft/284
hō'mō-graft

hypnotic/308
hip-not'ik

hypoglycemic/308
hī'pō-glī-sē'mik

hysterectomy/278
his'tĕr-ek'tŏ-mē

ileostomy/274
il'ē-os'tŏ-mē

intracorporeal lithotripsy/296
in'tră-kōr-pōr'ē-ăl lith'ō-trip-sē

laparoscopic surgery/308
lap'ă-rō-skop'ik sŭr'jĕr-ē

laparotomy/271
lap'ă-rot'ŏ-mē

laser surgery/300
lā'zĕr sŭr'jĕr-ē

mammoplasty/291
mam'ō-plas-tē

mastectomy/277
mas-tek'tŏ-mē

mastopexy/288
mas'tō-pek-sē

myringotomy/273
mir-in-got'ŏ-mē

narcotic/306
nar-kot'ik

nonsteroidal antiinflammatory drug (NSAID)/308
non'ster-oy'dăl an'tī-in-flam'ă-tōr-ē drŭg

oophorectomy/278
ō'of-ōr-ek'tŏ-mē

orchiopexy/288
ōr'kē-ō-pek'sē

paracentesis/281
par'ă-sen-tē'sis

percutaneous transluminal coronary angioplasty (PTCA)/292
pĕr'kyū-tā'nē-ŭs trans-lū'mĕn-ăl kōr'ŏ-nār-ē an'jē-ō-plas-tē

physical medicine and rehabilitation therapy/302
fiz'i-kăl med'i-sin and rē'hă-bil'i-tā'shŭn thār'ă-pē

physical therapy (PT)/303
fiz'i-kăl thār'ă-pē

physiotherapy/303
iz'ē-ō-thār'ă-pē

prostatectomy/278
pros'tă-tek'tŏ-mē

psychotherapy/302
sī'kō-thār'ă-pē

psychotropic drug/308
sī'kō-trō'pik drŭg

radiation therapy/302
rā'dē-ā'shŭn thār'ă-pē

reduction mammoplasty/291
rĕ-dŭk'shŭn mam'ō-plas-tē

rhinoplasty/290
rī'nō-plas-tē

salpingostomy/274
sal'ping-gos'tŏ-mē

salpingotomy/274
sal'ping-got'ŏ-mē

sedative/308
sed'ă-tiv

splenorrhaphy/294
splē-nōr'ă-fē

spondylosyndesis/283
spon'di-lō-sin-dē'sis

tenodesis/283
ten'ŏ-dē'sis

thoracocentesis/281
thōr'ă-kō-sen-tē'sis

thoracostomy/274
thōr'ă-kos'tŏ-mē

thoracotomy/272
thōr'ă-kot'ŏ-mē

thrombolytic agent/308
throm'bō-lit'ik ā'jĕnt

tracheostomy/274
trā'kē-os'tŏ-mē

tracheotomy/272
trā'kē-ot'ŏ-mē

transurethral resection of the prostate (TURP)/279
trans-yŭr-ē'thrăl rē-sek'shŭn of the pros'tāt

urostomy/275
yūr-os'tŏ-mē

vasectomy/278
vas-ek'tŏ-mē

vasoconstrictor/308
vā'sō-kŏn-strik'tŏr

vasodilator/308
vā'sō-dī'lā-tŏr

xenograft/285
zen'ō-graft

Examine Your Understanding

For the following terms, draw a line or lines to separate the prefixes (P), combining forms (CF), roots (R), and suffixes (S). Then, write the meaning of each component on the corresponding blank to define the term.

EXAMPLE

hyperlipemia

hyper/lip/emia

<u>above or excessive</u> / <u>fat</u> / <u>blood condition</u>

P   R   S

1. hysterectomy

     _____ / _____
           R   S

2. colocentesis

     _____ / _____
          CF   S

3. tracheostomy

     _____ / _____
          CF   S

4. glossorrhaphy

     _____ / _____
          CF   S

5. angioplasty

     _____ / _____
          CF   S

6. arthrodesis

     _____ / _____
          CF   S

7. salpingotomy

     _____ / _____
          CF   S

8. lithotripsy

     _____ / _____
          CF   S

9. autograft

     _____ / _____
          P   S

10. orchiopexy

     _____ / _____
          CF   S

Match the following diagnoses with surgeries.

11. _____ prostate cancer
12. _____ otitis media
13. _____ hernia
14. _____ colon cancer
15. _____ ascites
16. _____ tubal pregnancy
17. _____ macromastia
18. _____ nephrolithiasis
19. _____ breast cancer
20. _____ benign prostatic hyperplasia
21. _____ third-degree burn
22. _____ atherosclerotic buildup
23. _____ stomach cancer
24. _____ cholecystitis
25. _____ appendicitis
26. _____ cryptorchism
27. _____ pendulous breast
28. _____ torn tongue

a. mastopexy
b. appendectomy
c. angioplasty
d. cholecystectomy
e. glossorrhaphy
f. lithotripsy
g. orchiopexy
h. autograft
i. gastrectomy
j. colectomy
k. herniorrhaphy
l. abdominocentesis
m. myringotomy
n. mastectomy
o. transurethral resection of prostate
p. prostatectomy
q. salpingostomy
r. mammoplasty

Circle the meaning of the following prefixes.

29. *per-*
    a. across   b. abnormal   c. alongside of   d. by

30. *an-*
    a. half   b. without   c. with   d. deficient

31. *syn-*
    a. together   b. above   c. below   d. without

32. *hyper-*
    a. small   b. above   c. abnormal   d. large

33. *macro-*
    a. excessive   b. deficient   c. large   d. above

34. *para-*
    a. across   b. through   c. around   d. alongside of

35. *micro-*
   a. below   b. excessive   c. small   d. deficient

36. *hemi-*
   a. half   b. abnormal   c. around   d. small

37. *ec-*
   a. within   b. out   c. alongside of   d. below

38. *intra-*
   a. within   b. below   c. between   d. above

39. *anti-*
   a. within   b. excessive   c. opposed to   d. before

40. *contra-*
   a. with   b. against   c. toward   d. below

For each of the following, circle the combining form that corresponds to the meaning given.

41. muscle	*my/o*	*mast/o*	*arthr/o*
42. ovary	*hyster/o*	*orchi/o*	*oophor/o*
43. bile	*lith/o*	*chol/e*	*ur/o*
44. abdomen	*gastr/o*	*lapar/o*	*nephr/o*
45. joint	*arthr/o*	*my/o*	*vertebr/o*
46. chest	*trache/o*	*ven/o*	*thorac/o*
47. stomach	*abdomin/o*	*gastr/o*	*lapar/o*
48. urine	*ur/o*	*uter/o*	*metr/o*
49. eardrum	*rhin/o*	*myring/o*	*salping/o*
50. skin	*my/o*	*vas/o*	*cutane/o*

Write out the expanded term of each acronym or abbreviation.

51. CABG _____

   (hint: cardiovascular procedure)

52. TURP _____

   (hint: male genitourinary procedure)

53. OT _____

   (hint: rehabilitation profession)

54. PTCA _____

   (hint: cardiovascular procedure)

55. NSAID _____

    (hint: therapeutic drug class)

56. ESWL _____

    (hint: urinary procedure)

57. TPA or tPA _____

    (hint: thrombolytic agent)

58. LASER _____

    (hint: acronym for surgical instrument)

59. PT _____

    (hint: rehabilitation profession)

Match the following conditions to the class of drugs most commonly used in their treatment.

60. _____ pain   a. antiemetic

61. _____ vomiting   b. hypoglycemic

62. _____ fever   c. cathartic

63. _____ itch   d. antihistamine

64. _____ myocardial infarction   e. cardiotonic

65. _____ constipation   f. thrombolytic agent

66. _____ anxiety   g. antipyretic

67. _____ congestive heart failure   h. antihyperlipidemic

68. _____ high blood sugar   i. analgesic

69. _____ hypercholesterolemia   j. antipruritic

70. _____ urticaria (hives)   k. anxiolytic

Compare and contrast the following terms.

71. anticoagulant vs. thrombolytic _____

    _____

72. psychotropic vs. antipsychotic _____

    _____

73. vasoconstrictor vs. vasodilator _____

    _____

74. homograft vs. xenograft _____

    _____

75. intracorporeal lithotripsy vs. extracorporeal lithotripsy _____ __

_____

76. tracheotomy vs. tracheostomy _____

_____

Match the surgical terms with definitions.

77 _____ myringotomy   a. fixation of a testicle

78. _____ thoracostomy   b. incision in eardrum

79. _____ salpingostomy   c. excision of ovary

80. _____ oophorectomy   d. creation of an opening in uterine tube

81. _____ paracentesis   e. surgical repair of nose

82. _____ orchiopexy   f. creation of an opening in the chest

83. _____ rhinoplasty   g. puncture for aspiration of the abdomen

Complete the following sentences.

84. Electrocautery is an electrosurgical instrument used to _____ bleeding areas by burning the tissue.

85. Cryosurgery destroys tissue by _____ it.

86. Arthroscopic surgery is a procedure using an instrument called a/an _____ to examine, diagnose, and repair from within a joint.

87. Laser is commonly applied to _____ tissues because of its precision in depth and diameter.

88. Laparoscopic surgery is referred to as _____ _____ surgery because of the small incision that is made.

89. An expectorant is a drug that breaks up mucus and promotes _____.

90. A hypnotic is an agent that induces _____.

91. A diuretic increases the secretion of _____.

92. An anesthetic is used to temporarily block transmission of nerve conduction to produce a loss of _____.

93. Treatment of disease with chemical agents that destroy selected cells or impair their ability to reproduce is called _____therapy.

94. Psychotherapy uses verbal and nonverbal interaction with patients to treat diseases of the _____.

95. Radiation therapy uses ionizing _____ to impede the proliferation of abnormal cells.

96. The physician who specializes in physical medicine and rehabilitation therapy is called a/an _____.

97. Pharmacotherapy describes the treatment of disease using _____.

98. Therapy to regain or improve functions in areas of self-care and activities of every-day living is performed by _____ therapists.

99. Exercise, hydrotherapy, and therapeutic ultrasound are methods commonly used by _____ therapists.

100. Speech-language therapy involves diagnosis, treatment, and prevention of _____ disorders.

MEDICAL RECORD EXERCISES

Medical Record 6-1

Chart Notes

You first read about Larry Phelps in the Meet the Patient vignette at the beginning of this chapter. Medical Record 6-1 (pages 326-327) is a series of three progress notes written by Dr. Derrick after first meeting with Mr. Phelps to schedule surgery, after the surgery and discharge, and after seeing Mr. Phelps in a follow-up 10 days later. Read the chart notes and answer the following questions.

Questions about Medical Record 6-1

1. Below are medical terms used in this record that you have not yet encountered in the text. Underline each term where it appears in the record and, using a medical dictionary, define the term below.

   sterility _____

   genitalia _____

   vas (vas deferens) _____

   scrotum _____

   infiltrated _____

   cauterized _____

   suture _____

   semen _____

   ejaculation _____

   ecchymoses _____

   epididymides _____

   induration _____

2. The medical record suggests that Mr. Phelps signed which of the following before surgery?

   a. last will and testament
   b. consent form
   c. application to sperm bank
   d. none of the above

3. In your own words, without using medical terminology, briefly summarize the procedure that Dr. Derrick performed. _____
   _____
   _____

4. Complications of the surgery included which of the following?

    a. sterility
    b. fever
    c. nausea
    d. bleeding
    e. all of the above
    f. none of the above

5. Translate the instruction for the immediate postoperative medication (how much, how often). _____

    _____

    _____

6. Which of the following were symptoms that Mr. Phelps reported to Dr. Derrick at his follow-up visit 10 days after surgery?

    a. fever
    b. bleeding
    c. pain in the scrotum
    d. impotence
    e. suture loosening

7. In your own words, define the diagnosis that Dr. Derrick made at the follow-up visit.

    _____

    _____

    _____

8. In the table below, translate Dr. Derrick's medication instructions after the follow-up visit.

Medication	Strength	How Often

CENTRAL MEDICAL GROUP, INC.

Department of Urology

201 Medical Center Drive • Central City, US 90000-1234 • PHONE: (012) 125-8888 • FAX: (012) 125-3434

PROGRESS NOTES

PHELPS, LAWRENCE

June 4, 20xx

SUBJECTIVE: This 31-year-old male desires vasectomy for sterility. He and his wife have two children. He states that another pregnancy would put his wife at health risk.

OBJECTIVE: Normal genitalia with single vas bilaterally.

ASSESSMENT: The procedure, goals and risks were thoroughly discussed with the aid of pictures. The vasectomy booklet and consent form were provided to the patient.

PLAN: Schedule bilateral vasectomy.

DL:ti   T:6/7/20xx

J. Derrick, M.D.
J. Derrick, M.D.

June 10, 20xx

PROCEDURE: Bilateral vasectomy.

The patient was placed supine on the table; and the scrotum was shaved, prepped, and draped in the usual fashion. The right testicle was grasped, and the right vas was brought to the skin and was infiltrated with 1% Xylocaine. The vas was freed through a small incision. A segment was resected, and the ends were cauterized and tied with 3-0 silk suture. The skin was closed with 4-0 chromic suture. The same procedure was repeated on the left. There were no complications or bleeding.

PLAN: The patient is discharged to the care of his wife with an Rx for Darvocet-N, 100 mg, 1 q 4 h p.r.n. pain. He has been given a post-vasectomy instruction sheet. He is asked to call if there are any problems. He was also instructed to submit a semen specimen for analysis after 15-20 ejaculations.

DL:ti   T:6/12/20xx

J. Derrick, M.D.
J. Derrick, M.D.

MEDICAL RECORD 6-1   Chart Notes

CENTRAL MEDICAL GROUP, INC.

Department of Urology

201 Medical Center Drive • Central City, US 90000-1234 • PHONE: (012) 125-8888 • FAX: (012) 125-3434

PROGRESS NOTES

PHELPS, LAWRENCE

June 20, 20xx

SUBJECTIVE: The patient has had pain in the right scrotum since surgery which became worse yesterday with pain in his right back. He states he has had no fevers, nausea, or vomiting.

OBJECTIVE: 1) Mild scrotal ecchymoses inferiorly. Normal testes and epididymides.
2) Small induration at left vasectomy site without tenderness.
3) Exquisitely tender 1.5 cm nodule at right vasectomy site; no induration in upper scrotum or cord.

ASSESSMENT: Probable small hematoma at right vasectomy site.

PLAN: Rx: Cipro 500 mg b.i.d. x 5 d
Darvocet-N 100 mg q 4 h p.r.n. pain
ibuprofen p.r.n.

RTO in one week.

DL:ti   T:6/22/20xx

J. Derrick, M.D.
J. Derrick, M.D.

Medical Record 6-2

Operative Report

In the Meet the Patient vignette earlier in this chapter, you learned about Alice Toohey's accident and emergency transport to the hospital, where she was admitted for surgical treatment of a broken ankle. Medical Record 6-2 (page 330) is the operative report, dictated by Dr. Ricardo Rodriguez after he performed the surgery. Read the report and answer the following questions.

Questions about Medical Record 6-2

1. 📖 Below are medical terms used in this record that you have not yet encountered in the text. Underline each term where it appears in the record and, using a medical dictionary, define the terms below.

   fracture _____

   dislocation _____

   malleolus _____

   sterile _____

   tourniquet _____

   curettage _____

   articular cartilage _____

   talus _____

   oblique _____

   fibula _____

   dressing _____

   splint _____

2. In your own words, without using medical terminology, briefly describe the preoperative diagnosis for Mrs. Toohey. _____

   _____

   _____

3. Put the following operative steps in the correct order by numbering them from 1 to 10.

   _____ a. radiograph of the screws that were too long

   _____ b. incision on the outer side of the ankle

   _____ c. plate placed onto fibula

   _____ d. sewing the incisions

_____ e. radiograph of satisfactory screw position

_____ f. towel clip positioned

_____ g. removal of medial hematoma

_____ h. removal of lateral hematoma

_____ i. placement of screw into lower tibia

_____ j. incision on the inner side of the right ankle

4. In this operation, the surgeon redid one step after using a diagnostic procedure to check whether that step was as effective as possible. In your own words, explain what Dr. Rodriquez changed, and why. _____

_____

_____

5. Describe the fracture lines in your own words.

medial malleolus _____

lateral malleolus _____

6. When Dr. Rodriquez examined the ankle after making the first incision, he found a problem that he could not and did not repair. In your own words, what had been destroyed in Mrs. Toohey's injury? _____

_____

_____

7. Which of the following actions did not occur in this operation?

a. washing the wound with antibiotic
b. taping the fracture line
c. drilling holes in the bone
d. stapling the skin closed

8. Describe Mrs. Toohey's condition when transferred to postanesthesia recovery (PAR) after the operation. _____

_____

_____

CENTRAL MEDICAL CENTER

211 Medical Center Drive • Central City, US 90000-1234 • PHONE: (012) 125-6784 • FAX: (012) 125-9999

OPERATIVE REPORT

DATE OF OPERATION: 10/19/20XX

PREOPERATIVE DIAGNOSIS: Trimalleolar fracture, right ankle/fracture dislocation.

POSTOPERATIVE DIAGNOSIS: Trimalleolar fracture, right ankle/fracture dislocation.

OPERATION PERFORMED: Open reduction and internal fixation of medial malleolus and lateral malleolus, right ankle.

ANESTHESIOLOGIST: K. Teglam, M.D.

ANESTHESIA: General.

DESCRIPTION OF OPERATION: After successful general anesthesia, the right lower extremity was prepped and draped in a sterile fashion. A pneumatic tourniquet was used in the case at 300 mmHg for 51 minutes. The medial side was opened first; the skin was incised, and this was carried down through the subcutaneous tissue down to the periosteum, which was incised enough at the fracture site for visualization of a large transverse medial malleolar fracture. A hematoma was evacuated by curettage and irrigation. Unfortunately, there was some debris within the joint which was articular cartilage destruction and damage on the talus.

Attention was then directed laterally where an incision was made and carried through the skin and subcutaneous tissue. The fracture was brought into full view very easily. The fracture was long and oblique. This was curetted of hematoma and irrigated, and, using a bone clamp, it was clamped in a reduced position. A 6-hole semitubular fibular-type plate was then bent to position and placed onto the fibula; and after predrilling, premeasuring, and pretapping, six cortical 3.5 mm diameter screws were used to hold the plate to the fractured fibula.

Attention was then directed medially. The fracture was reduced and held in place with a towel clip, and a 60 mm long malleolar screw was then inserted into the fragment into the distal tibia. X-rays revealed that three of the screws laterally were too long, and these were changed. The medial malleolus screw was also tightened down further. Repeat film revealed very satisfactory position of all the screws. The posterior malleolar fragment was felt to be adequately positioned. All the wounds were then irrigated with goodly amounts of antibiotic solution. Vicryl sutures, 0 and 2-0, were used to close the subcutaneous tissue on both sides; and staples were used for the skin. A bulky Jones dressing was applied with splints anteriorly and posteriorly.

The patient tolerated the procedure well and was transferred to the recovery room with stable vital signs.

R. Rodriguez, M.D.

RR: mb
D: 10/19/20xx
T: 10/20/20xx

OPERATIVE REPORT	PT. NAME:	TOOHEY, Alice M.
	ID NO:	IP-236701
	ROOM NO:	729
	ATT. PHYS:	R. RODRIGUEZ, M.D.

MEDICAL RECORD 6-2   Operative Report

Answers to Examine Your Understanding

1. hyster/ectomy
   <u>uterus</u> / <u>excision or removal</u>
      R   S

2. colo/centesis
   <u>colon (large intestine)</u> / <u>puncture for aspiration</u>
            CF   S

3. tracheo/stomy
   <u>trachea (windpipe)</u> / <u>creation of an opening</u>
            CF   S

4. glosso/rrhaphy
   <u>tongue</u> / <u>suture</u>
      CF   S

5. angio/plasty
   <u>vessel</u> / <u>surgical repair or reconstruction</u>
      CF   S

6. arthro/desis
   <u>joint</u> / <u>binding</u>
      CF   S

7. salpingo/tomy
   <u>uterine or fallopian tube</u> / <u>incision</u>
               CF   S

8. litho/tripsy
   <u>stone</u> / <u>crushing</u>
      CF   S

9. auto/graft
   <u>self</u> / <u>transfer</u>
      P   S

10. orchio/pexy
    <u>testis or testicle</u> / <u>suspension or fixation</u>
               CF   S

11. p	24. d	37. b
12. m	25. b	38. a
13. k	26. g	39. c
14. j	27. a	40. b
15. l	28. e	41. my/o
16. q	29. d	42. oophor/o
17. r	30. b	43. chol/e
18. f	31. a	44. lapar/o
19. n	32. b	45. arthr/o
20. o	33. c	46. thorac/o
21. h	34. d	47. gastr/o
22. c	35. c	48. ur/o
23. i	36. a	49. myring/o

50. cutane/o
51. coronary artery bypass graft
52. transurethral resection of the prostate
53. occupational therapy
54. percutaneous transluminal coronary angioplasty
55. nonsteroidal antiinflammatory drug
56. extracorporeal shock wave lithotripsy
57. tissue plasminogen activator
58. light amplification by stimulated emission of radiation
59. physical therapy or physiotherapy

60. i	64. f	68. b
61. a	65. c	69. h
62. g	66. k	70. d
63. j	67. e	

71. anticoagulant—prevents clotting of blood; thrombolytic—dissolves clots
72. psychotropic—all medications used to treat mental illness; antipsychotic—class of psychotropic drugs used to treat psychosis
73. vasoconstrictor—causes a narrowing of the blood vessels, thereby decreasing blood flow; vasodilator—causes dilation of the blood vessels, thereby increasing blood flow
74. homograft—transfer of tissue from one human to another; xenograft—graft of tissue from one species to another, such as animal to human
75. intracorporeal lithotripsy—technique using a lithotripter within an endoscope to directly pulverize a stone; extracorporeal lithotripsy—use of ultrasonic shock waves penetrated from outside the body to crush kidney stones
76. tracheotomy—incision in the trachea; tracheostomy—creation of an opening in the trachea

77. b	85. freezing	93. chemo
78. f	86. arthroscope	94. mind
79. d	87. delicate	95. radiation
80. c	88. key hole	96. physiatrist
81. g	89. coughing	97. drugs or medications
82. a	90. sleep	98. occupational
83. e	91. urine	99. physical
84. stop	92. sensation	100. communication

ANSWERS TO MEDICAL RECORD EXERCISE 6-1

1. See medical dictionary
2. b
3. The procedure was the removal of all or a segment of the vas deferens to produce sterility in the male.
4. f

5. Darvocet-N, 100 milligrams every four hours as needed for pain
6. c
7. Answers will vary. Apparently a small amount of blood seeped into tissue at the place where the right vasectomy was performed, causing a "blood tumor" to form.
8.

Medication	Strength	How Often
Cipro	500 milligrams	twice a day for five days
Darvocet-N	100 milligrams	every four hours as needed for pain
ibuprofen	not stated	as needed

ANSWERS TO MEDICAL RECORD EXERCISE 6-2

1. See medical dictionary.
2. Mrs. Toohey has a broken ankle in three places with separation of the ankle from the joint.
3. __8__ radiograph of the screws that were too long
  __3__ incision on the outer side of the ankle
  __5__ plate placed onto fibula
  __10__ sewing the incisions
  __9__ radiograph of satisfactory screw position
  __6__ towel clip positioned
  __2__ removal of medial hematoma
  __4__ removal of lateral hematoma
  __7__ placement of screw into lower tibia
  __1__ incision on the inner side of the right ankle
4. An x-ray showed that three of the screws placed on the outside of the ankle onto the fibula were too long, so they were removed and replaced with shorter ones.
5. medial malleolus—straight, horizontal line; lateral malleolus—long and slanted line
6. Cartilage within the ankle joint was destroyed, and there was also damage to the heel bone (talus).
7. b
8. She appeared to have tolerated the procedure well and had normal temperature, pulse, respirations, and blood pressure at the time she was moved to the postanesthesia recovery room.

APPENDIX A

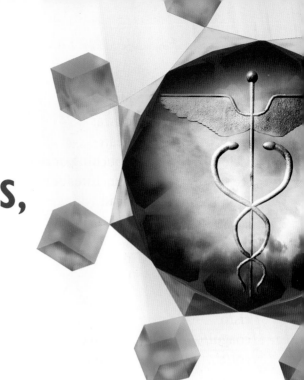

GLOSSARY OF PREFIXES, SUFFIXES, AND COMBINING FORMS

Term Component to English

Term Component	Meaning	Term Component	Meaning
a-	without	anxi/o	anxiety
ab-	away from	aort/o	aorta
abdomin/o	abdomen	append/o	appendix
acr/o	extremity or topmost	appendic/o	appendix
ad-	to, toward, or near	-ar	pertaining to
aden/o	gland	arteri/o	artery
adip/o	fat	arthr/o	joint
adren/o	adrenal gland	-ary	pertaining to
adrenal/o	adrenal gland	ather/o	fatty, or lipid, paste
-al	pertaining to	atri/o	atrium
-algia	pain	audi/o	hearing
allo-	other	aur/i	ear
alveol/o	alveolus (air sac)	auto-	self
an-	without	bi-	two or both
an/o	anus	bi/o	life
ana-	up, apart	bil/i	bile
angi/o	vessel	blephar/o	eyelid
ante-	before	brady-	slow
anti-	against or opposed to	bronch/o	bronchus (airway)

Term Component	Meaning
carcin/o	cancer
cardi/o	heart
-cele	pouching or hernia
-centesis	puncture for aspiration
cephal/o	head
cerebr/o	largest part of the brain
cervic/o	neck
chol/e	bile
chondr/o	cartilage
cis/o	to cut
coagul/o	clotting
col/o	colon (large intestine)
colon/o	colon (large intestine)
colp/o	vagina (sheath)
conjunctiv/o	conjunctiva
contra-	against or opposed to
corne/o	cornea
coron/o	circle or crown
cost/o	rib
crani/o	skull
crin/o	to secrete
cry/o	cold
cutane/o	skin
cyst/o	bladder or sac
cyt/o	cell
dacry/o	tear
de-	from, down, or not
dent/i	teeth
derm/o	skin
dermat/o	skin
-desis	binding
dia-	across or through
dips/o	thirst
duoden/o	duodenum
dys-	painful, difficult, or faulty

Term Component	Meaning
-e	noun marker
e-	out or away
-eal	pertaining to
ec-	out or away
-ectomy	excision or removal
electr/o	electricity
-emesis	vomiting
-emetic	pertaining to vomiting
-emia	blood condition
encephal/o	entire brain
endo-	within
enter/o	small intestine
epi-	upon
episi/o	vulva
erythr/o	red
esophag/o	esophagus
esthesi/o	sensation
eu-	normal
ex-	out or away
extra-	outside
fibr/o	fiber
gastr/o	stomach
-genesis	origin or production
-genic	pertaining to origin
gloss/o	tongue
glyc/o	sugar (glucose)
-graft	transfer
-gram	record
-graph	instrument for recording
-graphy	process of recording
gynec/o	female
hem/o	blood
hemi-	half
hepat/o	liver

Term Component	Meaning
herni/o	hernia
hetero-	different
hist/o	tissue
homo-	same
hormon/o	hormone
hydr/o	water
hyper-	above or excessive
hypn/o	sleep
hypo-	below or deficient
hyster/o	uterus
-ia	condition of
-iasis	formation or presence of
iatr/o	treatment
-ic	pertaining to
-icle	small
ile/o	ileum (third portion of small intestine)
immun/o	safe
inter-	between
intra-	within
ir/o	iris (colored circle)
irid/o	iris (colored circle)
isch/o	to hold back
-ism	condition of
-ist	one who specializes in
-itis	inflammation
-ium	structure or tissue
kerat/o	cornea
kyph/o	humpbacked
lacrim/o	tear
lapar/o	abdomen
laryng/o	larynx (voice box)
-lepsy	seizure
leuk/o	white
lingu/o	tongue

Term Component	Meaning
lip/o	fat
lith/o	stone
-logist	one who specializes in the study or treatment of
-logy	study of
lord/o	bent
lumb/o	loin (lower back)
lymph/o	clear fluid
-lysis	breakdown or dissolution
-lytic	pertaining to breakdown or dissolution
macro-	large
-malacia	softening
mamm/o	breast
-mania	condition of abnormal impulse toward or frenzy
mast/o	breast
megal/o	large
-megaly	enlargement
melan/o	black
men/o	month (menstruation)
mening/o	membrane (meninges)
meta-	beyond, after, or change
-meter	instrument for measuring
metr/o	uterus
metri/o	uterus
-metry	process of measuring
micro-	small
mono-	one
muscul/o	muscle
my/o	muscle

Term Component	Meaning	Term Component	Meaning
myel/o	bone marrow or spinal cord	para-	alongside of or abnormal
myring/o	eardrum or tympanic membrane	path/o	disease
		pector/o	chest
narc/o	stupor or sleep	-penia	abnormal reduction
nas/o	nose	per-	by
necr/o	death	peri-	around
neo-	new	-pexy	suspension or fixation
nephr/o	kidney	phag/o	eat or swallow
neur/o	nerve	pharyng/o	pharynx or throat
ocul/o	eye	phas/o	speech
odont/o	teeth	-phil	attraction for
-odynia	pain	phleb/o	vein
-ole	small	-phobia	condition of abnormal fear or sensitivity
-oma	tumor		
onc/o	tumor		
oophor/o	ovary	phot/o	light
ophthalm/o	eye	phren/o	diaphragm, mind
-opsy	process of viewing	plas/o	formation
opt/o	eye	-plasty	surgical repair or reconstruction
or/o	mouth		
orch/o	testis or testicle	-plegia	paralysis
orchi/o	testis or testicle	-pnea	breathing
orchid/o	testis or testicle	pneum/o	air or lung
ortho-	straight, normal, or correct	pneumon/o	air or lung
		-poiesis	formation
-osis	condition or increase	poly-	many
		post-	after
oste/o	bone	pre-	before
ot/o	ear	pro-	before
-ous	pertaining to	proct/o	rectum and anus
ov/i	egg	prostat/o	prostate gland
ov/o	egg	psych/o	mind
ovari/o	ovary	-ptosis	falling or downward displacement
ox/o	oxygen		
pan-	all	pulmon/o	lung
pancreat/o	pancreas	pyret/o	fever

Term Component	Meaning
quadri-	four
radi/o	ray or radiation
rect/o	rectum
ren/o	kidney
retin/o	retina
rhin/o	nose
-rrhage	to burst forth (usually blood)
-rrhagia	to burst forth (usually blood)
-rrhaphy	suture
-rrhea	discharge
salping/o	uterine or fallopian tube
sarc/o	flesh
schiz/o	split
scler/o	hard or sclera
scoli/o	twisted
-scope	instrument for examination
-scopy	process of examination
semi-	half
sigmoid/o	sigmoid colon
somn/o	sleep
son/o	sound
-spasm	involuntary contraction
sperm/o	sperm
spermat/o	sperm
spin/o	thorn
spir/o	breathing
splen/o	spleen
spondyl/o	vertebra
squam/o	scale
-stasis	stop or stand
sten/o	narrow
steth/o	chest

Term Component	Meaning
stomat/o	mouth
-stomy	creation of an opening
sub-	below or under
super-	above or excessive
syn-	together or with
tachy-	fast
test/o	testis or testicle
therm/o	heat
thorac/o	chest
thromb/o	clot
thym/o	thymus gland or mind
thyr/o	thyroid gland (shield)
thyroid/o	thyroid gland (shield)
-tic	pertaining to
tom/o	to cut
-tomy	incision
ton/o	tone or tension
tonsill/o	tonsil
trache/o	trachea (windpipe)
trans-	across or through
tri-	three
-tripsy	crushing
troph/o	nourishment or development
tympan/o	eardrum
-ule	small
ultra-	beyond or excessive
uni-	one
ur/o	urine
ureter/o	ureter
urethr/o	urethra
urin/o	urine
uter/o	uterus

Term Component	Meaning
vagin/o	vagina
varic/o	swollen, twisted vein
vas/o	vessel
vascul/o	vessel
ven/o	vein
ventricul/o	ventricle (belly or pouch)

Term Component	Meaning
vertebr/o	vertebra
vesic/o	bladder or sac
vulv/o	vulva
xeno-	strange or foreign
-y	condition or process of

English to Term Component

Meaning	Term Component
abdomen	abdomin/o, lapar/o
abnormal	para-
abnormal reduction	-penia
above	hyper-, super-
across	dia-, trans-
adrenal gland	adren/o, adrenal/o
after	post-, meta-
against	anti-, contra-
air	pneum/o, pneumon/o
air sac	alveol/o
airway	bronch/o
all	pan-
alongside of	para-
alveolus	alveol/o
anus	an/o
anus and rectum	proct/o
anxiety	anxi/o
aorta	aort/o
apart	ana-
appendix	append/o, appendic/o

Meaning	Term Component
around	peri-
artery	arteri/o
atrium	atri/o
attraction for	-phil
away	e-, ec-, ex-, exo-
away from	ab-
before	ante-, pre-, pro-
belly	ventricul/o
below	hypo-, sub-
bent	lord/o
between	inter-
beyond	meta-, ultra-
bile	chol/e, bil/i
binding	-desis
black	melan/o
bladder	cyst/o, vesic/o
blood	hem/o, hemat/o
blood condition	-emia
bone	oste/o
bone marrow	myel/o
both	bi-
brain	cerebr/o
brain, entire	encephal/o

Meaning	Term Component	Meaning	Term Component
brain, largest part	cerebr/o	crown	coron/o
breakdown	-lysis	crushing	-tripsy
breast	mast/o, mamm/o	death	necr/o
breathing	-pnea, spir/o	deficient	hypo-
bronchus	bronch/o	development	troph/o
by	per-	diaphragm	phren/o
cancer	carcin/o	different	hetero-
cartilage	chondr/o	difficult	dys-
cell	cyt/o	discharge	-rrhea
cerebrum	cerebr/o	disease	path/o
change	meta-	dissolution	-lysis
chest	pector/o, steth/o, thorac/o	down	de-
		downward displacement	-ptosis
circle	coron/o	duodenum	duoden/o
clear fluid	lymph/o	ear	aur/i, ot/o
clot	thromb/o	eardrum	tympan/o, myring/o
clotting	coagul/o		
cold	cry/o	eat	phag/o
colon	col/o, colon/o	egg	ov/i, ov/o
condition	-osis	electricity	electr/o
condition of	-ia, -ism, -y	enlargement	-megaly
condition of abnormal fear or sensitivity	-phobia	entire brain	encephal/o
		esophagus	esophag/o
		excessive	hyper-, super-, ultra-
		excision	-ectomy
condition of abnormal impulse toward or frenzy	-mania	extremity	acr/o
		eye	ocul/o, opt/o, ophthalm/o
conjunctiva	conjunctiv/o	eyelid	blephar/o
contraction, involuntary	-spasm	falling	-ptosis
		fallopian tube	salping/o
		fast	tachy-
cornea	corne/o, kerat/o	fat	adip/o, lip/o
correct	ortho-	fatty paste	ather/o
creation of an opening	-stomy	faulty	dys-
		female	gynec/o

Meaning	Term Component	Meaning	Term Component
fever	pyret/o	joint	arthr/o
fiber	fibr/o	kidney	nephr/o, ren/o
fixation	-pexy	large	macro-, megal/o
flesh	sarc/o	large intestine	col/o, colon/o
foreign	xeno-	largest part of the brain	cerebr/o
formation	plas/o, -iasis, -poiesis		
four	quadri-	larynx	laryng/o
from	de-	life	bi/o
gland	aden/o	light	phot/o
glucose	glyc/o	lipid paste	ather/o
half	hemi-, semi-	liver	hepat/o
hard	scler/o	loin	lumb/o
head	cephal/o	lower back	lumb/o
hearing	audi/o	lung	pneum/o, pneumon/o, pulmon/o
heart	cardi/o		
heat	therm/o	many	poly-
hernia	herni/o, -cele	membrane	mening/o
hormone	hormon/o	meninges	mening/o
humpbacked	kyph/o	menstruation	men/o
ileum (third portion of small intestine)	ile/o	mind	psych/o, phren/o
		month	men/o
		mouth	or/o, stomat/o
		muscle	my/o, muscul/o
incision	-tomy	narrow	sten/o
increase	-osis	near	ad-
inflammation	-itis	neck	cervic/o
instrument for examination	-scope	nerve	neur/o
		new	neo-
instrument for measuring	-meter	normal	eu-, ortho-
		nose	nas/o, rhin/o
instrument for recording	-graph	not	de-
		noun marker	-e
involuntary contraction	-spasm	nourishment	troph/o
		one	mono-, uni-
iris (colored circle)	ir/o, irid/o	one who specializes in	-ist

Meaning	Term Component	Meaning	Term Component
one who specializes in the study or treatment of	-logist	process of viewing	-opsy
		production	-genesis
		prostate gland	prostat/o
opening, creation of an	-stomy	puncture for aspiration	-centesis
		radiation	radi/o
opposed to	anti-, contra-	ray	radi/o
origin	-genesis	record	-gram
other	allo-	rectum	rect/o
out	e-, ec-, ex-, exo-	rectum and anus	proct/o
outside	extra-		
ovary	oophor/o, ovari/o	red	erythr/o
oxygen	ox/o	removal	-ectomy
pain	-algia, -odynia	retina	retin/o
painful	dys-	rib	cost/o
pancreas	pancreat/o	sac	cyst/o, vesic/o
paralysis	-plegia	safe	immun/o
pertaining to	-al, -ar, -ary, -eal, -ic, -ous, -tic	same	homo-
		scale	squam/o
pertaining to breakdown or dissolution	-lytic	sclera	scler/o
		seizure	-lepsy
		self	auto-
pertaining to origin	-genic	sensation	esthesi/o
		sheath	vagin/o, colp/o
pertaining to vomiting	-emetic	shield	thyr/o, thyroid/o
		sigmoid colon	sigmoid/o
pharynx	pharyng/o	skin	derm/o, dermat/o, cutane/o
pouch	ventricul/o		
pouching	-cele	skull	crani/o
presence of	-iasis	sleep	hypn/o, narc/o, somn/o
process of	-y		
process of examination	-scopy	slow	brady-
		small	-icle, -ole, -ule, micro-
process of measuring	-metry		
		small intestine	enter/o
process of recording	-graphy	softening	-malacia

Meaning	Term Component
sound	son/o
speech	phas/o
sperm	sperm/o, spermat/o
spinal cord	myel/o
spleen	splen/o
split	schiz/o
stand	-stasis
stomach	gastr/o
stone	lith/o
stop	-stasis
straight	ortho-
strange	xeno-
structure	-ium
study of	-logy
stupor	narc/o
sugar	glyc/o
surgical repair or reconstruction	-plasty
suspension	-pexy
suture	-rrhaphy
swallow	phag/o
swollen, twisted vein	varic/o
tear	lacrim/o, dacry/o
teeth	dent/i, odont/o
tension	ton/o
testicle	test/o, orchi/o, orchid/o
testis	test/o, orchi/o, orchid/o
thirst	dips/o
thorn	spin/o
three	tri-
throat	pharyng/o
through	trans-
thymus gland	thym/o

Meaning	Term Component
thyroid gland	thyr/o, thyroid/o
tissue	hist/o, -ium
to burst forth (usually blood)	-rrhage, -rrhagia
to cut	tom/o, cis/o
to hold back	isch/o
to or toward	ad-
to secrete	crin/o
together	syn-
tone	ton/o
tongue	lingu/o, gloss/o
tonsil	tonsill/o
topmost	acr/o
trachea	trache/o
transfer	-graft
treatment	iatr/o
tumor	onc/o, -oma
twisted	scoli/o
two	bi-
tympanic membrane	myring/o
under	sub-
up	ana-
upon	epi-
ureter	ureter/o
urethra	urethr/o
urine	ur/o, urin/o
uterine tube	salping/o
uterus	uter/o, hyster/o, metr/o, metri/o
vagina	vagin/o, colp/o
vein	ven/o, phleb/o
ventricle (belly or pouch)	ventricul/o
vertebra	vertebr/o, spondyl/o

Meaning	Term Component	Meaning	Term Component
vessel	angi/o, vas/o, vascul/o	white	leuk/o
voice box	laryng/o	windpipe	trache/o
vomiting	-emesis	with	syn-
vulva	vulv/o, episi/o	within	endo-, intra-
water	hydr/o	without	a-, an-

APPENDIX B

ABBREVIATIONS AND SYMBOLS

Abbreviations and symbols that appear in red font are considered "Dangerous Abbreviations" and should not be used. The preferred use is noted in brackets ([ ]). Those included on the official JCAHO "Do Not Use" list are marked by an asterisk (*).

Abbreviation or Symbol	Meaning	Abbreviation or Symbol	Meaning
ā	before	AU	both ears [spell out *both ears*]
A	anterior; assessment		
A&W	alive and well	BCC	basal cell carcinoma
a.c.	before meals	b.i.d.	twice a day
AD	right ear [spell out *right ear*]	BMP	basic metabolic panel
		BP	blood pressure
ad lib.	as desired	BPH	benign prostatic hypertrophy; benign prostatic hyperplasia
ADHD	attention-deficit/ hyperactivity disorder		
alb	albumin	BRP	bathroom privileges
ALT	alanine aminotransferase (enzyme)	BS	blood sugar
		BUN	blood urea nitrogen
		Bx	biopsy
a.m.	before noon	c̄	with
AP	anterior-posterior	C	Celsius; centigrade
AS	left ear [spell out *left ear*]	C&S	culture and sensitivity
		CABG	coronary artery bypass graft
AST	aspartate aminotransferase (enzyme)	CAD	coronary artery disease

Abbreviation or Symbol	Meaning
CAM	complementary and alternative medicine
cap	capsule
CAT	computed axial tomography
CBC	complete blood count
cc	cubic centimeter [use the metric equivalent *mL*]
CC	chief complaint
CCU	coronary (cardiac) care unit
CHF	congestive heart failure
cm	centimeter
CMP	comprehensive metabolic panel
CNS	central nervous system
c/o	complains of
CO_2	carbon dioxide
CP	chest pain
CSF	cerebrospinal fluid
CT	computed tomography
cu mm	cubic millimeter
CVA	cerebrovascular accident
d	day
DC, D/C	discharge; discontinue [spell out *discharge* or *discontinue*]
DM	diabetes mellitus
DTR	deep tendon reflex
Dx	diagnosis
ECG	electrocardiogram
echo	echocardiogram
ECU	emergency care unit

Abbreviation or Symbol	Meaning
EEG	electroencephalogram
EGD	esophagogastroduodenoscopy
EKG	electrocardiogram
EMG	electromyogram
ENT	ear, nose, and throat
ER	emergency room
ESWL	extracorporeal shock wave lithotripsy
ETOH	ethyl alcohol
F	Fahrenheit
FH	family history
fl oz	fluid ounce
g	gram
GI	gastrointestinal
gm	gram
gr	grain
gt	drop
gtt	drops
GYN	gynecology
h	hour
H&P	history and physical
HCT or Hct	hematocrit
HDL	high-density lipoprotein
HEENT	head, eyes, ears, nose, and throat
HGB or Hgb	hemoglobin
hpf	high-power field
HPI	history of present illness
h.s.	bedtime [spell out *bedtime*]
Ht	height
HTN	hypertension
Hx	history

Abbreviation or Symbol	Meaning
ICU	intensive care unit
ID	intradermal
IM	intramuscular
IMP	impression
IP	inpatient
ISMP	Institute for Safe Medication Practices
IV	intravenous
JCAHO	Joint Commission on Accreditation of Healthcare Organizations
kg	kilogram
L	liter
Ⓛ	left
L&W	living and well
lb	pound
LDL	low-density lipoprotein
LLQ	left lower quadrant
lpf	low-power field
LUQ	left upper quadrant
m	meter
ⓜ	murmur
MCH	mean cell hemoglobin
MCHC	mean cell hemoglobin concentration
MCV	mean cell volume
MD	medical doctor
mg	milligram
MI	myocardial infarction
ml or mL	milliliter
mm	millimeter
mm³	cubic millimeter
MRI	magnetic resonance imaging
NAD	no acute distress

Abbreviation or Symbol	Meaning
NKDA	no known drug allergy
noc.	night
NPO	nothing by mouth
NSAID	nonsteroidal antiinflammatory drug
O	objective information
OB	obstetrics
OD	right eye [spell out *right eye*]
OH	occupational history
OP	outpatient
OR	operating room
ORIF	open reduction, internal fixation
OS	left eye [spell out *left eye*]
OT	occupational therapy
OU	both eyes [spell out *both eyes*]
oz	ounce
p̄	after
P	plan; posterior; pulse
PA	posterior-anterior
PACU	postanesthetic care unit
PAR	postanesthetic recovery
p.c.	after meals
PE	physical examination; pulmonary embolism
per	by or through
PERRLA	pupils equal, round, and reactive to light and accommodation
PET	positron-emission tomography

Abbreviation or Symbol	Meaning
pH	potential of hydrogen (measure of the acidity or alkalinity of urine)
PH	past history
PI	present illness
PID	pelvic inflammatory disease
p.m.	after noon
PLT	platelet
PMH	past medical history
p.o.	by mouth
post-op or postop	postoperative
PR	per rectum
pre-op or preop	preoperative
p.r.n.	as needed
pt	patient
PT	physical therapy
PTA	percutaneous transluminal angioplasty
PTCA	percutaneous transluminal coronary angioplasty
PTSD	posttraumatic stress disorder
PV	per vagina
Px	physical examination
q	every
q.d.*	every day, daily [spell out *every day* or *daily*]
qh	every hour
q2h	every 2 hours
q.i.d.	four times a day

Abbreviation or Symbol	Meaning
q.o.d.*	every other day [spell out *every other day*]
qt	quart
R	respiration
®	right
RBC	red blood cell; red blood count
RLQ	right lower quadrant
R/O	rule out
ROS	review of symptoms
RRR	regular rate and rhythm
RTC	return to clinic
RTO	return to office
RUQ	right upper quadrant
Rx	recipe; prescription
$\bar{s}$	without
S	subjective information
SC	subcutaneous [spell out *subcut* or *subcutaneously*]
SCC	squamous cell carcinoma
SH	social history
Sig:	label; instruction to patient
SL	sublingual
SOB	shortness of breath
SPECT	single-photon emission computed tomography
SpGr	specific gravity
SQ	subcutaneous [spell out *subcut* or *subcutaneously*]
SR	systems review

Abbreviation or Symbol	Meaning
s̄s̄	one-half [use *one-half* or ½]
STAT	immediately
sub-Q	subcutaneous [spell out *subcut* or *subcutaneously*]
suppos	suppository
Sx	symptom
T	temperature
tab	tablet
t.i.d.	three times a day
tPA or TPA	tissue plasminogen activator
Tr	treatment
TURP	transurethral resection of the prostate
Tx	treatment; traction
UA	urinalysis
UCHD	usual childhood diseases
US or U/S	ultrasound
VS	vital signs
WBC	white blood cell; white blood count
WDWN	well-developed and well-nourished
wk	week

Abbreviation or Symbol	Meaning
WNL	within normal limits
Wt	weight
x	times; for
x-ray	radiography
y/o or y.o.	year old
yr	year
♀	female
♂	male
#	number; pound
°	degree; hour
↑	increased
↓	decreased
∅	none; negative
×	times; for
>	greater than [spell out *greater than*]
<	less than [spell out *less than*]
ı̄	one
ı̄ı̄	two
ı̄ı̄ı̄	three
ı̄v	four
I, II, III, IV, V, VI, VII, VIII, IX, and X	uppercase Roman numerals 1–10

APPENDIX C

COMMONLY PRESCRIBED DRUGS

The following alphabetical list of commonly prescribed drugs (trade and generic) is based on a listing of the most frequently dispensed prescriptions in the United States during 2007. The classification and major therapeutic uses for each are also provided. Trade drug names begin with a capital letter; the generic names accompany them in parentheses. All generic names are set in lowercase.

Name	Classification	Major Therapeutic Uses
Actos (pioglitazone)	oral antidiabetic	type 2 diabetes mellitus
Advair Diskus (salmeterol and fluticasone)	bronchodilator and antiinflammatory combination	asthma
albuterol aerosol	bronchodilator	asthma, chronic bronchitis
alprazolam	anxiolytic, sedative, hypnotic	anxiety
Altace (ramipril)	antihypertensive	hypertension, congestive heart failure
amlodipine besylate	antihypertensive; antianginal, antiarrhythmic	hypertension, angina pectoris, cardiac arrhythmias
amoxicillin	antibiotic	bacterial infections
atenolol	antihypertensive; antianginal, antiarrhythmic	hypertension, angina pectoris, cardiac arrhythmias
azithromycin	antibiotic	bacterial infections

Name	Classification	Major Therapeutic Uses
Celebrex	nonsteroidal antiinflammatory drug (NSAID)	pain, arthritis
Cephalexin	antibiotic	bacterial infections
Crestor (rosuvastatin)	antihyperlipidemic	hyperlipidemia (hypercholesterolemia, hypertriglyceridemia)
Cymbalta (duloxetine hydrochloride)	antidepressant	depression
Diovan (valsartan)	antihypertensive	hypertension
Effexor XR (venlafaxine)	antidepressant	depression
Fosamax (alendronate)	bone resorption inhibitor	osteoporosis
Furosemide	diuretic	hypertension, edema related to congestive heart failure (CHF) or renal failure
hydrochlorothiazide	diuretic	hypertension, edema related to congestive heart failure (CHF) or renal failure
hydrocodone and acetaminophen	narcotic and nonsteroidal antiinflammatory drug (NSAID); analgesic and antipyretic combination	moderate to severe pain
Lantus (insulin glargine)	insulin, antidiabetic	types 1 and 2 diabetes mellitus
Levaquin (levofloxacin)	antibiotic	bacterial infections
levothyroxine sodium	thyroid hormone	hypothyroidism
Lexapro (escitalopram)	antidepressant	depression
Lipitor (atorvastatin)	antihyperlipidemic	hyperlipidemia (hypercholesterolemia, hypertriglyceridemia)
lisinopril	antihypertensive	hypertension
metformin	oral antidiabetic	type 2 diabetes mellitus
metoprolol	antihypertensive, antiarrhythmic, antianginal	hypertension, angina pectoris, cardiac arrhythmias

Name	Classification	Major Therapeutic Uses
Nasonex (mometasone)	steroid (antiinflammatory, immunosuppressant)	allergic rhinitis
Nexium (esomeprazole)	gastric acid secretion inhibitor	peptic ulcer disease, gastroesophageal reflux disease
Norvasc (amlodipine besylate)	antihypertensive, antianginal	hypertension, angina pectoris
oxycodone and acetaminophen	narcotic and nonsteroidal antiinflammatory drug (NSAID); analgesic and antipyretic combination	moderate to severe pain
Plavix (clopidogrel)	antiplatelet agent	clot prevention
prednisone	steroid (antiinflammatory, immunosuppressant)	inflammation, immunological disorders, allergy
Premarin (conjugated estrogens)	estrogen derivative	hormone replacement
Prevacid (lansoprazole)	gastric acid secretion inhibitor	peptic ulcer disease, gastroesophageal reflux disease
Protonix (pantoprazole)	gastric acid secretion inhibitor	peptic ulcer disease, gastroesophageal reflux disease
propoxyphene napsylate and acetaminophen	narcotic and nonsteroidal antiinflammatory drug (NSAID); analgesic and antipyretic combination	mild to moderate pain
Risperdal (risperidone)	antipsychotic	psychoses (e.g. schizophrenia)
Seroquel (quetiapine)	antipsychotic	psychoses (e.g. schizophrenia)
sertraline hydrochloride	antidepressant	depression
simvastatin	antihyperlipidemic	hyperlipidemia (hypercholesterolemia, hypertriglyceridemia)
Singulair (montelukast)	leukotriene-receptor antagonist (bronchodilator)	asthma, allergic rhinitis

Name	Classification	Major Therapeutic Uses
Synthroid (levothyroxine sodium)	thyroid hormone	hypothyroidism
Toprol-XL (metoprolol)	antihypertensive, antiarrhythmic, antianginal	hypertension, angina pectoris, cardiac arrhythmias
trazodone	antidepressant	depression
TriCor (fenofibrate)	antihyperlipidemic	hyperlipidemia (hypercholesterolemia, hypertriglyceridemia)
Vytorin (ezetimibe and simvastatin)	antihyperlipidemic	hyperlipidemia (hypercholesterolemia, hypertriglyceridemia)
warfarin, sodium	anticoagulant	thromboembolic disorders
Zetia (ezetimibe)	antihyperlipidemic	hyperlipidemia (hypercholesterolemia, hypertriglyceridemia)
Zyrtec (cetirizine)	antihistamine	allergy

Data from:

Top 200 Prescription Drugs of 2007, Pharmacy Times, May, 2008, http://www.pharmacytimes.com/issues/articles/2008-05_003.asp

Stedman's Medical Dictionary for the Health Professions and Nursing, 6th edition, Appendix listing of Commonly Prescribed Drugs and Their Applications. Baltimore: Lippincott Willams & Wilkins, 2008

FIGURE CREDITS

Cluster of erythrocytes. LifeART image copyright © 2009 Lippincott Williams & Wilkins. All rights reserved.

Female reproductive system, ovary, fallopian tube, uterus, and vagina. Asset provided by Anatomical Chart Co.

Medical assistant photo from Kronenberger J, Durham LS, Woodson D. *Lippincott Williams & Wilkins' Comprehensive Medical Assisting.* 3rd ed. Baltimore: Lippincott Williams & Wilkins, 2008.

Dental hygienist photo courtesy of the National Dental Hygienists' Association, Tampa, FL.

Radiologic technologist photo courtesy of the American Society of Radiologic Technologists, Albuquerque, NM.

Medical biller/coder photo courtesy of the American Academy of Professional Coders, Salt Lake City, UT.

Pharmacy technician photograph copyright © Keith Brofsky/Photodisc-Health & Medicine 2/Getty Images.

FIGURE 4-1   From Rubin E, Farber JL. *Pathology.* 3rd ed. Philadelphia: Lippincott Williams & Wilkins, 1999.

FIGURE 4-3   From Goodheart HP. *Goodheart's Photoguide of Common Skin Disorders.* 2nd ed. Philadelphia: Lippincott Williams & Wilkins, 2003.

FIGURE 4-4   From Weber J, Kelly J. *Lippincott's Learning System: Health Assessment in Nursing.* Philadelphia: Lippincott Williams & Wilkins, 1997:188.

FIGURE 4-11   From Goodheart HP. *Goodheart's Photoguide of Common Skin Disorders.* 2nd ed. Philadelphia: Lippincott Williams & Wilkins, 2003.

Nursing assistant photo courtesy of the National Association of Health Care Assistants, Joplin, MO.

Occupational therapist photograph copyright © Keith Brofsky/Photodisc-Health & Medicine 2/Getty Images.

FIGURE 5-2   Reprinted with permission from Erkonen WE, Smith WL. *Radiology 101: Basics and Fundamentals of Imaging*. Philadelphia: Lippincott Williams & Wilkins, 1998.

FIGURE 5-3   Courtesy of Orange Coast College Cardiovascular Technology Program, Costa Mesa, CA.

FIGURE 5-4   Courtesy of VIASYS Respiratory Care.

FIGURE 5-5   Endoscope and fiberoptics courtesy of Olympus America, Inc., Lake Success, NY.

FIGURE 5-6   Courtesy of VIASYS Respiratory Care.

FIGURE 5-8   Courtesy of Deutsches Roentgen-Museum, Remscheid-Lennep, Germany.

FIGURE 5-9   **A.** Inset, courtesy of Orange Coast College, Costa Mesa, CA. **B.** Courtesy of Toshiba America Medical Systems, Inc. **C.** Courtesy of West Coast Radiology Center, Santa Ana, CA.

FIGURE 5-10   **A.** Courtesy of ADAC Laboratories, a Philips Medical Systems Company, Bothell, WA. **B.** Courtesy of Newport Diagnostic Center, Newport Beach, CA.

FIGURE 5-11   **A.** Inset, courtesy of Mission Imaging Center, Mission Viejo, CA. **B.** Courtesy of Philips Medical Systems, Bothell, WA.

FIGURE 5-12   **B.** Courtesy of Sanford Schulwolf, sanfordphoto.com, and Seimens Medical Solutions, Inc., Ultrasound Division, Mountain View, CA. **C.** Courtesy of Dr. Saied M. Tohamy.

FIGURE 5-13   **A.** From Ratcliff KM. Esophageal foreign bodies. *Am Fam Physician*. 1991;44:827. **B.** Courtesy of William Brandt, M.D.

Medical transcriptionist photograph © John Cumming/Iconica Collection/Getty Images.

Diagnostic medical sonographer photograph © Keith Brofsky/Photodisc-Health & Medicine 2/Getty Images.

Clinical laboratory technologist photograph © Keith Brofsky/ Photodisc-Health & Medicine 2/Getty Images.

Auscultation photo from Pillitteri A. *Maternal and Child Nursing*. 4th ed. Philadelphia: Lippincott Williams & Wilkins, 2003.

FIGURE 6-10   **A.** PTCA courtesy of Medtronic Interventional Vascular, San Diego, CA.

FIGURE 6-12   **B.** Courtesy of ACMI Corporation, Southborough, MA.

FIGURE 6-14   From Goodheart HP. *Goodheart's Photoguide of Common Skin Disorders*. 2nd ed. Philadelphia: Lippincott Williams & Wilkins, 2003.

FIGURE 6-15   Photo courtesy of Lumenis, Inc.

FIGURE 6-16   Courtesy of Lumenis, Inc.

Surgical technologist photo courtesy of the Association of Surgical Technologists, Littleton, CO.

Emergency medical technician photo courtesy of Arthur Hsieh, Piedmont, CA.

Massage therapist photo from Braun MB, Simonson SJ. *Introduction to Massage Therapy*. 2nd ed. Baltimore: Lippincott Williams & Wilkins, 2007.

Athletic trainer photo on Student Resource CD from Anderson MK, Hall SJ, Parr GP. *Foundations of Athletic Training: Prevention, Assessment, and Management*. 4th ed. Baltimore: Lippincott Williams & Wilkins, 2008.

Nutritionist photo on Student Resource CD courtesy of the National Association of Nutrition Professionals, Danville, CA.

INDEX

Note: An *f* following a page number indicates a figure.

A

a-, 27, 149, 306, 335, 345
ab-, 27, 335, 340
Abbreviations, 347–351
   error prone, 112–113
   in history and physical, 98–102
   medical care facilities, 113–114
   patient care, 114–115
   pharmaceutical, 116–119
   prescription, 124–126
   in progress notes, 98–102
   units of measure, 117–118
Abdomen, 60
   anatomic and clinical
     divisions of, 76, 77f, 78–79
   examination of, 271
Abdominal cavity, 74, 76
Abdominal paracentesis, 281
abdomin/o, 60, 215, 280, 335, 340
Abdominocentesis, 281
Abduction, 72, 72f
Acral, 27
acr/o, 33, 166, 335, 341, 344
Acromegaly, 167, 167f
Acrophobia, 181
Actos (pioglitazone), 353
Acupuncture, 303
Acute, 192
ad-, 27, 335, 342, 344
Adduction, 72, 72f
aden/o, 50, 173, 335, 342
Adenocarcinoma, 178
adip/o, 31, 335, 341
Adipose tissue, 33
Adrenal gland, 52
adrenal/o, 50, 340
adren/o, 50, 335, 340

Advair Diskus (salmeterol and
   fluticasone), 353
Affective disorders, 165
Agranulocytes, 44
-al, 7, 27, 214, 335, 343
Alanine aminotransferase
   (ALT), 245
Albumin, 245, 250
albuterol aerosol, 353
-algia, 148, 335, 343
Alkaline phosphatase, 245
allo-, 284, 335, 343
alprazolam, 353
Altace (ramipril), 353
Alveoli, 47
alveol/o, 45, 335, 340
Alzheimer disease, 165
Amenorrhea, 185
amlodipine besylate, 353
Amniocentesis, 281–282, 282f
Amniotic fluid, 281
Amniotic sac, 281
amoxicillin, 353
an-, 27, 149, 306, 335, 345
ana-, 27, 335, 340, 344
Analgesics, 306, 308, 309, 354, 355
Anatomic position, 66–70, 67f
Anatomic terms related to body
   structures, 28–30, 29f
Anatomy
   gross, 30
   macroscopic, 30
Ancillary reports, 103, 111
Anemia, 158, 247
Anesthesiologist's report, 103, 111
Anesthetics, 306, 308
Aneurysms, 189, 189f
angi/o, 8, 38, 215, 289, 335, 345

Angiograms, 216–217
Angiography, 219
Angioplasty, 291, 302
an/o, 57, 223, 335, 340
Anorexia, versus anorexia
   nervosa, 165
Anorexia nervosa, 165
Antacids, 306, 309
ante-, 27, 335, 340
Anterior, 68, 69
Anterior-posterior, 68, 69
anti-, 306, 335, 340, 343
Antianginals, 306, 309, 314, 353,
   354, 355, 356
Antianxiety agents, 306, 309
Antiarrhythmics, 307, 310, 353,
   354, 356
Antibiotics, 307, 310, 353, 354
Anticoagulants, 307, 310, 356
Anticonvulsants, 307, 310
Antidepressants, 307, 310, 354,
   355, 356
Antidiabetics, 307, 310, 353, 354
Antiemetics, 307, 310
Antifungals, 307, 310
Antihistamines, 307, 311, 356
Antihyperglycemics, 308, 313
Antihyperlipidemics, 307, 354,
   355, 356

Antihyperlipids, 313
Antihypertensives, 307, 311, 353, 354, 355, 356
Antiinflammatories, 307, 311
Antiplatelet agents, 355
Antipruritics, 307
Antipsychotics, 308, 313, 355
Antipyretics, 307, 311, 354, 355
Antiseptics, 307, 311
Antispasmodics, 307, 311
Antithyroid drugs, 307, 311
Antivirals, 307, 312
Anus, 58
Anxiety disorders, 165, 180
anxi/o, 306, 335, 340
Anxiolytics, 306, 309, 353
Aortic valve, 39
aort/o, 38, 335, 340
Aphagia, 156
Aphasia, 155
Apnea, 181
Apothecary system, 116, 117
  abbreviations for, 117–118
  measures of, 119
Appendectomy, 277, 301
Appendicitis, 162
appendic/o, 160, 335, 340
Appendix, 18, 162
append/o, 275, 335, 340
-ar, 27, 335, 343
Arrhythmias, 154
Arteries, 41
arteri/o, 38, 168, 215, 335, 340
Arterioles, 41
Artery bypass graft, 285, 286f
Arthralgia, 150
Arthritis, 161
arthr/o, 33, 150, 223, 280, 335, 342
Arthrocentesis, 282
Arthroplasty, 290, 290f
Arthroscopy, 226, 301
-ary, 27, 335, 343
Ascites, 281
Aspartate aminotransferase (AST), 245
Aspiration, 281
Assessment, 96
atenolol, 353
ather/o, 168, 335, 341, 342
Atherosclerosis, 170–171
Atherosclerotic buildup, 171, 285

atri/o, 38, 335, 340
Atrium, 39
Atrophy, 190
Attention-deficit/hyperactivity disorder (ADHD), 165
audi/o, 227, 335, 342
Audiometer, 228
Audiometry, 229
Auditory tube, 28
Augmentation mammoplasty, 291
aur/i, 54, 335, 341
Auricle, 56
Auscultation, in physical examination, 221
Autism, 165, 188
auto-, 149, 215, 284, 335, 343
Autograft, 284
Autopsy, 232
Ayurveda, 304
Ayurvedic diet, 303
azithromycin, 353

B
Bacteria, 18
Bacterial meningitis, 49
Bacteriuria, 251
Barium as contrast medium, 238
Basal cell carcinoma, 176, 176f
Basal layer, 32
Basic metabolic panel (BMP), 242, 246
Basophils, 244, 247
Bathroom privileges (BRP), 116
Benign, 192
Benign prostatic hyperplasia, 279
bi-, 27, 149, 215, 335, 340, 344
Bicuspid valve, 40
Bilateral salpingectomy, 278
bil/i, 57, 335, 340
Bilirubin, 245, 249, 250
bi/o, 230, 306, 335, 342
Bioelectromagnetic-based therapy, 304
Biofield therapy, 304
Biologically based practices, 304
Biopsy, 230
  endoscopic, 231–232
  incisional, 231
  needle, 232
  renal, 232
  types of, 231–232, 231f
Bipolar disorder, 164

Bladder, 60, 153
blephar/o, 182, 335, 341
Blepharoptosis, 182, 182f
Blepharospasm, 187
Blood, 42
  components of, 42f
  terms relating to, 5
Blood and lymph system, 28, 41–45, 42f
Blood chemistry, 242, 246
  panels, 242
  tests, 245
Blood count, 246
Blood culture, 242, 246
Blood indices, 243, 247
Blood pressure (BP), 116
Blood sugar, 242
Blood tests, 241–247
Blood urea nitrogen (BUN), 245
Blood vessels, 38, 41
Body cavities, 74–76, 75f
  abdominal, 74
  cranial, 74
  pelvic, 74
  thoracic, 74
  vertebral, 74
Body movements, 71–74, 72f
  abduction, 72
  adduction, 72
  dorsiflexion, 73
  eversion, 73
  extension, 72
  flexion, 72
  inversion, 73
  plantar flexion, 73
  pronation, 73
  rotation, 73
  supination, 73
Body planes, 67–68, 67f, 69
  coronal or frontal plane, 68
  sagittal plane, 68
  transverse plane, 68
Body positions, 70–71
  decubitus, 71
  erect, 71
  prone, 71
  recumbent, 71
  supine, 71
Body structures, anatomic terms related to, 28–30, 29f
Body systems, 28
Body weight, 118

Bone resorption inhibitor, 354
Bones, 36
brady-, 149, 335, 343
Bradycardia, 154
Bradypnea, 181
Brain, 48, 74
    midsagittal view of, 48*f*
Brand names, 122, 123–124
Breast, 65
Breve, 15
Bronchioles, 47
Bronchitis, 161
bronch/o, 45, 159, 223, 306, 335, 340, 341
Bronchodilators, 307, 312, 353
Bronchogenic, 159
Bronchoscope, 225, 225*f*
Bronchoscopy, 225*f*
Bronchospasm, 187
Bronchus, 47, 159
Bulimia nervosa, 165

C
Calcium, 245
Calculus, 174
Capillaries, 41
Capsule, 119
carcin/o, 173, 336, 341
Cardiac care unit, 114
Cardiac catheterization, 299
cardi/o, 8, 38, 154, 215, 306, 336, 342
Cardiomegaly, 167
Cardiomyopathy, 191
Cardiotonics, 307, 312
Cardiovascular system, 28, 38–41, 39*f*
Cartilage, 36
Cathartics, 307, 312
Caudal, 70
-cele, 148, 336, 342, 343
Celebrex, 354
Cells, 28, 29, 30
-centesis, 270, 336, 343
Centimeter, 118
Central nervous system (CNS), 48*f*
Cephalalgia, 151, 193
Cephalexin, 354
cephal/o, 150, 336, 342
Cephalodynia, 151
Cerebral embolism, 188, 189*f*

cerebr/o, 47, 187, 336, 340, 341, 342
Cerebrovascular accident, 188, 189*f*
Cerebrum, 48
Cervical dysplasia, treatment for, 298*f*
Cervical vertebra, 27
cervic/o, 33, 336, 342
Cervix, 27, 65
Chemical names, 122, 124
Chemotherapy, 302, 305
Chest pain, 116
Chief complaint, 96
Chiropractic medicine, 304
chol/e, 57, 173, 275, 336, 340
Cholecyst, 174, 277
Cholecystectomy, 277, 301
Cholecystitis, 277
Cholelithiasis, 174, 277, 295
chondr/o, 33, 163, 336, 341
Chondromalacia, 163
Chronic, 192
Circulation, 41
    coronary, 41
    pulmonary, 41
    systemic, 41
cis/o, 230, 336, 344
Clinical laboratory technologist, 241
Clinical resume, 103
Clinical summary, 103, 111
coagul/o, 306, 336, 341
Cognitive disorders, 165
Colectomy, 277
col/o, 57, 273, 336, 341, 342
colon/o, 57, 222, 273, 336, 341, 342
Colonoscope, 223
Colonoscopy, 226
Colostomy, 274
colp/o, 63, 160, 336, 343, 344
Combining forms, 5, 7, 10, 28
Combining vowels, 4–5, 7, 12
Commonly prescribed drugs, 353–356
Complains of, 96
Complementary and alternative medicine (CAM), 303–304
Complete blood count (CBC), 242, 244, 246
Comprehensive metabolic panel (CMP), 242, 243*f*, 246

Computed axial tomography (CAT), 233
Computed tomography (CT), 219, 233, 234*f*, 239–240
Computer technology, 239
Condyloma, 18
Condylomata, 18
Conjunctiva, 55
conjunctiv/o, 54, 336, 341
Consultation reports, 103, 111
Contact dermatitis, 160*f*
contra-, 306, 336, 340, 343
Contrast medium, 238, 239*f*, 241
Cornea, 55
corne/o, 54, 336, 341
Coronal plane, 67*f*, 68, 69
Coronary arteries, 293*f*
Coronary artery disease, 171, 171*f*
Coronary care unit, 114
Coronary circulation, 41
coron/o, 38, 336, 341
Corrections to medical records, 129–130
cost/o, 33, 336, 343
Cranial cavity, 74, 76
crani/o, 33, 336, 343
Cranium, 36
Creatine, 245
Crestor (rosuvastatin), 354
crin/o, 50, 336, 344
Crushing, 295
cry/o, 298, 336, 341
Cryosurgery, 298, 298*f*, 300
Cryptorchidism, 288, 288*f*
Cubic centimeter, 119
Cuspid, 40
cutane/o, 31, 289, 336, 343
Cymbalta (duloxetine hydrochloride), 354
cyst/o, 60, 152, 223, 336, 340, 343
Cystocele, 153, 153*f*
Cystoscopy, 226
cyt/o, 41, 168, 336, 341
Cytology, 29, 30

D
dacry/o, 54, 336, 344
Dacryocyst, 55
Date, recording, on medical records, 130–131
de-, 149, 336, 341, 342

Decongestants, 307, 312
Decubitus, 71
Degeneration, 192
Degenerative disease, 192
Dental hygienist, 56, 59
dent/i, 57, 336, 344
Dermatitis, contact, 160*f*
dermat/o, 31, 160, 336, 343
Dermatologist, 33
Dermatology, 33
Dermis, 32, 32*f*, 33
derm/o, 31, 336, 343
-desis, 270, 336, 340
Developmental disorders, 165
dia-, 149, 336, 340
Diabetes mellitus, 156–157, 250
Diagnosis, 96, 148, 192
Diagnostic imaging, 233
    computed tomography, 233,
        234*f*, 239–240
    contrast medium in, 238, 239*f*,
        241
    magnetic resonance imaging,
        236, 237*f*
    nuclear medicine imaging,
        234–235, 235*f*, 240
    radiography, 233, 233*f*,
        238–239
    sonography, 236, 238*f*, 240
Diagnostic medical sonographer,
    236
Diagnostic tests, 103
Diarrhea, 185
Diet, Ayurvedic, 303
Differential count, 243–244
Differential diagnosis, 97
Diovan (valsartan), 354
dips/o, 154, 336, 344
Directional terms, 68, 69
    anterior, ventral, 68
    anterior-posterior, 68
    distal, 68
    inferior, caudal, 68
    lateral, 68
    medial, 68
    posterior, dorsal, 68
    posterior-anterior, 68
    proximal, 68
    superior, cephalic, 68
Discharge, 116
Discharge abstract, 103, 109*f*, 111
Discharge summary, 103, 111

Diseases
    common terms related to,
        191–194
    usual childhood, 96
Disposition, 97
Distal, 68, 69, 70
Diuretics, 307, 311, 354
Dorsiflexion, 72*f*, 73, 74
Drugs
    commonly prescribed, 353–356
    forms of, 119–120
    names of, 122
    therapeutic classifications of,
        305–314
Duct, 9
duoden/o, 223, 336, 341
dys-, 149, 336, 341, 343
Dysmenorrhea, 185
Dysphagia, 156
Dysphasia, 155
Dysplasia, 176
Dysrhythmia, 154
Dysthymia, 155
Dystrophy, 190–191

E
e-, 27, 336, 340, 343
-e, 27, 336
-eal, 27, 214, 336, 343
Ear, 54*f*, 56
Eardrum, 272–273
Eating disorders, 165
ec-, 275, 336, 340, 343
Echocardiogram, 217, 217*f*
-ectomy, 7, 270, 336, 341, 343
Ectopic pregnancy, 274
Effexor XR (venlafaxine), 354
electr/o, 215, 298, 336, 341
Electrocardiogram (ECG), 216,
    216*f*, 220
Electrocardiograph, 220
Electrocautery, 298, 298*f*, 301
Electroencephalograph, 220
Electrolytes, 245
Electromyogram (EMG), 216
Electromyograph, 220
Electronic health records,
    128–129
Electrosurgery, 298, 300
Embolism, 188, 188*f*
Embolus, 188
Emergency care unit (ER), 114

Emergency medical technicians,
    287
-emesis, 336, 345
-emetic, 306, 336, 343
-emia, 3, 7, 148, 336, 340
encephal/o, 47, 215, 336, 340,
    341
endo-, 27, 149, 215, 298, 336,
    345
Endocardium, 40
Endocrine system, 28, 50–53, 51*f*
Endometriosis, 170
Endometritis, 162
Endometrium, 64
Endorectal, 218
Endoscope, 223, 224, 299
Endoscopic biopsy, 231–232
Endoscopy, 224, 301
    lower, 226
    upper, 225
Endovaginal, 218
Energy medicine, 304
ENT, 56
enter/o, 8, 57, 186, 336, 343
Enterospasm, 187
Eosinophils, 44, 244, 247
epi-, 27, 149, 336, 344
Epidermis, 32, 32*f*
Epigastralgia, 151
Epigastric region, 78
Epilepsy, 175
episi/o, 63, 336, 345
Eponyms, 28
Erect position, 71
erythr/o, 41, 178, 336, 343
Erythrocytes, 42, 246
Erythrocytopenia, 179
esophag/o, 8, 57, 215, 336, 341
Esophagogastroduodenoscopy,
    226
Esophagoscope, 225
Esophagoscopy, 225
Esophagus, 58
Essential hypertension, 102
esthesi/o, 306, 336, 343
Estrogen, 53
Estrogen derivatives, 355
Etiology, 192
eu-, 149, 336, 342
Eustachian tube, 28
Eustachio, Bartolomeo, 28
Eversion, 72*f*, 73, 74

ex-, 27, 215, 336, 340, 343
Exacerbation, 192
Excision, 276
exo-, 27, 340, 343
Expectorants, 308, 312
Extension, 72, 72f
extra-, 295, 336, 343
Extracorporeal shock wave
    lithotripsy (ESWL), 295–296
Eyes, 54f, 55–56

F
Fallopian tubes, 28, 64–65, 274
Fallopius, Gabrielle, 28, 65
Family history, 96
Febrile, 192
Females
    reproductive system in, 63–66,
        63f
    sterilization of, 299
Fetus, 64
fibr/o, 173, 336, 342
Fibroma, 177
Fibromyoma, 177
Fixation, 287, 289
Flexion, 72, 72f
Fluids, 119
Fosamax (alendronate), 354
Frontal plane, 67f, 68, 69
Fungus infections, 310
Furosemide, 354

G
Gallbladder, 277
Gall stones, 277, 295
Gamma rays, 234–235, 240
Gastralgia, 151
Gastrectomy, 278
Gastric acid secretion inhibitor,
    355
Gastric resection, 278
gastr/o, 8, 57, 150, 223, 275, 336,
    344
Gastrointestinal system, 28,
    56–58, 57f
Gastroscopy, 225–226
Generalized anxiety disorders
    (GAD), 165
Generic names, 122, 123–124
-genesis, 27, 336, 343
-genic, 148, 336, 343
Gestational diabetes, 156

gloss/o, 57, 292, 336, 344
Glossorrhaphy, 294
Glucose, 245, 250
Glycemia, 157–158
glyc/o, 157, 336, 344
Gonorrhea, 186
Graft, 284
-graft, 270, 336, 344
Gram, 118
-gram, 214, 336, 343
Granulocytes, 44
-graph, 214, 336, 342
-graphy, 214, 336, 343
Gross anatomy, 30
gynec/o, 63, 336, 341
Gynecology, 66

H
Head, eyes, ears, nose, and throat
    (HEENT), 96
Health care professionals
    clinical laboratory technologist,
        241
    dental hygienist, 59
    diagnostic medical sonogra-
        pher, 236
    emergency medical technicians,
        287
    massage therapists, 304
    medical assistant, 50
    medical biller/coder, 110
    medical transcriptionist, 227
    nursing assistants, 151
    occupational therapists, 166
    pharmacy technician, 123
    radiologic technologist, 97
    surgical technologist, 276
Health care provider's plan, 97
Health care records
    history and physical, 94, 95f,
        96–97
    medical facilities and patient
        care abbreviations, 112–115
    patient care records, 94
    progress notes, 97–98, 98f
Health Insurance Portability and
    Accountability Act (HIPAA),
    129
Heart, 38–39, 39f
Heart valves, 39–40
hemat/o, 8, 41, 340
Hematocrit (HCT or Hct), 242

Hematology, 42
hemi-, 183, 275, 336, 342
Hemicolectomy, 277
Hemiplegia, 183
hem/o, 8, 41, 336, 340
Hemoglobin (HGB or Hgb), 242,
    246
Hemolysis, 250
Hemopoiesis, 42
Hemorrhage, 184
Hepatitis, 162
hepat/o, 57, 160, 336, 342
Hepatomegaly, 167
Hernia, 152, 294
    hiatal, 152
    inguinal, 152
herni/o, 292, 337, 342
Hernioplasty, 294
Herniorrhaphy, 294
hetero-, 284, 337, 341
Heterograft, 285
Hiatal hernia, 152
Histamines, 307, 311
hist/o, 337, 344
Histology, 29, 30
History, 96
    family, 96
    past, 96
    of present illness, 96
    social, 96
History and physical, 94, 95f,
    96–97, 103, 104–105f, 110
    abbreviations used in, 98–102
Homeopathic medicine, 304
homo-, 284, 337, 343
Homograft, 284
Hooke, Robert, 29
Hormones, 52
    thyroid, 354, 356
hormon/o, 50, 337, 342
Hospital records, 103, 110–111
Human anatomy, 30
hydr/o, 152, 337, 345
Hydrocele, 152, 153f
hydrochlorothiazide, 354
hydrocodone and
    acetaminophen, 354
hyper-, 3, 8, 27, 149, 289, 337,
    340, 341
Hyperglycemia, 158, 313
Hyperlipemia, 6, 7, 157
Hyperlipoproteinemia, 6

Hypermastia, 291
Hypertension, 102
   essential, 102
   persistent, 102
   primary, 102
   secondary, 102
Hypertensives, 311
Hyperthyroidism, 187
Hypertrophy, 190
Hyphens, placement of, 31
hypn/o, 306, 337, 343
Hypnotics, 308, 312, 353
hypo-, 8, 27, 149, 289, 337, 340, 341
Hypochondriac regions, 78
Hypogastric region, 79
Hypoglycemia, 158
Hypoglycemics, 308, 313
Hypomastia, 291
Hypothyroidism, 187
Hypoxemia, 158
Hysterectomy, 278, 294
hyster/o, 63, 275, 337, 344

I
-ia, 148, 337, 341
-iasis, 148, 337, 342, 343
iatr/o, 159, 337, 344
Iatrogenic, 159
-ic, 7, 27, 148, 337, 343
-icle, 27, 337, 343
ile/o, 273, 337, 342
Ileostomy, 274–275
Immune, 44–45
immun/o, 41, 337, 343
Impression, 96
Incision, 271
Incisional biopsy, 231
Index, 18
Infarct, 173
Inferior, 68, 69, 70
Inflammation, 160–162
   characteristics of, 160
Informed consent, 103, 111
Inguinal hernia, 152
Inguinal region, 79
Injections, 121
Inpatient, 114
Inspection in physical
   examination, 221
Insulin, 58, 156, 354
Integrative medicine, 303

Integumentary system, 28, 31–33, 32f
Intensive care unit, 114
inter-, 27, 337, 340
Interatrial septum, 40
Interventricular septum, 40
intra-, 295, 337, 345
Intramuscular injection, 121
Intravenous injection, 121
Inversion, 72f, 73
Ionizing radiation, 238, 239
irid/o, 54, 337, 342
Iris, 55
ir/o, 54, 337, 342
Ischemia, 159, 172
isch/o, 157, 168, 337, 344
Islets of Langerhans, 156
-ism, 148, 337, 341
-ist, 27, 214, 337, 342
-itis, 7, 148, 337, 342
-ium, 27, 337, 344

J
Joint Commission on
   Accreditation of Healthcare
   Organizations (JCAHO), 112
   Do Not Use List of abbreviations,
   112–113, 347

K
kerat/o, 54, 337, 341
Ketones, 247, 250
Kidneys, 30, 52, 60
Kidney stones, 295
Kilogram, 118
kyph/o, 168, 337, 342
Kyphosis, 168, 169f

L
Lacrimal gland, 55
Lacrimal sac, 55
lacrim/o, 54, 337, 344
Lantus (insulin glargine), 354
lapar/o, 223, 271, 337, 340
Laparoscope, 271, 299
Laparoscopy, 226
Laparotomy, 271
Large intestine, 58
laryng/o, 45, 163, 337, 342, 345
Laryngomalacia, 163
Larynx, 46
LASER, 300, 302

Laser surgery, 300, 300f
Lateral, 68, 69
Lateral position, 71
Laxatives, 312
Left upper quadrant, 79
-lepsy, 148, 337, 343
Leukemia, 158
leuk/o, 41, 157, 337, 345
Leukocytes, 43–44
   types of, 43–44
Leukocytopenia, 179
Leukocytosis, 170
Leukopenia, 179
Leukotriene-receptor antagonist
   (bronchodilator), 355
Levaquin (levofloxacin), 354
levothyroxine sodium, 354
Lexapro (escitalopram), 354
lingu/o, 57, 337, 344
Lipemia, 6
Lipidemia, 6
Lipid panel, 242
Lipitor (atorvastatin), 354
lip/o, 3, 8, 31, 157, 337, 341
Lips, 245
Liquid forms, 119
Liquid measures in apothecary
   system, 117
lisinopril, 354
Liter, 118
Lithiasis, 295
lith/o, 173, 295, 337, 344
Lithotripsy, 296f
   intracorporeal, 296, 296f
Lithotripter, 296
Localized, 192
-logist, 27, 214, 337, 343
-logy, 7, 27, 148, 214, 337, 344
lord/o, 168, 337, 340
Lordosis, 168, 169f
Lower endoscopy, 226
Lumbar puncture, 49, 66
Lumbar region, 79
Lumbar vertebra, 27
lumb/o, 33, 337, 342
Lumpectomy, 276
Lymphadenopathy, 191, 191f
lymph/o, 190, 337, 341
Lymphocytes, 44, 243
-lysis, 337, 341
-lytic, 306, 337, 343

M

macro-, 27, 149, 289, 337
Macrocytosis, 170
Macromastia, 291
Macron, 15
Macroscopic anatomy, 30
Magnetic resonance imaging, 236, 237f
-malacia, 149, 337, 343
Male reproductive system, 61–63, 61f
Malignant, 192
Mammary glands, 65
mamm/o, 63, 215, 337, 341
Mammogram, 216, 217f
Mammoplasty, 291
  augmentation, 291
  reduction, 291
Mania, 164
-mania, 337, 341
Manic depression, 164
Manipulative and body-based practices, 304
Massage therapists, 304, 305
Massage therapy, 302, 303, 304
Mastectomy, 277
mast/o, 63, 275, 337, 341
Mastopexy, 288
Mean cell hemoglobin (MCH), 243
Mean cell hemoglobin concentration (MCHC), 243
Mean cell volume (MCV), 243
Medial, 68, 69, 70
Medical assistants, 50
Medical biller/coder, 110
Medical care facilities, abbreviations for, 113–114
Medical errors, 112
Medical orders, 124
Medical records
  corrections to, 129–130
  recording date and time on, 130–131
Medical terminology, 1–23
  combining forms in, 5, 7, 10, 28, 31
  combining vowels in, 4–5, 7
  defined, 2
  defining, through word structure analysis, 8–10
  prefixes in, 4, 5, 6, 7, 26, 27–28

roots in, 4, 5, 6, 7
  exceptions to the rule, 9
rules for forming and spelling, 12–14
rules of pronunciation, 14–16
singular and plural forms, 16–18
spelling, 31
suffixes in, 4, 5, 6, 7, 26, 27
  diagnostic, 11
  general, 11
  role of, in defining, 10–11
  surgical, 11
  symptomatic, 11
term components, 3, 7, 26–28
Medical transcriptionist, 227
Meditation, 304
megal/o, 166, 337, 342
-megaly, 149, 337, 341
melan/o, 31, 173, 337, 340
Melanocytes, 32, 32f, 177
Melanoma, signs of, 177f
Meninges, 48, 49
Meningitis, 49
  bacterial, 49
  viral, 49
mening/o, 47, 337, 342
men/o, 184, 337, 342
Menorrhagia, 184
Menstruation, 64
Mental healing, 304
Mental illness, 165
meta-, 149, 337, 340, 341
Metastasis, 9, 17, 178
Meter, 118
-meter, 214, 337, 342
metformin, 354
metoprolol, 354
Metric system, 116–117, 118–119
  abbreviations for, 117
metri/o, 160, 337, 344
metr/o, 63, 160, 275
Metrorrhagia, 184
-metry, 214, 337, 343
micro-, 27, 149, 289, 337, 343
Microcytosis, 170
Microlithiasis, 174
Micromastia, 291
Microscope, 29, 30, 222
Military time, 130
Milligram, 118
Milliliter, 118

Millimeter, 118
Mind-body medicine, 304
Mitral valve, 40
mono-, 27, 337, 342
Monocytes, 44, 243, 247
Monosyllables, 15
Mood disorders, 165
Mouth, 58
muscul/o, 33, 150, 337, 342
Musculoskeletal system, 28, 33, 34–35f, 36–37
Myalgia, 151
myel/o, 33, 47, 150, 338, 340, 344
my/o, 33, 150, 215, 289, 337, 342
Myocardial infarction, 173
Myocardium, 40, 309
Myodynia, 151
Myoma, 177
Myometrium, 64
Myoplasty, 290
myring/o, 54, 271, 338, 341, 344
Myringotomy, 272–273

N

narc/o, 173, 306, 338, 343, 344
Narcolepsy, 175
Narcotics, 306, 309, 354, 355
nas/o, 45, 160, 184, 223, 289, 338, 342
Nasonex (mometasone), 355
Nasopharyngoscopy, 224–225
Naturopathic medicine, 304
necr/o, 164, 338, 341
Necromania, 164
Necrophobia, 181
Necrosis, 172
Needle biopsy, 232
neo-, 150, 338, 342
Neoplasia, 176
Neoplasm, 176
nephr/o, 60, 168, 230, 295, 338, 342
Nephrolithiasis, 174, 295
Nephrologist, 61
Nephroptosis, 182
Nephrosis, 170
Nervous system, 28, 47–49, 48f, 74
neur/o, 47, 168, 338, 342
Neurology, 49
Neurosis, 169

Neutrophils, 44, 243, 247
Nexium (esomeprazole), 355
Nitrite, 249, 251
Nitroglycerin, 309
No acute distress (NAD), 96
No known drug allergies (NKDA), 96
Nonsteroidal antiinflammatory drugs, 308, 313, 354, 355
Norvasc (amlodipine besylate), 355
Nose, 46
Nuclear medicine imaging, 234–235, 235*f*, 240
Nurse's notes, 103, 107*f*, 110
Nursing assistants, 151

O
Objective information, 96
Obsessive-compulsive disorder, 165
Obstetrics, 66
Occlusion, 172, 172*f*
Occult blood urine, 248
Occupational history, 96
Occupational therapists, 166
Occupational therapy, 302, 303
Ocular, 55
ocul/o, 54, 338, 341
odont/o, 57, 338, 344
-odynia, 148, 338, 343
-ole, 27, 338, 343
-oma, 149, 338, 344
onc/o, 173, 338, 344
Oncology, 178
Oophorectomy, 278
Oophoritis, 162
oophor/o, 50, 63, 160, 275, 338, 343
Open reduction, internal fixation (ORIF), 289
Operating room, 114
Operative reports, 103, 108*f*, 111, 297*f*
Operative suffixes, 270, 271
    Greek origins of, 294
Operative terms, 270–302
Ophthalmic, 55
ophthalm/o, 54, 222, 338, 341
Ophthalmologist, 229
Ophthalmoscope, 222, 223, 224

Ophthalmoscopy, 224
-opsy, 214, 338, 343
Optic, 55
opt/o, 54, 228, 338, 341
Optometrists, 229
Optometry, 228–229
Oral antidiabetics, 353, 354
Oral prophylaxis, 59
orchid/o, 50, 62, 338, 344
orchi/o, 50, 62, 287, 338, 344
Orchiopexy, 288
orch/o, 50, 62, 338
Organs, 28, 30
or/o, 57, 338, 342
ortho-, 150, 338, 341, 342, 344
Orthopnea, 181
-osis, 149, 338, 341, 342
Ostealgia, 150
oste/o, 8, 33, 150, 338, 340
Osteodynia, 150
Osteoma, 177
Osteomalacia, 163
Osteopathic medicine, 304
Osteopenia, 179
Osteoporosis, 179, 180*f*
Osteosarcoma, 177
Ostomies, 274–275, 275*f*
Otalgia, 151
Otitis externa, 161
Otitis media, 273
ot/o, 54, 150, 222, 338, 341
Otodynia, 151
Otology, 56
Otorhinolaryngology, 56
Otorrhea, 185
Otoscope, 222, 223
Otoscopy, 224
-ous, 27, 338, 343
Outpatient, 114
Ovaries, 17, 53, 64
ovari/o, 50, 63, 275, 338, 343
Over-the-counter (OTC) drugs, 122
ov/i, 63, 338, 341
Oviduct, 9
Ovigenesis, 64
ov/o, 63, 338, 341
Ovum, 17, 64
ox/o, 8, 157, 338, 343
oxycodone and acetaminophen, 355

P
Palpation in physical examination, 221
pan-, 27, 338, 340
Pancreas, 52–53, 58
pancreat/o, 50, 57, 338, 343
Pancytopenia, 179
Panic disorder, 165
para-, 8, 27, 183, 280, 338, 340
Paracentesis, 281
Paralysis, 183
Paraplegia, 183
Parathyroid glands, 53, 120*f*
Parenteral route of administration, 120, 121
Paroxysm, 189
Past history, 96
Past medical history, 96
Patella, 28
path/o, 190, 230, 338, 341
Pathologist, 30, 230, 232
Pathology, 30
Pathology reports, 103
Patient care, abbreviations for, 114–115
Patient care records, 94
    history and physical, 94, 95*f*, 96–97
pector/o, 33, 338, 341
Pelvic cavity, 74, 76
Pelvic floor relaxation, 153*f*
Pelvic inflammatory disease (PID), 162
-penia, 149, 338, 340
per-, 289, 338, 341
Percussion in physical examination, 221
Percutaneous transluminal angioplasty (PTA), 291
Percutaneous transluminal coronary angioplasty (PTCA), 291, 293*f*, 299
peri-, 8, 28, 338, 340
Pericarditis, 10
Pericardium, 40
Persistent hypertension, 102
-pexy, 270, 338, 342, 344
phag/o, 154, 338, 341, 344
Pharmaceutical abbreviations and symbols, 116–119
Pharmacotherapy, 305–314
Pharmacy technician, 123

Pharyngitis, 161
pharyng/o, 45, 160, 223, 338, 343, 344
Pharynx, 46
phas/o, 154, 338, 344
-phil, 27, 338, 340
Phlebitis, 162
phleb/o, 38, 160, 338, 344
Phlebotomist, 245
Phlebotomy, 242, 245
Phobia, 165, 180
-phobia, 149, 338, 341
phot/o, 180, 338, 342
Photophobia, 180
phren/o, 154, 338, 341
Physiatrists, 305
Physical, 96
Physical examination, 96
  methods of
    auscultation, 221
    inspection, 221
    palpation, 221
    percussion, 221
Physical medicine, 302
Physical therapists, 305
Physical therapy, 302, 303
Physician's orders, 103, 106f, 110
Physician's progress notes, 103, 110
Plantar flexion, 72f, 73, 74
plas/o, 173, 338, 342
-plasty, 270, 338, 344
Platelet count, 244, 247
Platelets, 44, 247
Plavix (clopidogrel), 355
-plegia, 149, 338, 343
Plural forms, 16–18
-pnea, 149, 338, 341
pneum/o, 45, 338, 340, 342
Pneumonia, 155, 161
Pneumonitis, 161
pneumon/o, 45, 154, 338, 340, 342
-poiesis, 27, 338, 342
poly-, 150, 215, 338, 342
Polydipsia, 156, 157
Polysomnography, 219, 220f
Polyuria, 156, 157
Positron emission tomography, 235, 235f, 240
post-, 28, 338, 340
Postanesthetic care unit, 116

Posterior, 68, 69
Posterior-anterior, 68, 69
Posttraumatic stress disorder (PTSD), 165
Pouching, 153, 153f
Prayer, 304
pre-, 27, 338, 340
prednisone, 355
Prefixes, 4, 5, 6, 7, 26, 27–28
Pregnancy
  ectopic, 274
  tubal, 274
Premarin (conjugated estrogens), 355
Preoperative H&P, 97
Prescription, 121, 122f, 123
  abbreviations on, 124–126
Present illness, 96
Prevacid (pantoprazole), 355
Primary accent, 15
Primary hypertension, 102
pro-, 27, 338, 340
Procedural suffixes, 214–215
proct/o, 223, 338, 340, 343
Proctoscope, 226
Proctoscopy, 226
Progesterone, 53
Prognosis, 192
Progressive, 192
Progress notes, 97–98, 98f
  abbreviations used in, 98–102
Prolonged ischemia, 172
Pronation, 72f, 73, 74
Prone position, 71
Pronunciation, rules of, 14–16
propoxyphene napsylate and acetaminophen, 355
Prostate cancer, treating, 278
Prostatectomy, 278
Prostate gland, 62–63
prostat/o, 62, 275, 338, 343
Proximal, 68, 69, 70
Pruritus, 311
psych/o, 338
Psychosis, 169
Psychotherapy, 302, 305
Psychotic disorders, 165
Psychotropic drugs, 308, 313
Ptosis, 182
-ptosis, 149, 341
Pulmonary artery, 40
Pulmonary circulation, 41

Pulmonary embolism, 188, 189f
Pulmonary function testing, 229
Pulmonary semilunar valve, 40
pulmon/o, 45, 187, 228, 338, 342
Pulmonologist, 230
Pulse, 116
Puncture, 281
Pupils equal, round, and reactive to light and accommodation (PERRLA), 96
pyret/o, 306, 338, 342

Q
quadri-, 183, 329, 342
Quadriplegia, 183

R
Radiation therapy, 302, 305
radi/o, 218, 329, 343
Radiographs, 221, 233, 233f
Radiography, 219, 233, 233f, 238–239
Radiologic technologist, 97
Radiology, 238
Radionuclide, 234, 240
Recommendation, 97
rect/o, 57, 152, 215, 329, 343
Rectocele, 153, 153f
Rectum, 58, 153
Recumbent position, 71
Red blood cells, 42
Red blood count (RBC), 242, 244, 246
Reduction mammoplasty, 291
Regulations and legal considerations, 128
Rehabilitation therapy, 302
Remission, 192
Renal biopsy, 232
Renal calculi, 174
ren/o, 60, 230, 295, 329, 342
Reproductive system, 28
  female, 63–66, 63f
  male, 61–63, 61f
Respiration, 116
Respiratory system, 28, 45–47, 46f
Retina, 55
retin/o, 54, 329, 343
Return to office, 116
Review of systems, 96
Rhinitis, 161
rhin/o, 45, 160, 184, 289, 329, 342

Rhinoplasty, 290
Rhinorrhea, 185
Ribs, 36
Rickets, 163
Right lower quadrant, 79
Right upper quadrant, 79
Risperdal (risperidone), 355
Roots, 4, 5, 6, 7
 exceptions to the rule, 9
 lip, 3
 protein, 3
Rotation, 72f, 73, 74
Routes of administration,
 119–120
-rrhage, 149, 329, 344
-rrhagia, 149, 329, 344
-rrhaphy, 270, 329, 344
-rrhea, 149, 329, 341
Rule out, 97

S
Sagittal plane, 67f, 68, 69
Salpingectomy, 278
 bilateral, 278
Salpingitis, 162
salping/o, 63, 160, 273, 329, 341,
 344
Salpingo-oophorectomy, 278
Salpingotomy, 274
sarc/o, 173, 329, 342
schiz/o, 154, 329, 344
Schizophrenia, 155, 165
Sclera, 55
scler/o, 54, 168, 329, 342, 343
Sclerosis, 170
scoli/o, 168, 329, 344
Scoliosis, 168–169, 169f
-scope, 27, 214, 270, 329, 342
-scopy, 214, 270, 329, 343
Scrotum, 53
Secondary hypertension, 102
Sedatives, 308, 314, 353
Seizure, 175
semi-, 28, 329, 342
Sepsis, 311
Septum, 40
 interatrial, 40
 interventricular, 40
Seroquel (quetiapine), 355
sertraline hydrochloride, 355
Shortness of breath, 116
Sigmoid colon, 226

sigmoid/o, 223, 329, 343
Sigmoidoscope, 226
Sigmoidoscopy, 226
Sign, 192
simvastatin, 355
Single photon emission computed
 tomography (SPECT), 235,
 235f, 240
Singulair (montelukast), 355
Singular forms, 16–18
Skeletal muscles, 34, 35f, 36
Skeleton, 34, 34f
Skin, 32, 32f
Skull, 36
Small intestine, 58
SOAP method of documentation,
 97–98, 98f
Social history, 96
sodium, 356
Solid forms, 119
somn/o, 218, 329, 343
son/o, 215, 329, 344
Sonogram, 217, 220
Sonograph, 220
Sonography, 219, 236, 238f, 240
Spasm, 186–187
-spasm, 7, 149, 329, 341, 342
Special senses, 53–56, 54f
Specific gravity (SpGr), 247, 249
Specific instructions for
 administration, 121, 122f
Speech-language therapy, 302, 303
Sperm, 62
spermat/o, 62, 329, 344
sperm/o, 62, 329, 344
Spinal cavity, 74
Spinal cord, 27, 48, 74
Spinal fusion, 283, 283f
Spinal tap, 49, 66
Spine, 36–37
spin/o, 33, 329, 344
-spir, 341
spir/o, 227, 329, 341
Spirometer, 228, 229
Spirometry, 229, 229f
Spleen, 45, 294
 ruptured, 294
splen/o, 41, 166, 292, 329, 344
Splenorrhaphy, 294
spondyl/o, 33, 168, 282, 329, 344
Spondylosis, 170
Spondylosyndesis, 283, 283f, 294

squam/o, 31, 329, 343
Squamous cell carcinoma, 176
Squamous cell layer, 33
-stasis, 149, 329, 344
sten/o, 168, 329, 342
Stenosis, 171, 172
Sternum, 36
Steroids (antiinflammatory,
 immunosuppressant), 355
steth/o, 222, 329, 341
Stethoscope, 222
Stoma, 273, 274
Stomach, 58, 78
Stomach cancer, treating, 278
stomat/o, 57, 329, 342
-stomy, 270, 329, 341, 343
Stroke, 188
sub-, 28, 329, 340, 344
Subcutaneous injection, 121
Subcutaneous tissue layer, 32, 32f
Subjective information, 96
Substance abuse disorders, 165
Suffixes, 4, 5, 6, 7, 26, 27
Sugar, 156
super-, 27, 329, 340, 341
Superior, 68, 69, 70
Supination, 72f, 73, 74
Supine position, 71
Suppository, 119, 121
Surgical procedures, 271
Surgical technologist, 276
Suspension, 287
Suturing, 292
Symbols, 347–351
Symptoms, 96, 148, 192
syn-, 282, 329, 344, 345
Syndrome, 192
Synthroid (levothyroxine
 sodium), 356
Systemic circulation, 41
Systems review, 96

T
Tablet, 119, 121
tachy-, 150, 329, 341
Tachycardia, 154
Teeth, 58
Temperature, 116
Tenodesis, 283
Term components, 3, 7, 26–28,
 335–345. *See also* Combining
 forms; Prefixes; Roots; Suffixes

Testes, 152. 153f
Testicle, 53, 62, 288
Testis, 53, 62, 288
test/o, 50, 62, 329, 344
Testosterone, 53, 62
Therapeutic drug classifications, 305–314
Therapeutic terms, 302–305
therm/o, 227, 329, 342
Thermometer, 228
Thoracentesis, 281
Thoracic cavity, 74, 76
Thoracic vertebra, 27
thorac/o, 33, 271, 329, 341
Thoracocentesis, 281
Thoracostomy, 274
Thoracotomy, 272
Thorax, 18, 36
Throat, 46
thromb/o, 41, 160, 306, 329, 341
Thrombocytes, 44, 179, 247
Thrombocytopenia, 179
Thrombolytic agents, 308, 314
Thrombosis, 172
Thrombus, 18, 172, 172f, 188
thym/o, 41, 50, 154, 329, 344
Thymus, 45, 52
thyr/o, 50, 329, 343, 344
Thyroid gland, 52, 53
Thyroid hormone, 354, 356
thyroid/o, 50, 187, 329, 343, 344
-tic, 148, 329, 343
Time, recording, on medical records, 130–131
Tissues, 28, 30
tom/o, 218, 271, 329, 344
Tomography, 219
-tomy, 7, 270, 329, 342
Tongue, 58, 294f
ton/o, 306, 329, 344
tonsill/o, 160, 329, 344
Topical administration, 121
Topical forms, 120
Total knee arthroplasty, 290f
Trachea, 272, 274
    blockage of, 272
trache/o, 45, 163, 271, 329, 344, 345
Tracheomalacia, 163
Tracheostomy, 272f
Tracheotomy, 272, 272f, 274

Trade name, 122
Traditional Chinese medicine, 304
trans-, 28, 215, 275, 289, 329, 340, 344
Transabdominal, 218
Transducers, 218
Transesophageal, 218
Transurethral resection of the prostate (TURP), 279, 280f
Transverse plane, 67f, 68, 69
trazodone, 356
tri-, 28, 329, 344
TriCor (fenofibrate), 356
Tricuspid valve, 40
-tripsy, 270, 329, 341
troph/o, 190, 329, 341, 342
Toprol-XL (metoprolol), 356
Tubal ligation, 299, 301
Tubal pregnancy, 274
Tumors, 176
Tympanic membrane, 28, 272
tympan/o, 54, 329, 341
Tympany, 56
Type I diabetes mellitus, 156, 157
Type 2 diabetes mellitus, 156, 157

U
-ule, 27, 329, 343
ultra-, 215, 329, 340, 341
Ultrasonography, 219
Ultrasound, 217, 220, 236, 240
Umbilical region, 79
uni-, 27, 329, 342
Units of measure, 116–119, 118–119
    abbreviations for, 117–118
Upper endoscopy, 225
ureter/o, 60, 329
Ureters, 60–61
Urethra, 60
urethr/o, 60, 329, 344
Urinalysis, 247, 248f, 249, 250
Urinary system, 28, 30, 59–61, 59f
Urine, 60
Urine culture and sensitivity (C&S), 249, 251
Urine tests, 247–251
urin/o, 329, 344
ur/o, 60, 154, 273, 329, 344
Urobilinogen, 249, 250
Urologist, 61
Urology, 61

Urostomy, 275
Usual childhood diseases (UCHD), 96
Uterine tube, 64–65
uter/o, 63, 160, 275, 329, 344
Uterus, 64

V
Vagina, 65
Vaginitis, 162
vagin/o, 63, 160, 215, 340, 343, 344
varic/o, 152, 340, 344
Varicocele, 152, 153f
vascul/o, 8, 38, 340, 345
Vas deferens, 62, 278, 279f
Vasectomy, 278, 279f
vas/o, 8, 38, 62, 275, 340, 345
Vasoconstrictors, 308, 314
Vasodilators, 308, 314
Vasospasm, 187
Veins, 41
Venipuncture, 242, 245
ven/o, 38, 160, 215, 340, 344
Venograms, 217
Ventricle, 39
ventricul/o, 38, 340, 343, 344
Venules, 41
Verruca, 17
Vertebra, 27, 48
    cervical, 27
    lumbar, 27
    thoracic, 27
Vertebral cavity, 74, 76
Vertebral column, 36
vertebr/o, 33, 168, 282, 340, 344
vesic/o, 60, 152, 223, 340, 343
Viral meningitis, 49
Virus, 18
Vital signs, 116
Voice box, 46
Vulva, 65
vulv/o, 63, 340, 345
Vytorin (ezetimibe and simvastatin), 356

W
warfarin, 356
Warts, 17
Weight measure in apothecary system, 117

White blood cells, 43, 44, 247

White blood count (WBC), 242, 244, 246

Whole medical systems, 304

Windpipe, 46–47, 272

Within normal limits (WNL), 96

Word structure analysis in defining medical terms, 8–10

X

xeno-, 284, 340, 342, 344

Y

-y, 27, 149, 340, 341, 343

Yoga, 304

Z

Zetia (ezetimibe), 356

Zyrtec (cetirizine), 356

P-1

a-
an-

P-2

ab-

P-3

ad-

P-4

allo-

P-5

ana-

P-6

ante-
pre-
pro-

P-7

anti-
contra-

P-8

auto-

P-9

brady-

P-10

de-

before

without

against, or opposed to

away from

self

to, toward, or near

slow

other

from, down, or not

up, apart

dia-

trans-

eu-

dys-

extra-

e-

ec-

ex-

exo-

hemi-

semi-

endo-

intra-

hetero-

epi-

homo-

normal

across or through

outside

painful, difficult, or faulty

half

out or away

different

within

same

upon

P-21

**hyper-
super-**

P-22

hypo-

P-23

inter-

P-24

macro-

P-25

meta-

P-26

micro-

P-27

**mono-, uni-
bi-
tri-
quadri-**

P-28

neo-

P-29

ortho-

P-30

pan-

small

above or excessive

one
two or both
three
four

below or deficient

new

between

straight, normal,
or correct

large

all

beyond, after,
or change

P-31

para-

P-36

sub-

P-32

per-

P-37

syn-

P-33

peri-

P-38

tachy-

P-34

poly-

P-39

ultra-

P-35

post-

P-40

xeno-

below or under	alongside of or abnormal
together or with	by
fast	around
beyond or excessive	many
strange or foreign	after

S-1

-al, -ar, -ary, -eal, -ic, -ous, -tic

S-6

-ectomy

S-2

**-algia
-odynia**

S-7

-emia

S-3

-cele

S-8

-genesis

S-4

-centesis

S-9

-genic

S-5

-desis

S-10

-graft

excision or removal

pertaining to
(adjectival endings)

blood condition

pain

origin or production

pouching or hernia

pertaining to origin

puncture for aspiration

transfer

binding

S-11

-gram

S-16

-icle

-ole

-ule

S-12

-graph

S-17

-ist

S-13

-graphy

S-18

-itis

S-14

-ia

-ism

S-19

-ium

S-15

-iasis

S-20

-lepsy

small

record

one who specializes in

instrument for recording

inflammation

process of recording

structure or tissue

condition of

seizure

formation or
presence of

S-21

-logist

S-26

-meter

S-22

-logy

S-27

-metry

S-23

-malacia

S-28

-oma

S-24

-mania

S-29

-opsy

S-25

-megaly

S-30

-osis

instrument for measuring	one who specializes in the study or treatment of
process of measuring	study of
tumor	softening
process of viewing	condition of abnormal impulse toward or frenzy
condition or increase	enlargement

S-31	S-36
-penia	**-plegia**
S-32	S-37
-pexy	**-pnea**
S-33	S-38
-phil	**-poiesis**
S-34	S-39
-phobia	**-ptosis**
S-35	S-40
-plasty	**-rrhage** **-rrhagia**

paralysis	abnormal reduction
breathing	suspension or fixation
formation	attraction for
falling or downward displacement	condition of abnormal fear or sensitivity
to burst forth (usually blood)	surgical repair or reconstruction

S-41

-rrhaphy

S-46

-stasis

S-42

-rrhea

S-47

-stomy

S-43

-scope

S-48

-tomy

S-44

-scopy

S-49

-tripsy

S-45

-spasm

S-50

-y

stop or stand	suture
creation of an opening	discharge
incision	instrument for examination
crushing	process of examination
condition or process of	involuntary contraction

CF-1

abdomin/o

lapar/o

CF-2

acr/o

CF-3

aden/o

CF-4

adip/o

lip/o

CF-5

angi/o

vas/o

vascul/o

CF-6

arthr/o

CF-7

ather/o

CF-8

aur/i

ot/o

CF-9

blephar/o

CF-10

carcin/o

joint

abdomen

fatty, or lipid, paste

extremity or topmost

ear

gland

eyelid

fat

cancer

vessel

CF-11

cardi/o

CF-16

crani/o

CF-12

cephal/o

CF-17

crin/o

CF-13

cervic/o

CF-18

cyst/o

vesic/o

CF-14

chol/e

bil/i

CF-19

cyt/o

CF-15

cost/o

CF-20

dent/i

odont/o

skull	heart
to secrete	head
bladder or sac	neck
cell	bile
teeth	rib

derm/o

dermat/o

cutane/o

gastr/o

encephal/o

gynec/o

enter/o

hem/o

hemat/o

erythr/o

hepat/o

esthesi/o

hist/o

stomach	skin
female	entire brain
blood	small intestine
liver	red
tissue	sensation

CF-31

hydr/o

CF-36

lingu/o
gloss/o

CF-32

hypn/o
somn/o

CF-37

lith/o

CF-33

iatr/o

CF-38

mast/o
mamm/o

CF-34

lacrim/o
dacry/o

CF-39

melan/o

CF-35

leuk/o

CF-40

my/o
muscul/o

tongue	water
stone	sleep
breast	treatment
black	tear
muscle	white

CF-41

myel/o

CF-42

narc/o

CF-43

nas/o
rhin/o

CF-44

necr/o

CF-45

nephr/o
ren/o

CF-46

path/o

CF-47

phag/o

CF-48

phas/o

CF-49

phot/o

CF-50

plas/o

disease

bone marrow or
spinal cord

eat or swallow

stupor or sleep

speech

nose

light

death

formation

kidney

CF-51

pneum/o
pneumon/o

CF-56

salping/o

CF-52

proct/o

CF-57

sarc/o

CF-53

psych/o

CF-58

scler/o

CF-54

pulmon/o

CF-59

spir/o

CF-55

pyret/o

CF-60

sten/o

uterine or fallopian tube

air or lung

flesh

rectum and anus

hard or sclera

mind

breathing

lung

narrow

fever

CF-61	CF-66
test/o **orch/o** **orchi/o** **orchid/o**	**tympan/o** **myring/o**

CF-62	CF-67
therm/o	**ur/o** **urin/o**

CF-63	CF-68
thorac/o **pector/o** **steth/o**	**ven/o** **phleb/o**

CF-64	CF-69
thromb/o	**vertebr/o** **spondyl/o**

CF-65	CF-70
troph/o	**vulv/o** **episi/o**

eardrum or tympanic membrane

testis or testicle

urine

heat

vein

chest

vertebra

clot

vulva

nourishment or development